Advancing Perioperative Practice

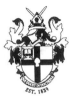

Advancing Perioperative Practice

EDITED BY

Mark Radford
Consultant Nurse (Perioperative Emergency Care)
Good Hope Hospital NHS Trust, UK, and
Visiting Lecturer (University of Central England in Birmingham)
Birmingham, UK

Bernie County
Workforce Development Manager
Pan Birmingham Cancer Network
Birmingham, UK

Melanie Oakley
Lead Advanced Practitioner PACU
South West London Elective Orthopaedic Centre
London, UK

Published in 2004 by:
Nelson Thornes Ltd
Delta Place
27 Bath Road
CHELTENHAM
GL53 7TH
United Kingdom

04 05 06 07 08 / 10 9 8 7 6 5 4 3 2 1

A catalogue record for this book is available from the British Library

ISBN 0 7487 5398 2

Page make-up and illustration by Pantek Arts Ltd

Printed in Great Britain by Ashford Colour Press

Contents

PREFACE

Advancing Perioperative Practice set out to be different. There is an abundance of standard perioperative texts that help the reader prepare for practice in the perioperative environment, but what about the needs of those *in practice*, those practitioners wishing to extend their knowledge and critical thinking abilities? This book has sought to bridge this gulf and provide experienced perioperative practitioners with challenging ideas to enhance their practice. The book also aims to provide inspiration to those in training or newly appointed in the perioperative environment, as to the wealth of practice opportunities available.

In order to achieve this, *Advancing Perioperative Practice* is an eclectic mixture of advanced theory and practice. This is drawn from a range of disciplines with valuable and pertinent insights that contribute the essence of perioperative care. The challenge for such a book is often integrating this knowledge successfully into realistic guidance for practitioners to use in every-day care delivery. The brief given to the expert contributors was to help redefine perioperative practice in the light of contemporary changes in health care. They have achieved this, challenging some of the traditional boundaries, and ensuring that the extra knowledge needed to deliver perioperative practice at a higher level is presented in a user-friendly and easily accessible manner.

Advancing Perioperative Practice is also a 'shop window' for other health-care practitioners whose roles have evolved as perioperative practice has developed to a new level of individual holistic care. This approach takes the subject beyond the traditional view, that the perioperative environment is technical and devoid of the essence of care.

The changing role of the nurse with particular reference to the perioperative environment sets the scene in **Chapter 1**. An exploration of the concept of professionalism is undertaken, with a discussion around whether perioperative nurses have the autonomy and unique knowledge base to truly be thought of as a profession. Nursing practice within the perioperative environment and the skills and knowledge that are inherent in it are analysed. The chapter culminates in a reflection on the future of care delivery and the nurse as a perioperative practitioner.

Chapter 2 compares and contrasts specialist and advanced practice highlighting the historical development in the perioperative arena. An evaluation of advanced perioperative roles is undertaken, including an explanation of the competencies of advanced practice. Practice exemplars are used to underpin discussions and reinforce good practice messages.

The principles of infection control related to perioperative practice are discussed in **Chapter 3**. The chain of infection and host-specific defence mechanisms are explained along with the role of blood-borne viruses. The health clearance of staff and what results mean are described. Standard Precautions and other infection control methods in the pre- and perioperative phase are also identified.

The anaesthetic practitioner's role in airway management and haemodynamic assessment is explored, along with induction and maintenance of anaesthesia. These are placed in the clinical context and consideration of potential hazards and the practitioner's role in supporting the patient is undertaken. Anaesthetic pharmacology is also discussed, along with the desired effects and potential complications. Finally a review of emergency situations concludes **Chapter 4**.

The principles of surgical nursing are the focus of **Chapter 5**. The topic is covered from an evidence-based practice point of view. Infection control specific to the intraoperative period is discussed. There is also an exploration of relevant equipment and how to handle it safely; this is achieved without creating an equipment catalogue. Patient care during the surgical phase is analysed, and the relevance of accurate documentation is highlighted.

In **Chapter 6,** we explore the recovery practitioner's role in managing the patient's airway, fluid balance and cardiovascular status. We highlight cardiac arrhythmias and the necessary interventions along with the management of cardiac arrests in the recovery unit. The evidence base for dealing with the problems of postoperative nausea and vomiting are also discussed.

Chapter 7 focuses on perioperative clinical management and the challenges of developing managerial decision making skills. The essential features of management are contrasted with the role of clinical practitioner. The limitations of effectiveness and how personal credibility is of paramount importance to success are also discussed. Comparisons between management and leadership are drawn and the key issue of whether leadership qualities are a pre-requisite to effective management are examined.

Consent and associated legal issues for perioperative nurses are the basis of **Chapter 8.** Examples from practice are used to demonstrate problems that can be encountered when obtaining consent. Who may give consent and who may obtain consent are explained along with the concept of defence.

What constitutes personal and professional development and how you achieve it is discussed in **Chapter 9.** Key terms are clarified along with the positive factors that enable the personal development of the practitioner. Support mechanisms and how they relate to individual points in a career are discussed. The chapter culminates in an explanation of how appraisal, personal development plans and career planning can be used to shape personal and professional development.

We hope that you find this book helpful and thought provoking, and that it will encourage you to analyse your practice and develop a greater contribution to perioperative care. We have enjoyed writing and editing this book and hope that you enjoy reading it.

Mark Radford, Bernie County
and Melanie Oakley

ACKNOWLEDGEMENTS

A big thank you to Helen for all your help.

Mark: Thanks to my wife and daughter, my parents and family; the perioperative staff at Good Hope Hospital NHS Trust; and to Dr Liz Walker, Mr Iain Whorton, Dr Alastair Williamson, Dr Paul Johnston, Mrs Anne Abbassi, Mr Alan Jewkes, and the late Mr Mike Crowson, FRCS.

Bernie: Thanks to Debbie; your practical support made it all possible. To Mom and Dad, whose support has never faltered. Finally Fiona and Jenny, who continue to challenge the way I think.

Melanie: Firstly I would like to thank my husband Pete and my daughter Phoebe who as always have been my rock. Also my parents and my sister Caroline, and yes I do expect you to read it cover to cover! Finally thanks Mark and Bernie, I have enjoyed working with you both.

CONTRIBUTORS

Bernie County
Workforce Development Manager
Pan Birmingham Cancer Network
Birmingham, UK

Pat A Hutchinson
Senior Infection Control Nurse
Walsall Hospitals NHS Trust
Walsall, UK

Melanie Oakley
Lead Advanced Practitioner PACU
South West London Elective Orthopaedic Centre
London, UK
Formerly Senior Lecturer
Kingston University and St George's Hospital
    Medical School
London, UK

Amanda Parker
Lead Nurse
Matron Critical Care Services
Queen Victoria Hospital NHS Trust
East Grinstead
Sussex, UK

Deborah A Pittaway
Senior Lecturer
School of Clinical Nursing
University of Central England
Birmingham, UK

Mark Radford
Consultant Nurse (Perioperative Emergency Care)
Good Hope Hospital NHS Trust, UK, and
Visiting Lecturer
University of Central England in Birmingham
Birmingham, UK

J Howard Shelley
Senior Operating Department Practitioner/
    Operating Department Information System
    Manager
Good Hope Hospital NHS Trust
Sutton Coldfield, UK

Christine Spiers
Senior Lecturer
Brighton University
Sussex, UK

1 THE CHANGING ROLE OF THE PERIOPERATIVE NURSE

Deborah A Pittaway

CHAPTER AIMS

- To explore the nurse's role within the perioperative environment
- To examine the professional role of the nurse
- To discuss nursing practice within the perioperative environment, including the knowledge and skills inherent within this role
- To evaluate the future of care delivery within the perioperative environment – the nurse as a 'perioperative practitioner'.

The 21st century has brought with it continued developments, innovations and changes to the role of the nurse in the UK today. Professional and government directives have both stretched and challenged the role of the nurse within every speciality (Department of Health [DoH] 1999a, 1999b, 2002a; English National Board [ENB] 1994, 2000; United Kingdom Central Council (UKCC) 1995, 1999a, 1999b). The advent of the specialist and consultant nurse roles and the emerging trend to an all-graduate profession has gathered momentum. These changes challenge professional beliefs and clinical practice, forcing nurses to justify, explain and most importantly account for their roles both individually and collectively. Nowhere perhaps has this role analysis been more evident than the scrutiny which the perioperative nurse[1] faces.

The role of the perioperative nurse has been under the spotlight for many years, forcing justification and rationalisation of this role (Bevan 1990; Brown 1994; Barker 1996; McGee 1997; Crawford 1999; Williams 2002). The introduc-

tion of, initially, the support worker and more recently the advent of the fully trained theatre practitioner or operating department practitioner (ODP) has led to a more immediate need for clarification of roles within theatre. The following discussion will seek to clarify the role of the perioperative nurse, exploring issues surrounding professionalism, the influence of surgical and anaesthetic advances and how the introduction of the theatre practitioner has challenged the traditionally held perception of the role of the perioperative nurse. The ability to manage these factors will enable the nurse to continue to provide patient care within the perioperative environment. However, the challenge will lie in the nurse's ability to justify and rationalise their practice in order to provide patient care. Such care could be described as evidence based or holistic care and consequently therein lies a further challenge to the perioperative nurse in that the theatre environment is often not conducive to delivery of holistic care. It is this that the perioperative nurse needs to question and explore in order to ensure their continued presence in this critical and often challenging environment.

THE PROFESSIONAL ROLE OF THE NURSE

Throughout history the role of the nurse has been challenged and questioned, and the issue of professional status and whether or not the nurse can be included in this elite band has been hotly debated (Morrall 2001). Sociological theory demonstrates a set of criteria deemed essential in order to be considered a member of a profession (Haralambros and Holborn 2000; Bowman 1995; Moloney 1992). The role of the perioperative nurse will be explored in relation to aspects of these essential criteria.

---

[1] The term 'perioperative nurse' will be used to describe the anaesthetic, scrub and recovery roles.

- A unique area of practice
- Autonomous practice
- A unique body of knowledge.

It is intended that remuneration and salaries will not be explored; they are seen as perhaps too controversial for discussion within the context of this chapter (DoH 2002a). Discussion around these topics is always sensed, but does not always necessarily alter or determine performance and in many cases is not always associated with the professional role. Herztberg (1959) describes these as the 'hygiene factors'.

- A unique area of practice implies a review and definition of the role performance of the nurse in the perioperative environment. The following discussion will question the development and uniqueness of the role.
- Autonomous practice involves autonomy, which according to Leddy and Mae Pepper (1998) means that 'one can perform one's total professional function on the basis of one's own knowledge and judgement – being recognised by others as having the right to do so' (p. 327). The extent to which a theatre nurse is able to deliver autonomous practice could be found within their Code of professional Conduct (Nursing and Midwifery Council [NMC] 2002). However, there are still legal, ethical and accountability issues that question the boundaries of nursing, particularly perioperative nursing.
- A unique body of knowledge has been described by Chinn and Kramer (1999) as knowledge that is in a form that can be shared or communicated with others. Subsequent discussion will quite possibly question the breadth, depth and uniqueness of the knowledge required of the perioperative nurse.

A UNIQUE AREA OF PRACTICE

So what exactly is the role of the perioperative nurse? Many have tried to explain, define and explore the role (Hind and Wicker 2000; McCloskey *et al.* 2001; Nightingale 1999;

Rothrock 1996). While these writers suggest wholly appropriate and correct definitions many within the profession, and indeed without, still find this role difficult to equate to the traditional role of the nurse seen in the more obvious settings of the ward or clinic environment. For many, the old vision of the 'surgeon's handmaiden' continues to be the prevailing image of the perioperative nurse.

For the first 60–70 years of the last century, in many instances this was probably a truism. Cleaning boots, laying out theatre greens, washing masks, sterilising equipment and ensuring a plentiful supply of good quality tea were among the daily chores facing the perioperative nurse. They were seen as essential for the smooth and indeed safe passage of the patient through the surgical experience. To a certain extent for some of these ritualistic practices there is indeed a certain amount of logic. But to most these practices beg the question: 'Does one have to be a nurse to carry out such tasks?' Certainly in many departments the more traditional roles of the nurse, for example the role of scrub nurse, is carried out most ably by qualified operating department practitioners. Similarly, non-nurses carry out roles within both the anaesthetic and recovery areas.

The notion of uniqueness in practice raises the question of the perioperative nurse's remit and whether or not this nurse can deliver holistic care. The early 1980s witnessed the emergence of 'total patient care', rather than the delivery of individual assigned tasks such as drug rounds, dressings and observations. An individual nurse would be responsible for all aspects of the patients' care, not just ensuring that the entire ward had had their bowels opened! If the nurse was unable to deliver any aspect of patient care then a more senior nurse supervised them in this role. What emerged was 'primary nursing' (Walton and Reeves 1996). This subsequently led to the role of the 'named nurse' who was responsible for the organisation and collation of care; someone who also ensured that the prescribed care was delivered (DoH 1991; Mackenzie 1998; NATN 1992). This did not mean a 24-hour cover by the named nurse, but rather the delegation of the delivery, in some cases, to other nurses in their absence. This co-ordinated approach to care delivery has similarities to 'team nursing' (Mackenzie 1998). With this some would suggest that nursing had come full circle.

The challenge now continues with the development of specialist roles. The allocation of such specialist roles within the team means that each is carrying out a different role, but all are essential to the patient. Once again it would appear care has become fragmented. Many are used to the 'tissue viability' nurse, the 'pain' nurse or the 'infection control' nurse, all contributing to an aspect of the patient's care. Clinical discussions with these specialists all reveal a fear that by their very roles they are deskilling more generalist nurses. Once again parallels within the perioperative environment can be drawn. Discussions in the clinical area reveal a worrying trend: 'I am a scrub nurse and I do not do recovery' and equally 'I'm a recovery nurse and I do not circulate'. This sort of debate and discussion can only be avoided or limited within the team when all can undertake care delivery of all aspects of perioperative practice. Multiskilling emerges and with this the term 'skill mix' (Mackenzie 1998).

Skill mix identifies the requisite skills required to carry out the job in question. The grading structure of the 1990s sought to define this even further. However, it was often difficult to define all aspects of a job, and in particular draw the boundaries between what is and what is not part of an individual's job. This is of particular importance where a patient's needs are at stake. Many nurses did not view their work as just specific to a small group of patients only, but felt they needed to continue to care for others who required assistance also. Parallels can be drawn within the theatre environment where some perioperative nurses have been prepared to take on other roles within the team to ensure quality patient care (Marson and Hartlebury 1992).

However, this whole issue of skill mix and total patient care has again opened the wider debate of 'what is the role of the nurse?' This brings one back to the notion of the perioperative nurse as 'handmaiden' or 'skilled practitioner'. In relation to this, there is a need to continue to identify the skills that are required of the 'good' perioperative nurse.

It is possible to compile such a list of the skills. Indeed recent discussions with qualified nurses working in the perioperative environment revealed many: tenacity, intuition, calm in a crisis, cheerful, sense of humour, quick thinking and reflective were just a few that were listed. Often these skills will be in relation to the specific area of theatre practice: roles within the anaesthetic environment; the scrub role; and the role in the recovery of patients. Often these are further defined into roles for the nurse, the operating department practitioner and the support worker. The division of the roles, areas and a preoccupation with the need to perform role tasks have further compounded a move away from holistic patient care delivery and have ensured within some units the apparent fragmentation of patient care. Quite often the traditional 'scrub' role is still seen as the main role for perioperative nurses. Indeed in some units it is the only role for nurses. More recently the advent of the preregistration Diploma (HE) Operating Department Practice has further confused and disorientated perioperative nurses and in many instances care areas have become even more difficult to articulate.

Anaesthetic developments too have influenced much of the developments in the role of the perioperative nurse. The 1970s witnessed a new dawn in anaesthesia with the advent of the intensive care unit (ICU). Here it was the anaesthetist who came into his own, no longer seen as the poor relation of the surgeon, but rather the expert. The critical care environment is one where it is often the intensivist who can make the difference to patient outcome. With this development in ICUs came the continued development in surgical anaesthesia and with this came the need for specialist practitioners to assist with the administration of anaesthesia in theatre. The role of the operating department assistant (ODA) had been created to assist with ever more complex anaesthetic practice, along with other new and exciting roles for the nurse in ICU.

With the emergence of this new role of ODA came a challenge to the traditional role of perioperative nurse. Very quickly the anaesthetic assistant role became vital to the smooth running of the theatre list. Often lists were cancelled if an ODA was not available, since it was perceived that available nurses could not provide the skilled assistance now required by the anaesthetist. For many perioperative nurses this was difficult, since they had provided this support previously. In many units the anaesthetists' preference for the ODA, who was qualified to assist in the anaesthetic room, quickly became the expected and accepted practice. Certainly in the last few years Association guidelines clearly stipulate the minimum requirements for assistance to the anaesthetist (AAGBI 1998).

The City and Guilds Course 752 became the preferred qualification for the anaesthetic assistant and indeed many anaesthetists refused to work with nurses if they did not hold this qualification. While the role of the ODA emerged, the Joint Board for Clinical Nursing Studies (JBCNS), that approved educational course for nurses, had developed specialist courses for theatre nurses. The JBCNS 176 Course in Operating Department Nursing and the JBCNS 182 Course in Anaesthetic Nursing were being delivered in many schools of nursing across the country. These post-basic courses were seen as the choice for some nurses wanting to develop the skills necessary to deliver care in the operating department, be it in the role of scrub or anaesthetic nurse. However, for the majority of nurses it was still the number of cases scrubbed for and complexity of surgery involved in, which appeared to be the only prerequisite for development and advancement within a career structure. While it is recognised that experience can never be viewed as a waste of time, it is equally important that this experience should be nurtured, developed and supported with a sound educational input. The problem for many qualified nurses working in the perioperative environment was that the impetus for educational development in tandem with clinical skill development was lacking. Possibly this could be blamed on the scarcity of these programmes at

the time, but equally there appeared to be a culture where clinical experience and years of service were the only requirements for progress, development and promotion. For many nurses this has become an issue, particularly given the recent developments in relation to the government's 'Agenda For Change' document (DoH 2002a).

So is it possible for the perioperative nurse to define the particular area of practice and also address the issue of delivering holistic care? Chinn and Kramer (1999) suggest that 'wholism' is based on the theory that a being cannot be reduced to single parts, it is rather the sum of these interrelated parts. Therefore while it would indeed seem that it is important for the nurse in theatre to deliver holistic care, clearly it may not always be practically possible to do so, particularly in the perioperative environment. The delivery of holistic care should be closely related to the situation and the operative procedure the patient requires including psychological and social care. This notion encompasses the need for the nurse to know the patient and make an assessment of their need in the preoperative period. However, consider the converse of this. Is it really necessary to know the patient in order to deliver the expert care required during surgery? Many would argue 'no' and certainly if other critical care areas are examined, do the nurses working in these areas always 'know' the patient? Certainly in the early hours of caring for the unconscious critically ill road traffic accident victim, the ICU nurse would have very little opportunity to know the patient. Much of the 'knowing' of the patient as a person would not begin until there was some dialogue with a family member. It would be doubtful that this not 'knowing' the patient prevented the ICU nurse from providing expert care. The relationship with the patient develops rather through continued contact and over time. Unfortunately the perioperative nurse does not always have this opportunity of seeing and developing a rapport with a patient or their relatives over a period of time. If the perioperative nurse was required to meet the holistic needs, particularly the psychological and social needs, it would appear that they must go beyond the confines of the theatre department in order to ensure it is possible to form a relationship with the patient. A challenge for many.

The notion of preoperative visiting has been in existence since the 1960s and its value and worth in relation to care delivery has been debated consistently since (Kalideen 1991; Wicker 1995; Martin 1996; Crawford 1999; Williams 2002). The term preoperative visiting is often confusing. Discussions reveal different objectives. Some suggest a 'getting to know you chat' while others reveal that the 'visit' should be much more than this and encompass an assessment of patient need both physical and psychological. It is this assessment that is crucial and which enables the perioperative nurse to carry out the four stages of the nursing process as a foundation for holistic care (Rothrock 1996). See Box 1.1 for the four stages of the nursing process.

Preoperative assessment of patients enables the perioperative nurse to meet with, make an assessment and subsequently develop the early stages of a plan of care specific and uniquely for that individual patient. Assessment will allow the perioperative nurse to make a risk assessment identifying those patients, for example, at risk from pressure sore development, inadvertent hypothermia, deep vein thrombosis or those predisposed to postoperative problems, such as nausea and vomiting, or respiratory distress. Patient anxiety can also be identified and reassurance given appropriately, drawing on and liaising with ward colleagues and medical staff to ensure the reduction of anxiety levels in the patient rather than the heightened anxiety feared by many. This should ensure that the patient has as positive an experience as is possible (Dimond 1994). Given sufficient time and enthusiasm the possibilities to enhance the quality of care delivery by the perioperative nurse are endless.

The benefits of the practice are well-documented (Wicker 1995; White and Coleman 1999; Welsh 2000). However, in many units perioperative nurses are still prepared to deliver care without ever setting eyes on the patient. Medical colleagues would certainly not consider the delivery of anaesthesia and the performing of surgery without making some assessment of the patient (Crawford 1999). So it would seem that the perioperative nurse, in contrast to medical colleagues, is often caring for the patient without any initial contact. Interestingly, this fact could actually support the uniqueness of the perioperative nurse role as being able to care for the patient at a specific period in time while carrying out a series of specific functions or skills. This would indeed challenge the whole notion of holistic care! Interestingly this preoccupation with preoperative visiting does not seem to be an issue for the emerging profession of operating department practitioners (Williams 2002).

The apparent difficulties with preoperative visiting and subsequent assessment of patients appears to mainly centre on the issue of time (White and Coleman 1999). Clinical discussions with colleagues reveal real concern regarding the ability of some perioperative nurses to actually have a conversation with a patient for fear of saying the wrong thing. This fear is further compounded in some areas where there is an apparent reluctance by surgeons and anaesthetists to 'allow' the perioperative nurse to visit 'their' patient. Indeed Williams (2002) cites an incident where an anaesthetist positively discouraged and prevented the practice altogether for fear of overload of the patient.

The preoccupation with time is for many perioperative nurses a reality. The nurse in the perioperative environment has become a facilitator of a service, rather than a caring and autonomous professional (Williams 2002). What appears to have taken precedence for many is the variety of essential tasks assigned to the perioperative nurse. Quite possibly it is not essential for a qualified perioperative nurse to carry out

Box 1.1 The nursing process involves four stages:

- Assessment
- Planning
- Implementation
- Evaluation

many of these essential tasks. Checking and ordering equipment, preparation of theatre, anaesthetic or recovery areas could possibly be carried out by other qualified and competent personnel. The emergence of the support worker qualified through the National Vocational Qualification (NVQ) framework could quite possibly enable the perioperative nurse to relinquish some of these essential but non-caring duties (Moore 2002).

Much of this preoccupation with these essential tasks appears to be dictated by the perioperative nurses' understanding of their role. For many these are the very tasks that define their role and direct patient care. This preoccupation is bound up with the perioperative nurses' perception of their accountability and autonomy which is linked to their unique role; a very real and challenging aspect of the role, but one that does question the place of holistic nursing within a theatre environment. This will be discussed further in the following section.

AUTONOMOUS PRACTICE

Autonomous can be defined as having the freedom to act independently. This would imply that for a practitioner to be autonomous they would be acting independently within the team.

For the perioperative nurse this means acting within the specified activities of the profession. The previous discussion has highlighted the complexities of the perioperative nurse's role; autonomous practice would appear to require a specific defined set of essential functions or tasks. Within the theatre environment these can be defined to specific areas of care delivery: the role of the anaesthetic assistant; the 'scrub' role; and the role within the postanaesthetic area. Implicit in the discussion of autonomous practice are issues of professional accountability, and also the legal and ethical requirements.

Professional accountability centres on the scope of practice of the perioperative nurse. It is crucial therefore to define the roles and boundaries of nursing in the perioperative environment.

THE ANAESTHETIC ROLE

The anaesthetic role in many areas is very much a supportive role to the anaesthetist, with the preparation of a safe environment and the provision of 'skilled' assistance in relation to care of the patient and the administration of anaesthesia. This involves the preparation of both the anaesthetic and operating rooms and in some areas the drawing up under supervision of anaesthetic and adjunct drugs for anaesthesia. At present the prescription and administration of anaesthetic drugs remains the domain of the anaesthetist; it is however worth noting the emerging issues of nurse-prescribing which might well alter the accountability and practice of this. This is under review in England at the present time. In other countries the nurse anaesthetist might perform the function of both prescribing and administering anaesthetics and is therefore accountable in their own right for this function (Hind and Wicker 2000). The Association of Anaesthetists and the Royal College of Anaesthetists (AAGBI and RCA 1996), in England, are working with the changing workforce programme from the modernisation agency to develop non-medical anaesthetic roles. Six pilot sites have commenced the early implementation of these role developments. The reduction of junior doctors' hours and the impending shortfall in anaesthetic registrars has hastened this process. Such a role will not be viewed lightly and issues surrounding accountability, autonomy and education will require a clear vision and resolution before becoming mainstream. Certainly in the UK, prior to this becoming a role for anyone other than the anaesthetist, a recognised scheme of education is being developed. This development cannot be viewed in isolation and many wider issues are also under the spotlight, for example the issues of nurse-prescribing (DoH 1998, 1999, 2001).

In the case of the perioperative nurse and administration of anaesthetics, clearly lines of accountability and professional liability need to be addressed prior to any change in the present role. Reducing numbers of junior doctors and the current development of roles in pre-assessment, first assistant and surgical practitioner may well lead to the expansion of the perioperative nurse's role as a necessity, in order to meet patient needs. Such needs are seen as crucial to the issue of nurse-prescribing, and indeed to any expansion of the nurse's role within the anaesthetic process. Consequently concern is raised with regard to the delivery of 'nursing care'; one cannot help wondering who will actually deliver 'care' if we are all so busy undertaking someone else's job.

The anaesthetic role in some trusts has moved beyond theatre. Many anaesthetic assistants, nurses and ODPs make up the team required to respond to cardiac arrest calls. They also provide essential support in some major injury units and indeed the role is now being seen as essential in some ICUs, particularly with the transport of critically ill and ventilated patients. Developments in this area of care are exciting and offer challenging career opportunities for the perioperative nurse and ODPs. The development of generic transferable critical care core skills will also see continued developments in this area and perhaps even transferability of skills across a variety of critical care settings.

THE SCRUB ROLE

In many units the scrub nurse's role has been abused – on the one hand being described by many as 'the monkey' and on the other being permitted to carry out the responsible roles of 'first' or 'surgeon's assistant' (Boss 2002). In the past the 'scrub' role was seen as one of the most important of the nurse's roles in the perioperative environment, the old style scrub sister ruling the roost in many departments. This has continued in some units with little or no research basis or evidence to support it or the surrounding activity of a theatre environment. Interestingly in some units this is now seen as the only role for the nurse. While the role is crucial to the safety and therapeutic needs of the patient undergoing a surgical procedure, it is much more than the ability to stand at the table, and count and hand instruments. The potential for development in this role is tremendous; it should and in some instances does encompass much wider issues, for example:

- The checking of consent to surgery and the ascertaining validity through liaison and collaboration with medical teams. Appreciating, understanding and ensuring that ethical and moral codes are adhered to.
- The preparation and maintenance and monitoring of an environment which is safe, not just for the patient, but also for other members of staff.
- Maintenance of this safe environment throughout the operative procedure, ensuring such aspects as temperature monitoring, safety during positioning, prevention of tissue or nerve damage and maintenance of a sterile field.
- The maintenance of accurate records that reflect patient care delivery while in the perioperative environment.
- Moving beyond the theatre walls to develop roles within such areas as tissue viability and infection control teams.

This is only a snapshot of what is possible for the scrub role. What in many cases is so frustrating is that these nursing activities are indeed carried out, but are often not actually recorded. There is little or no evidence from documentation in some areas that any 'nursing' or 'caring' activity has actually taken place. When speaking to many perioperative nurses undertaking the scrub role, they can often recite a list of activities contributing to the holistic needs of the patients, but fail to record them anywhere. To the outsider, and this often includes others in the nursing profession, omission can only lead to one conclusion, which is that the care did not actually take place! The nurse in this instance is in direct breach of the profession's guidelines for the maintenance of records (UKCC 1998). Perioperative nurses are often shocked by this, but continue to feel powerless to affect change in this area. If there were documentation of actions and a record of who carried them out, it might help to clarify the role the perioperative nurse and in particular the role of the 'scrub' nurse. It would appear that while the nurse has been functioning in the 'scrub' role other personnel within the departments have developed their roles. These developments further compound the issue of unique, autonomous practice for the perioperative nurse (NMC 2002).

New roles within the traditional scrub area have emerged in the last ten years. The nurse as the first assistant to the surgeon is one. Many traditional 'scrub' nurses have viewed this as a way forward for their career and certainly interest in the development of programmes to support this role is growing (Biggins 2002). Once again the cynic would perhaps argue that this is yet again a way of shoring up the shortfall in junior doctors, not a way of enhancing nursing care (McKenna 1993; Greenhalgh 1994; Woodhead 1995; Pearce 2003). In contrast, others view the role as a way of ensuring the provision of experts who provide quality care based on sound educational theory (Biggins 2002). The latter will not be possible, though, until *all* carrying out this role, rather than doing it because there is no one else to, undergo a designated educational programme of study. This will ensure that these roles, unlike others in the perioperative environment, are taken seriously and not viewed as those learned 'on the job'. This may prevent repetition of problems in terms of misconceptions and confusion regarding roles, which is so often witnessed in the perioperative environment.

If administered correctly these new roles present the perioperative nurse with a unique position in which she/he can truly affect patient care. The role of the surgical practitioner, in particular, will enable the perioperative nurse to combine the necessary diagnostic and checking procedures with the provision of psychological support for the patient, so often lacking in the busy assessment process. It would allow for holistic care, while also creating autonomous practice. This role is one emerging as a driving force in the field of day case surgery and in some trusts the role has further developed to encompass the role of the 'emergency pre-assessment clinician'. These are exciting roles for the perioperative nurse.

Tissue viability services and wound healing teams are another area in which the traditional role of 'scrub nurse' is being developed. The perioperative nurse can, through consultation with specialists in wound healing, select appropriate dressings, ensuring that the application of the correct dressing is made at the outset, rather than the application of the 'one the surgeon has always used', even when the nurse is fully aware of the inappropriateness of it! The development of specialist knowledge in this area will ensure a positive outcome and avoid unnecessary pain and suffering for the patient. In some trusts perioperative nurses are utilised as a resource in the management of wounds for all patients. This has done much to raise the profile of the perioperative nurse in the wider hospital setting.

The infection control role is similarly developing, perioperative nurses taking the lead in the provision of infection control services. The incidence of nosocomial infection is an ever-rising figure (DoH 2002b). Here the perioperative nurse can affect a positive outcome of care by the education of staff and adherence to infection control policy, through linking with the infection control team to develop strategies to limit cross infection. The in-depth knowledge gained 'on the job' is supplemented and enlarged by study and research in this specialist field. Discussions with clinical colleagues reveal a rise in the numbers of perioperative practitioners undertaking specialist studies in this area. This creates a perioperative nurse with a unique area of practice rather than the 'holistic' or generic nurse. This could be considered as more specific, but other developments may be creating a generic perioperative nurse.

Combining two or more roles within the perioperative environment is now commonplace for new nurse recruits to theatre. Many are combining the role of scrub nurse with that of anaesthetic nurse, having undergone post-basic education in the area. These courses ensure that the nurses are competent. For many, this allows them to combine the highly technical aspects of the roles, with the ability to communicate with the awake patient, providing expert assistance with the provision of both physical and psychological care in order to support the needs of the patient. These needs are also met by combining the role of scrub nurse with that of the recovery nurse.

It would seem that there is a role for the scrub nurse in providing holistic care for the patient, but in many instances this requires a monumental shift in the way in which some traditional 'scrub' nurses view their role. It is whether they can make this shift that will ultimately decide whether or not the scrub role remains. The additional question that follows is whether the scrub role remains the domain of the nurse or a scrub assistant. Is the role specific to nursing, and should nurses fulfil specific roles or become generic practitioners, covering all aspects of theatre work in a holistic approach to patient care?

THE POST-ANAESTHESIA ROLE

To many the most obvious environment for the perioperative nurse to deliver patient care is in the post-anaesthesia or recovery unit. Certainly it is the area where most nursing students on allocation to theatre feel most 'at home' and able to apply previously taught principles to the care of a patient. Traditionally this has always been the exclusive role of a nurse. However, with the introduction of NVQ care modules and the extended post-anaesthesia placement experience for those undertaking the Dip (HE) ODP programmes, this too is now not always strictly the case. Certainly in many trusts, ODPs now actively contribute to the service and in some areas lead the care provision in the post-anaesthetic phase.

The role of recovery nurse is becoming more and more challenging. The complexity of surgery performed is constantly developing and the need to operate on more critically ill patients has become the norm in many units. Consequently the clinical skills required of the recovery nurse have advanced to ensure a safe and effective recovery from these complex and lengthy procedures. This resulted in a natural progression to the provision of high-dependency care for these patients with increasing postoperative dependence. Many are now utilising these skills to continue this dependent care beyond the confines of the recovery

unit. Surgical and anaesthetic techniques have ensured that the needs of these patients have far exceeded merely supporting the patient's jaw until awake or ensuring that regular observations of vital signs are performed and recorded. The role of the perioperative nurse in recovery is now much more about the ability to manage the critically ill patient in a non-ICU environment. This undoubtedly places many new responsibilities on the recovery nurse, not least acquiring the clinical skills in order to care for these highly dependent patients. Many recovery nurses are undergoing specialist education in areas such as ICU and high-dependency nursing; others are building on their theatre experience and undertaking post-basic programmes in anaesthetic nursing.

Without this specialist input and attainment of specialist skills like the scrub nurse, the recovery nurse is in danger of becoming only able to deliver a snapshot of the patient's needs, knowing little of the anaesthetic techniques required or the intraoperative surgical management. However, like many scrub nurses, the recovery nurse is recognising the need to develop as an 'all rounder' in perioperative practice.

As alluded to earlier, multiskilling for the recovery nurse is not just confined to the theatre doors. The recovery role, as with roles performed by the anaesthetic and scrub nurse, has moved into the wider hospital arena. In some trusts the provision of high-dependency units (HDU) as well as recovery units has meant that recovery nurses are required to staff such areas and provide the 24-hour care required for these patients. With the move toward the provision of such services in high dependency and intensive care, the ability of the recovery nurse to translate and transfer skills is fast becoming a requirement of the role. As highlighted previously, the generic critical care role is fast becoming a reality. The Comprehensive Critical Care document (DoH 2000) has shifted the boundaries of care for the critical care patient further. This drive will see further development in the management of highly dependent patients within the walls of the operating department. What is again crucial is that perioperative nurses or practitioners working in this area are equipped with the necessary clinical skills to enable them to care for such highly dependent patients. Equally it will be important to ensure that there are sufficient numbers of appropriately qualified staff to cope with demand. This will require careful and meticulous workforce planning on the behalf of theatre manages and project team leaders.

Another role that has emerged over the last ten years for the recovery nurse beyond the scope of the perceived, 'traditional' role is their contribution to the delivery of an acute pain service in many hospitals. The report by the Royal College of Surgeons and College of Anaesthetists (1990) highlighted the need to provide a quality pain service within all hospitals. The recovery nurse has played in many instances a pivotal role in the provision of postoperative pain relief for surgical patients and indeed in some areas they actively contribute to the delivery of care to those patients in non-acute or chronic settings. Such roles are exciting and will ensure clinical development for the perioperative nurse.

A UNIQUE BODY OF KNOWLEDGE

In order to carry out the roles discussed in the previous section, it is necessary to examine the knowledge base and question the uniqueness of this for the perioperative nurse. The care of the patient in this critical time of surgery is served by the knowledge provided by so many disciplines. Clearly, it is extremely difficult to compartmentalise such care provision. As a profession, over the last 20–30 years, nursing has been striving to develop a body of knowledge that is unique to nursing. The developing body of knowledge has given rise to the creation of nursing theory that has attempted to describe and identify the complexity of nursing (Chinn and Kramer 1995; Edwards 2001).

This challenge has not just been for the perioperative nurse. Each speciality in nursing is endeavouring to achieve a body of knowledge discreet only to them. While the pursuit of evidence to support practice is to be applauded, the quest to develop uniqueness of knowledge has in some instances been complicated, if not impossible. The ultimate purpose of nursing has been to address patient needs, which are many and varied. The knowledge that is required to address these complex needs has been drawn from other disciplines, such as psychology, sociology, physiology and even medicine. This fact alone illustrates that nursing knowledge cannot ever be entirely unique. The uniqueness of nursing could be said to come in the 'care' aspect. However, this too could be questioned since the ability to 'care' is clearly not unique to the nurses' role. The challenge remains to identify the uniqueness while selecting from other disciplines the skills in order to address the complexity of patient needs.

Identifying knowledge has led to research development and the provision of evidence to support practice has become a requirement for the perioperative nurse. The advent of clinical governance and the provision of clinically effective care are now essential, and trusts throughout the country are all striving to ensure compliance with government requirements (DoH 1997). The perioperative environment is perhaps under its brightest spotlight.

Care delivery in the perioperative environment is being scrutinised both internally and externally. Some find this intrusive and threatening, while other perioperative nurses and practitioners are excited by the opportunities to develop new practices and enhance those already existing within their units.

The existence of research material specifically created by perioperative nurses has been limited. Access to funds specifically set aside for nursing research can be difficult and the time available to seek out such monies is again limiting for many nurses (Funk *et al.* 1991; Polit *et al.* 2001). The last few years have seen a reduction in the workforce in theatre and recruitment, as in many areas of nursing and health care, is low. Retention of existing staff is also an issue; this further compounds the manpower shortage in theatre (Hay Group 1999; Hind and Wicker 2000). This has meant that the remaining staff have struggled to provide a service with a depleted workforce. The need for professional development and education studies has in consequence been given a low priority in some units (West 1994). However, despite these very real challenges, there is still a need to explore and develop the practice of the perioperative nurse and the need to examine the care required by the patients in their care.

THE ROLE OF RESEARCH TO INFORM PERIOPERATIVE PRACTICE

Research has been described by Polit and Hungler (1995) as a 'systematic inquiry that uses orderly scientific methods to answer questions or solve problems' (p. 652).

This indicates the importance for perioperative nurses to endeavour to identify areas of practice for research and the setting of quality indicators for practice guidance. Some perioperative nurses find it difficult to even identify aspects of their work worthy of research. This is in many instances understandable. The culture in some units has been a little limiting in its approach to research and professional development. For others this has not been the case. Perioperative nurses have extensively explored areas such as pressure relief, the management of patient temperature in the theatre environment, aspects of information giving and the provision of preoperative assessment (Reid 1997; McNeil 1998; Scott 1998). However, there are still so many aspects of the patient experience that could be improved or enhanced by evidence to support practice, for example through bench marking and standard setting (Audit Commission 2000). Interestingly, even with evidence to support practice development and enhancement, care still falters. A prime example from practice is preoperative assessment by the perioperative nurse. While 'the body of knowledge' has indicated that the practice is a positive one for the patient, still the incidence of preoperative assessment in many units remains low (Williams 2002). Clearly, the perioperative nurse needs to be exploring why this is so.

While the pursuit of evidence to support practice is to be applauded, the quest to constantly develop uniqueness of knowledge has in some cases made the profession lose sight of what the patient's needs and wants are. In many nursing roles aspects of essential nursing care have been lost to the development of specialist skills. This is not unique to the perioperative nurse; other specialisms too have witnessed an erosion of nursing care provision. In many areas care perceived as the domain of the 'nurse' is carried out by the HCA, with the nurse occupied with managerial tasks. Recent developments in the media have interestingly highlighted the state of hospital wards and how the role of ensuring cleanliness should return to the ward sister. While this may result in a cleaner environment for patients, how will the sister have made time available to carry out this role reversal? Like most things it will have been added to their already busy schedule, taking them still further away from direct patient care. This type of role erosion is all too often witnessed in theatre.

The pursuit of knowledge to underpin and support practice must be seen as one of the many priorities within theatre departments; not just research for research sake, but also something seen as the pursuit of academics seeking to make a name for themselves. Research borne out of patient need and care development should be encouraged and actively supported with time and money. This might seem fanciful and typical of an academic, but the pursuit of excellence in practice must be encouraged even in the current and ever-continuing crisis in the NHS. If the perioperative nurse or indeed any nurse decides to settle for second best then they are advocating the delivery of second rate care for the patient. The collaboration between units and universities needs to be fostered and developed through a variety of schemes. It should not be the academic alone conducting research, but schemes should also assist and support those less experienced in the clinical area, in order to enable them to carry out studies in the 'real' environment. This will have a twofold effect. Firstly and most importantly, the patient will receive the 'best possible' care and secondly the practitioner will be meeting both professional requirements and also growing personally.

THE FUTURE, THE PERIOPERATIVE NURSE AND THE EMERGENCE OF THE PERIOPERATIVE PRACTITIONER

At the outset the challenges facing the perioperative nurse were outlined and it has emerged that this new century has witnessed new challenges to the role of the perioperative nurse. Throughout this chapter it has been difficult not to describe the nurse as a perioperative 'practitioner'. However, the remit was to discuss the changing role of the nurse in the perioperative environment and this necessitated the exploration of the nurses' role in some isolation. Clearly this is not a true reflection of most theatre departments. While many are still staffed by a majority of nurses, a large number too are staffed with operating department practitioners. The move has been toward a common title to prevent confusion among staff and make the transition to common pay spines more simplistic (DoH 2002a). This has meant changes for all staff in the area, but perhaps most for the 'nurse'. The loss of the title has for some been hard to bear. It is somehow seen as synonymous with the ability to 'care' and has presented serious consequences for some nurses in terms of re-registration with the NMC. The ability to meet and rise to these challenges will ultimately decide the future of the nurses' role in theatre.

The rapidly developing role of the ODP will undoubtedly present the greatest challenge for the perioperative nurse. Many former ODP training schools have or are amalgamating with universities. They are developing diploma level courses, degree programmes and seeking to link and develop programmes along a generic critical care route. These are exciting times for the ODP, creating new pathways and at last a programme of post-qualification development so often lacking for them within the clinical arena. The Association of Operating Department Practitioners (AODP) have worked tirelessly for these developments, much as nurses have done in the past. We are assured also that professional registration for the ODP is imminent and previous barriers to their progression are slowly being eroded. This will result in the emergence of yet another autonomous, professionally accountable practitioner. These issues will force those nurses wishing to pursue careers in theatre to examine, identify and clarify their roles. This may mean the pursuance of specialist roles within the context of surgical/critical care, for example, the roles highlighted within the discussion thus far: first assistant; surgical practitioner; acute pain management; infection control; and other roles within the critical care environments. These changes will require the perioperative nurse to undertake academic study in order to ensure that practice is underpinned with the appropriate theoretical knowledge, and will require the development of new clinical skills. This will undoubtedly require commitment and present individual challenges to the perioperative nurse.

To conclude this opening discussion, I would like to share the following personal observation and thoughts. All too often I have witnessed professional snobbery and confrontation in the perioperative environment. The debate and counter-debate regarding who is the best practitioner to provide the much needed care required by the patient, somehow seems to actually take precedence over the delivery of any care at all. The roles for *all* working within the perioperative environment have changed. The future for all working in this dynamic environment is exciting. However, to continue the futile debate regarding who is best to deliver care is foolhardy and will only perpetuate existing and long-standing problems such as recruitment and retention difficulties. So, the challenge to all perioperative practitioners will be to set aside some of these issues so often recounted and to really seek to analyse the nursing or caring contribution to be made for the patients in their care. I anticipate that there will be a continued role for the perioperative nurse, but this will rest on the individual's and the profession's tenacity and a continued desire to pursue professional goals. This clearly will only be achieved by the delivery of a quality patient-centred service.

REFERENCES

Association of Anaesthetists of Great Britain and Ireland (AAGBI), Royal College of Anaesthetists (RCA) (1996) *Anaesthesia in Great Britain and Ireland. A physician only service*. London: AAGBI and RCA.

Association of Anaesthetists of Great Britain and Ireland (AAGBI), Royal College of Anaesthetists (RCA) (1998). *The anaesthetic team*. London: AAGBI and RCA.

Audit Commission (2000) *Getting better all the time: making benchmarking work*. London: Audit Commission.

Barker M (1996) Should there be a nursing presence in the operating theatre? *British Journal of Theatre Nursing* 5(18): 1134–1137.

Bevan PG (1990) *A report on the utilisation and maintenance of operating theatres*. London: HMSO.

Biggins J (2002) The role of the RNSA in colorectal surgery. *British Journal of Perioperative Nursing* 12(6): 222–226.

Boss S (2002) Expanding the perioperative role. The surgeons' assistant. *British Journal of Perioperative Nursing* 12(3): 105–113.

Bowman M (1995) *The Professional Nurse: Coping with Change Now and the Future*. New York: Chapman and Hall.

Brown A (1994) Theatre nursing. The fight for survival. *Nursing Standard* 8(20): 31–34.

Chinn PL and Kramer MK (1995) *Theory and Nursing: A Systematic Approach*, 4th edn. New York: Mosby.

Chinn PL and Kramer MK (1999) *Theory and Nursing: Integrated Knowledge Development*, 5th edn. London: Mosby.

Crawford B (1999) Highlighting the role of the perioperative nurse – is preoperative assessment necessary? *British Journal of Theatre Nursing* 9(7): 319–322.

Department of Health (1991) *Patient Charter*. London: HMSO.

Department of Health (1997) *The new NHS – modern and dependable*. London: DoH.

Department of Health (1998) Review on prescribing, supply and administration of medicine. A report on the supply and administration under group protocols. London: DoH.

Department of Health (1999a) *Making a difference: strengthening the nursing midwifery and health visiting contribution to health and healthcare*. London: DoH.

Department of Health (1999b) *Continuing professional development: quality in the new NHS*. London: DoH.

Department of Health (2000) *Comprehensive critical care. A review of adult critical care services*. London: DoH.

Department of Health (2001) *Consultation on proposals to extend nurse prescribing*. London: DoH

Department of Health (2002a) *Agenda for change*. London: DoH.

Department of Health (2002b) *Getting ahead of the curve*. London: DoH.

Dimond B (1994) Legal aspects of role expansion. In: Hunt G and Wainwright P (eds) *Expanding the Role of the Nurse – The Scope of Professional Practice*. Oxford: Blackwell.

Edwards SD (2001) *Philosophy of Nursing. An Introduction*. New York: Palgrave.

English National Board for Nursing, Midwifery and Health Visiting (ENB) (1994) *Creating lifelong learners: pre-registration guidelines*. London: ENB.

English National Board for Nursing, Midwifery and Health Visiting (ENB) (2000) *Education in focus: strengthening pre-registration nursing and midwifery education*. London: ENB.

Funk SG, Champagne MT, Weise RA and Tornquist EM (1991) Barriers to using research findings in practice: The clinician's perspective. *Applied Nursing Research* 4: 90–95.

Greenhalgh & Co. (1994) *The interface between junior doctors and nurses: a research study for the Department of Health*. London: HMSO.

Haralambros M and Holborn M (2000) *Sociology. Themes and Perspectives*. London: Harper Collins.

Hay Group (1999) Report on nursing shortage study. *Nebraska Nurse* 32(2): 17.

Hertzberg F (1959) *The Motivation of Work*. New York: Wiley.

Hind M and Wicker P (2000) *Principles of Perioperative Practice*. London: Harcourt.

Kalideen D (1991) The case for pre-operative visiting. *British Journal of Theatre Nursing* 1(5): 19–21.

Leddy S and Mae Pepper J (1998) *Conceptual Bases of Professional Nursing*, 4th edn. Pennsylvania: Lippincott-Raven.

Mackenzie J (1998) (ed) *Ward Management in Practice*. Edinburgh: Churchill Livingstone.

Marson S and Hartlebury M (1992) *Managing People*. London: Macmillan.

Martin D (1996) Preoperative visits to reduce patient anxiety: a study. *Nursing Standard* 10: 23.

McCloskey DJ and Kennedy GH (2001) *Current Issues in Nursing*, 6th edn. New York: Mosby.

McGee P (1997) Theatre nurses face elimination. *British Journal of Nursing* 1(11): 535–536.

McKenna G (1993) Caring is the essence of nursing practice. *British Journal of Nursing* 2(1): 72–75.

McNeil BA (1998) Address the problems of inadvertent hypothermia in surgical patients. Part 1 and 2. *British Journal of Theatre Nursing* 8(4): 8–14 and 8(5): 25–33.

Moloney MM (1992) *Professionalization of Nursing. Current Issues and Trends*, 2nd edn. Pennsylvania: Lippincott.

Moore S (2002) Changing the workforce. *British Journal of Perioperative Nursing* 12: 6.

Morrall P (2001) *Sociology and Nursing*. New York: Routledge.

National Association of Theatre Nurses (NATN) (1992) *The named nurse in the operating department*. Harrogate: NATN.

Nightingale K (1999) *Understanding Perioperative Nursing*. London: Arnold.

Nursing and Midwifery Council (NMC) (2002) *Code of professional conduct*. London: NMC.

Pearce L (2003) Handing over. *Nursing Standard* 16(36): 33–37.

Polit DF and Hungler BP (1995) *Nursing Research Principles and Methods*. Pennsylvania: Lippincott.

Polit DF, Beck CT and Hungler BP (2001) *Essentials of Nursing Research Principles: Methods, Appraisal and Utilization*, 5th edn. New York: Lippincott.

Reid J (1997) Meeting the informational needs of a patient in a day surgery setting. An exploratory level study. *British Journal of Theatre Nursing* 7(4): 19–24

Rothrock JC (1996) *Perioperative Nursing Care Planning*, 2nd edn. New York: Mosby.

Scott E (1998) Hospital pressure sores as an indicator of quality. *British Journal of Theatre Nursing* 8(5): 19–24.

The Royal College of Surgeons of England and the College of Anaesthetists (1990) *Pain after surgery. Report of the working party of the commission of the provision of surgical services*. London: RCS.

United Kingdom Central Council for Nursing, Midwifery and Health Visiting (UKCC) (1995) *Prep and you. maintaining your registration*. London: UKCC.

United Kingdom Central Council for Nursing, Midwifery and Health Visiting (UKCC) (1998) *Guidelines for records and record keeping*. London: UKCC.

United Kingdom Central Council for Nursing, Midwifery and Health Visiting (UKCC) (1999a) *Fitness for practice: The UKCC Commission for Nursing and Midwifery Education*. London: UKCC.

United Kingdom Central Council for Nursing, Midwifery and Health Visiting (UKCC) (1999b) *A higher level of practice: a report of the consultation on the UKCC's proposals for a regulatory framework for post registration clinical practice*. London: UKCC.

Walton J and Reeves M (1996) *Management in the Acute Ward*. Wilts: Mark Allen.

Welsh J (2000) Reducing patient stress in theatre. *British Journal of Perioperative Nursing* 10(6): 321–327.

West BJ (1994) Caring: the essence of theatre nursing. *British Journal of Theatre Nursing* 3(9): 15–24.

White J and Coleman M (1999) Preoperative visits in Wales. B*ritish Journal of Theatre Nursing* 9(10): 472–479.

Wicker P (1995) Preoperative visiting: making it work. *British Journal of Theatre Nursing* 5(7): 16–19.

Williams M. (2002) Preoperative visiting – an urban myth? *British Journal of Perioperative Nursing* 12(5): 168.

Woodhead K (1995) Assisting the surgeon: the dilemma for nurses. *Nursing Standard* 10(3): 53–55.

2 ADVANCED AND SPECIALIST PERIOPERATIVE PRACTICE

Mark Radford

CHAPTER AIMS

- To define concepts of specialist and advanced perioperative practice
- To describe the historical development of perioperative advanced practice
- To explain competencies of advanced practice
- To evaluate effectiveness of perioperative advanced practice roles
- To introduce Practice Exemplars of perioperative specialist and advanced practice.

INTRODUCTION

Modern health care has changed radically in the last few decades; the UK in particular has seen changes in the economic, political and professional landscape in which it delivers health care. Perioperative practice has lagged behind in development and role innovation and this has led to what Barker (1996) describes as a 'watershed' in the very existence of perioperative practice. Nothing but a radical redirection is required by perioperative practitioners to focus upon holistic care and empowerment of the patient.

Advanced and specialist perioperative practitioner roles can provide the innovation required to rejuvenate perioperative practice, and may go further to help define the essence of perioperative practice itself. This possibility is important as the current stagnation of perioperative philosophy, research and clinical practice has led to professional isolation, particularly of the perioperative nurse from the mainstream of nursing culture.

This chapter will aim to both enhance knowledge and enable the comparison through critical evaluation of the emerging advanced practitioner

concepts in perioperative care. It will chart the development and influences of current perioperative roles, placing them in organisational and professional context. A detailed examination of the skills and competencies required by an advanced perioperative practitioner (APP) will be undertaken, using practice exemplars to highlight new ways of working in the modern perioperative setting.

ADVANCED, ADVANCING AND SPECIALIST PRACTICE – WORKING TOWARDS A DEFINITION

Finding a workable definition of advanced and specialist practice has been particularly problematic. Much of the published work from academics and professional bodies has left confused messages as to the function of many new roles. There is a great deal of evidence that exists to aid our understanding of current trends and developing theory, although much of it is anecdotal, opinion-based, biased or full of professional rhetoric.

The main problem is that both medical and nursing organisations have been unable to pinpoint whether advanced practice roles in general are responding to new clinical needs of patients, identifying missed opportunities in care, or the gradual withdrawal of a professional group from an aspect of physical or psychological care. Such 'withdrawal from the bedside' and then 're-engineering' of traditional roles has occurred at all levels and can go some way to explain the explosion of specialist nurse and paramedic roles in acute hospital settings. Dunn (1997) feels that this link between evolutionary advanced practice and the institutional requirements of health care is overwhelming, and in the case of advanced and specialist practice has mostly been achieved by the medical influence over other health professionals. These influences will be tackled in further detail later in the chapter.

Specialist practitioner

Although this chapter will concentrate on the development of advanced practice in the perioperative setting, analysing the differences between advanced and specialist practice is helpful in clarifying the role. Specialist practitioners are involved in more complex decision making than their general professional colleagues. However the core competencies are subtly different from those of advanced practitioners. They will be expected to be expert in their sphere of clinical influence, be involved in teaching, research and audit, providing leadership as either a manager or role model at local level.

One could argue, and many have, that all perioperative practitioners fit the description of a specialist. Indeed Hamric *et al.* (1996) had encountered this problem in the US, a country with a long history of development in this area, where she suggested that specialisation involves concentration in a selected clinical field, which has occurred over years of development. Perioperative practitioners work *within a speciality* and are therefore not specialists. However, within perioperative practice there are practitioners who will work at a higher and more specialist level, such as postoperative acute pain specialists. The United Kingdom Central Council's (UKCC 1994) definition of specialist practice helps define this better, in that:

specialist practitioners will demonstrate higher levels of clinical decision making and will be able to monitor and improve standards of care through the supervision of practice, clinical nursing audit, developing and leading practice, contributing to research, teaching and supporting professional colleagues.

UKCC (1994) p. 11

Legitimisation of this role has occurred over many years, mainly built on the work of the American author Benner (1984). From a UK perspective, Castledine (1995) has been vocal in identifying the specialist nursing role, when he suggested that the specialist nurse should:

explore new knowledge about the nature of nursing, integrate new medical treatment and technology into holistic nursing care, continue to integrate and understand the increasing and complex knowledge being developed in the biological and social sciences, satisfy the curiosity of the committed, intelligent, creative and sensitive nurse.

Castledine (1995) p. 264

Advanced and advancing practice

In identifying a definition it is useful to disengage two important phrases, *advanced* and *advancing practice*. There are subtle differences between those practitioners that are *advanced* in terms of their practice and those that are *advancing* professional practice. Historically, it is simple to identify those who have challenged the very essence of nursing practice to evolve its professional status to a higher level, such as Nightingale, Orem, and Roper. Time is a great leveller and what is now advancing practice will over time no longer be seen as the forefront of developments and will become embedded in professional roles, as new models supersede them.

Advancing practice has always been linked to the knowledge and skills interface that exists between nursing and medicine. Critics, particularly in nursing, continue in trying to understand the unique influence that nursing has over patient care to reject the recognition that nursing and medicine share much in terms of knowledge and outlook. For example, Manley (1997) suggests that roles taking on previously medical-orientated tasks such as initiating diagnostic investigations and clinical examination are not advancing their own professional knowledge base. What may distinguish the two is not necessarily particular knowledge, skills and competencies, but vision, leadership, and a willingness to use it. In perioperative care such attributes would be essential against a background of underdevelopment of perioperative care philosophy, high service pressures, under funding of education and working in organisations that remain dominated by surgeons and anaesthetists. Despite perioperative practice being burdened with this patriarchal atmosphere, it must be remembered that surgery and anaesthesia can only be performed by a multidisciplinary team. Therefore advancing perioperative practice can be achieved by developing new interprofessional roles that challenge traditional boundaries of care, in collaboration with medicine and recognition of common knowledge.

The UKCC definition of advanced practitioner in the early 1990s suggested that the advanced practitioner was concerned with:

adjusting the boundaries for the development of future practice, pioneering and developing new roles responsive to changing needs and with advanced clinical practice, research and education to enrich the profession as a whole.

UKCC (1994)

McGee (1998) identifies that this definition was a step forward in recognising that these roles require considerable professional knowledge and expertise, supported by professional qualification through cumulative education and professional maturity. This important view reflects the developmental qualities that experience can bring to the advanced practitioner. In support, Hamric *et al.* (1996) identifies that those who try to lead this process, such as physicians' assistants or nurse anaesthetists (CRNA), are often alienated from mainstream nursing culture, although widely accepted in the medical world.

McGee (1998), who is influenced by the work of Hamric *et al.* (1996), identifies that advanced practice is multifaceted and integrates a whole host of skills and competencies added to the individual's personal qualities, stating that:

Advanced practice is about what drives the individual, what motivates them ... Being an advanced practitioner is therefore as much about individual characteristics as professional expertise.

McGee (1998) p. 178

It is clear from the literature that a great deal of ambiguity remains as to the definition of advanced and specialist practice. A unanimous definition is unlikely to be reached until a complete advanced practice framework has emerged and clarification should be made by the practitioners themselves through evaluation and research rather than by academics or managers.

INFLUENCES IN THE DEVELOPMENT OF THE ADVANCED PRACTICE FRAMEWORK

There have been major political, social and economic changes leading to a general review of the health-care agenda. It is easy to identify that the global changes in health care can be seen in terms of increasing clinical knowledge, increased use of technology and a growing specialisation of both medicine, nursing and AHP's roles.

Castledine (1998) emphasises that nursing has been increasingly drawn into a gradual specialisation. The proliferation of specialist nursing forums such as National Association of Theatre Nurses (NATN) and British Anaesthetic and Recovery Nurses Association (BARNA) are testimony to this. However, Castledine identifies that a distinction must be drawn between the specialisation *in* nursing and the specialisation *of* nursing. The latter is determined by external influences, both in society and medicine.

Technological advances in surgery and anaesthesia are often the catalyst for the future development of perioperative roles. Such developments are well-documented; Wicker and Strachan (2001) state:

Changes in the organisation of the NHS, changing demographics and the social trends and a constantly evolving technical environment ... the way in which operating departments will be managed, planned and staffed also has widespread implications for the future role of (perioperative) practitioners.

Wicker and Strachan (2001) p. 29

In essence what they highlight is that a new breed of practitioner will be required to function in this arena. Perioperative practice will have to develop new skills and competencies, both clinically, academically and professionally to meet these challenges. The current professional climate has evolved to include advanced practice as a pivotal concept, and will be the practitioner that will confront the problems of a modern health service.

Technological advances only partly represent the whole picture. Other developments have challenged the traditional boundaries of medical power and autonomy in the UK, with far-reaching political consequence for nursing and AHPs. Conflicts between medicine and other health professionals, particularly nursing, are increasing. There is growing realisation that health-care provision is a sickness-focused service being delivered to a powerless patient by a centrally controlled and increasingly politically motivated medical profession. Using nursing as an example, this power differential can be explained through gender and the issue of occupations. Denny (1999) found that the development of nursing as an organised occupation is characterised by caring being perceived as women's work. Indeed early writers such as Hughes (1951) had linked the emergence of nursing to the role women played in the patriarchal home of Victorian Britain, reinforcing biological femininity and natural order within the home dominated by Victorian values. This subordinated nurses to the male dominated division of labour, confirming what feminists had understood for some time. Such patriarchal attitudes are remarkably resilient in contemporary health care, including the perioperative environment. The role women play in society and consequently the caring professions has changed positively over the last 30 years, particularly in terms of work and career, thus allowing women to assert their places in the professional workforce. Such positive philosophy permeated nursing, and challenges were made to the traditional role of the nurse in the health-care organisation. This is also true in the case of AHPs.

ADVANCED PERIOPERATIVE PRACTICE – EXTENDED AND EXPANDED TRADITIONAL ROLES, PIONEERS OR PROFESSIONAL NO MAN'S LAND?

In light of the previous section, the above question is important, as roles can now develop beyond the traditional boundaries independently of medical agreement. It is clear that the developments in the nurse–doctor interface will need realignment in the light of such contemporary evidence. Economic factors have also been very influential, particularly in the US where Bigbee (1996) identified that advanced practice developed out of the need for skills in rural areas, where medical staff were difficult to recruit.

The UK picture is quite different, with far greater medical involvement in the definition and work of advanced practice. The development of specialist nursing centred upon areas of medical specialisation – infection control, acute pain, stoma care and colorectal surgery. Each was headed by a medical consultant and the nurse took his or her place within the negotiated order of the 'team'. This system reflects both the dominant patriarchal model and the bureaucratic enforcement of the division of labour. What is important for the APP in this setting is to understand how this order is enforced and to what extent learned competencies can ensure that their voice is heard. Unless challenged, this structure with its negotiated order ensures that the APP serves to administer just to the 'emotional workload', a view supported by Thibodeu and Hawkins (1994) who established that the APP apply holism within a traditional medical model, relying mainly on psychosocial information. These roles often have very little legitimate power for the individual and may require strategies such as collaboration and consultancy to overcome this. The threat that this has generated to medical authority is clear as Hay (1994) a consultant surgeon writes:

Nursing has undergone a dangerous quasi-intellectualism over the last few years. Clinical autonomy has become the goal, self-improvement the spur and the service to the patient has become the abandoned policy of yesterday.
                                    Hay (1994) p. 42

Behind the rhetoric lies an important statement of the attitude within the medical profession that continues to contribute to the impression that nurses and AHPs are still subordinate to them, despite many changes to the social and healthcare landscape. Role developments do not need to remain static and controlled in such a way.

The role and function of many nurses and AHPs has often been guided by the Department of Health or organisational bodies such as the British Medical Association (BMA), General Nursing Council and Royal College of Nursing (RCN). For example the Briggs Report (DHSS 1972) examined those areas where nursing and medicine overlapped, with the recommendation that any task to be undertaken by a nurse should be part of their post-registration education and training. The guidelines issued by the Department of Health in 1977 (DHSS HC77[22]) to Health Authorities provided the legal and practical framework, including certification and additional education required to perform these extended roles.

Two important factors in the 1980s and 1990s finally brought the issue to a head. Firstly, the growing realisation that doctor numbers were declining and there would be a shortfall of specialists, coupled with the debate raging over junior doctor's hours and training. Secondly, the fact that nursing and AHPs truly lacked a positive clinical career structure. For nursing, the 1990s saw a barrage of policy, which focused on the perspective of role change. Key to this was the UKCC documents, the Scope of Professional Practice (UKCC 1992b) and Code of Professional Conduct (UKCC 1992a), changing the focus for nurses from one of dependence, subordination and medical delegation, to independence, autonomy and responsibility. Autonomy and accountability are recurring themes in the concept of advanced practice that will be explored in detail later in the chapter. However, unsurprisingly at the same time the calls for a reduction in junior doctors' hours (NHSME 1991) under the new deal arrangements and changes to medical speciality training under the Calman Hine system (Ham *et al.* 1998; DoH 1993) left many with the impression that these changes had been forced upon nursing, and well-orchestrated to ensure acceptance by both nursing and medicine. Despite attempts to maintain a nursing focus, a lack of political power saw nurses gradually take on tasks that were previously the domain of medicine.

This begs an important question, what is the difference between an expanded and extended role? The difference is in historical semantics, in that extended roles were those tasks delegated by medical practitioners and not learnt during pre-registration training. After 1992, they became expanded, although they were packaged to include a positive nursing focus. Such rationalisation of roles and task allocation is evident in the perioperative literature. Brennan (1999) makes the distinction between these when examining how they became part of the perioperative practitioner's repertoire, suggesting that expanded roles are more flexible, proactive and patient-focused.

However for each individual patient undergoing surgery, a set plan of care must be completed with both physical and psychological elements. The importance of this for APPs must be that they impact on this care process and not collect delegated medical tasks, unless they are useful in fulfilling the needs of the patient. Therefore, APPs should augment the process rather than be defined by certain tasks and roles. For example, in Exemplars 2.1 and 2.2 – to work as part of the team, assessment may be completed by the anaesthetist or APP; if a task such as clinical examination or ECG interpretation is not complete, then either can perform this function and then share in the decision making process. It can be argued that it is this model that is truly holistic and it is explored in much more detail on p. 23, through collective clinical knowledge. When training to take on additional tasks, the appropriate expert must be found to facilitate this; it may mean tutoring from a doctor for clinical examination skills, nutritionist for postop feeding regimes, or physiotherapist for pre- and postoperative exercises.

PRACTICE EXEMPLAR 2.1: ADVANCED PERIOPERATIVE PRACTICE IN EMERGENCY SURGERY

An increasing proportion of the NHS activity is emergencies, both medical and surgical. Such activity is spread between many specialities, and many professional groups. The processes involved in getting these patients the appropriate care are often complex, and can be disjointed and subject to delay. This creates frustration for patients who require information on their treatment progress, plus problems for clinicians and the organisation.

The creation of operating theatres dedicated to emergency surgery has occurred in many NHS hospitals; there are high activity, high cost facilities that due to the nature of the workload are difficult to plan and co-ordinate effectively.

An advanced perioperative role in pre-assessment was collaboratively developed to shape and manage the emergency and trauma surgical workload. An APP was equipped with skills in physical preoperative assessment and by evaluation of the patient's condition was able to co-ordinate the care process between A&E, the wards, and through to the operating theatre to ensure rapid access to surgery. With these skills, the nurse is not only able to co-ordinate the surgical care

process, but support the anaesthetic, surgical, and nursing teams in prioritisation, and optimisation of the patient condition, including initiating investigation and prompting further treatment. This has also afforded the opportunity to develop the professional nurse's role in the management of emergency patients through training and education in patient management:

- Management of specific patient group – emergency patient admissions through casualty, including minor gynaecological, general plus orthopaedic trauma, general surgery.
- APP of an interdisciplinary team of consultant anaesthetist, registrar and senior house officer.
- The relationship with the team is one of 'consultancy' rather than supervision.
- A team role of holistic patient care. An individual role of:
  - Preoperative assessment and optimisation of condition for surgery and anaesthetic (advanced health assessment). Initiate investigations where appropriate.
  - Postoperative evaluation, follow-up, health promotion and patient education.

THE NURSE/AHP CONSULTANT

The falling public confidence of the medical profession, and new initiative in releasing the potential of nurses and AHPs, was the cornerstone policy in re-evaluating the NHS. From the point of advanced practice, in the early 1990s the UKCC and DoH details were still in draft form. However, the government documented the creation of 'Nurse and AHP Consultants' at the 'Nurse 1998 Awards', who in the words of Tony Blair would have 'the same status within nursing that medical consultants have within their profession' (DoH 1998a). This set a benchmark of expectation for the public and medical staff of what these practitioners intended to do in prac-

tice. Firm plans for 'nurse consultant' were left until the publication of the next White Paper, 'Making a Difference' (DoH 1998b), which had an emphasis entirely on the nursing profession in the NHS. Although well-presented, it had been quickly collated and had less to do with the nursing agenda than with the political timetable. However, in a sense it acted as a catalyst for a variety of organisations to commit to the concept. Ultimately the nurse consultant was placed at the top of the pile of professional expertise mirroring that of the medical profession, providing an extended clinical career ladder (see Figure 2.1).

The issue of academic preparation for such roles has been widely debated. In the US, the link between advanced practice and a high level of

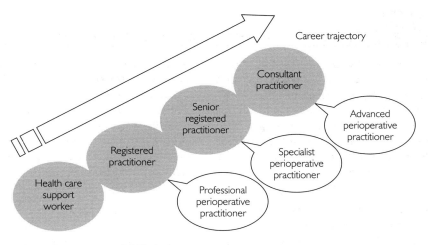

Figure 2.1 Career pathway for nurse post (NHS plan)

academic achievement is well-established, and often acts as a descriptor to the status of the practitioner. The same has been suggested in the UK context by Wicker and Strachan (2001) and Radford (2000). The American Society of PeriAnaesthesia Nurses (ASPAN) provided the following position statement in 1996:

An advanced practitioner must

- Possess a minimum of a Masters degree in Nursing.
- Integrate the role components of clinical practice, education, research, management, leadership and consultation.
- Function in a collegiate relationship with nurses, physicians, CRNAs, nurse midwives and other health-care providers.

CURRENT PERIOPERATIVE TRENDS

What does this mean for the future of perioperative practice? The cumulative specialisation both *in* and *of* nursing, coupled with the fundamental 'biomedical and task-orientated' models of the early 1980s made it very difficult for perioperative practice to fit with the modern perception and definition of what was a caring profession. With perioperative practice, ultimately entwined with what is perceived as an interventional biomedical model, rather than the health promotion focus, it

was not viewed as holistic. As has been well-documented in Chapter 1, the introduction of the specialist operating department assistant (ODA), initially a technical role, in the late 1970s by Lewin (DHSS 1970) and the later re-evaluation by Bevan (NHSME 1989), into operating theatre practice furthered the argument about the lack of holism in perioperative practice. The implication for perioperative nurses was that with the addition of care planning, recovery skills and drug administration under the NVQ system which created the operating department practitioner (ODP), conflicts occurred in the operating theatre as to who had the sole right of care delivery.

The ODP was a very powerful catalyst in changing attitudes towards skills mix in the operating theatre (see Chapter 1). The concentration of managerial efforts looked to rationalise the use of the multiskilled practitioner. Such pressures further polarised views between professional organisations; indeed BARNA ran two provocatively entitled debates during their national conference of 1997 and 1999 – 'the nurse's place is in the anaesthetic room and the ODP should be consigned to the scrub role' and 'the specialist versus multiskilled practitioner debate'. The result of the latter was overwhelming support for further specialisation by scrub, anaesthetic and recovery roles. The undertones of this went against the established position of flexible staffing from organisations and other professional bodies such as NATN and AODP. In terms of advanced practice debate, the ODP has been left out of service developments, an opportunity largely ignored by the DoH and NHS Trusts, although a NVQ framework to level 5 exists.

Advanced perioperative practice has seen little movement in the last two decades, although Castledine (1998) had recognised that specialist anaesthetic roles had developed in the 1970s, with Millington (1976) who worked in an expanded capacity within an anaesthetic team. The role was mostly delegated responsibilities such as preoperative visits, IV therapy and postoperative pain techniques. The lack of forward movement in enhanced roles for practitioners in the anaesthesia team has been because the debate is interlocked with the issue over nurse anaesthesia. Nurse anaesthesia was without support as a concept within the UK medical profession (Reilly *et al.* 1996), until recently when anaesthetic bodies have accepted the role within a European training framework and it is currently under development with the Modernisation Agency Workforce Confederation. Other role development from the surgical perspective has been attempted, including the most publicised role developed by Suzanne Holmes (1994), who started as the cardiac surgeon's assistant at the Radcliffe Hospital, Oxford. Initially her role was very interventional, harvesting veins for bypass grafting, and her clinical results proved very positive when compared to medical colleagues. However, her role changed later to include preoperative assessment and counselling, plus discharge liaison and postoperative issues. Despite the change in emphasis, the role has been criticised as paramedical, or described as physician's assistant (Castledine 1998), although it has been vociferously defended by the practitioners themselves.

Despite the arguments, the proliferation of surgical assistant posts accelerated with support from professional bodies. The 1998 document 'Perioperative Nursing: The Future', sponsored by NATN, RCN and BARNA effectively rubber-stamped the posts, but was clear to distinguish that two levels of such assistants existed, the nurse as the first assistant (NATN 1993), and the nurse as a surgeon's assistant (NATN 1994). Brennan (1999) identifies the differences between the two: the surgeon's assistant is able to undertake operative procedures under supervision, although others recognise that they have now evolved to be able to undertake indirect supervised sessions. The first assistant plays a less proactive role and mainly assists in retraction and suturing. The medical profession has accepted such role development, as they are able to maintain an element of control of future capabilities through training and accreditation, and in some respects perpetuates the patriarchal relationships that have existed previously.

Very few perioperative roles in the UK have been established at consultant level; by 2001 only two out of 451 existed which mainly concentrated in elective preoperative assessment and have a role in continuing professional education. Most of these developmental and pioneering roles will act as templates for a future generation of practitioners. It is important that a diverse range of strategies are employed to identify the role and skills required to complete the job, before perioperative practice is lumbered with politically and clinically sanitised advanced practice roles. Now more than at any point in the history of perioperative practice is a debate worth generating to establish the pioneering and advancing nursing roles to the wider nursing arena.

A CONCEPTUAL MODEL OF ADVANCED PERIOPERATIVE PRACTICE

This model of advance practice requires someone who has vision and depth of clinical understanding to challenge the model of care delivery with critical thinking, providing patients with holistic health assessment and to augment their care process with advanced interventions, both physical and psychological. This definition incorporates several key features that are important. Firstly, that the APP must have vision and experience in the current care setting, with a broader understanding of the organisational context that their role will play. The APP must have the ability to challenge existing practice and rituals, with both autonomy and collaborative strategies. Secondly, such strategies are dynamic and are not limited to their own professional knowledge or skills boundaries. Therefore the APP can intervene therapeutically at any point in the care process dependent on their clinical experience and ability. This allows for the possibility that as experience grows, so their role may change and produce positive outcomes for the patients they care for.

There are many facets to the advanced perioperative practitioner. Those that are most important are described in detail here, such as direct expert practice and the use of collective clinical knowledge, collaboration and consultancy, professional leadership and clinical change agent skills, coaching and guiding patients through the perioperative and evaluation through research and audit.

DIRECT CLINICAL PRACTICE

Central to advanced practice models is direct clinical practice. UK nurse consultant posts have a minimum of 50% of their time devoted to clinical work. Key to any model of clinical perioperative practice must be the care process rather than the acquisition of a few new specialist clinical skills, or tasks. It is not these skills, such as taking bloods and reading the ECG, that make the role advanced, but as we have seen in this chapter the method in which they are utilised.

With the surgical patient, the care process will have many pre-determined stages that are dealt with by a different health-care professional. The preoperative phase sees a concentration on assessment, investigation and preparation to gain a greater understanding of the patient's physical and psychological health. In many cases this information is collected separately by each professional involved in their care, with little cross-referencing of clinical findings. Challenging this traditional model will help the APP take a greater involvement in the care process. To enable the practitioner to participate more directly in clinical decision making requires a

wider understanding, in terms of medicine and perioperative care issues, but also the confidence and ability to intervene and make decisions based upon a collective knowledge gained through advanced health assessment.

COLLECTIVE PATIENT KNOWLEDGE IN THE CARE PROCESS

The issue of collective knowledge for the APP is vitally important. It is clear from the literature that demarcations exist between professional groups, based upon hierarchical and often archaic perceptions of role and experience. For example, a junior staff nurse on a preoperative visit may identify that a patient requires an ECG, but is unable to perform the task. However, the senior nurse may perform the test, but would not be able to make an interpretative diagnosis or report findings to the medical team. Such situations occur many times in the care process of a surgical patient. The focus for the APP is to challenge this, both in terms of direct intervention and the role as consultant and advocate. For the APP will be guided by their experience and competence, and this will influence their consultative style.

For example, using Practice Exemplar 2.2, they would be involved during preoperative assessment, in the clinic or ward setting. The team of medical consultant, junior doctors, and APP would feed information on the patient's condition into the collective pool, based either on a notes or care pathway record. If during routine examination by the APP a heart murmur was heard, the APP could initiate further investigation and report back findings for wider discussion with the surgical team. The same would apply in the postoperative phase, if during routine follow-up it is noticed that that the surgical drain is full with largely fresh blood-stained fluid. Any practitioner should initiate investigation to ensure that the component of care process is complete (see Figure 2.2).

This process is fundamental in providing holistic care, and such interventions must remain dynamic, because by allocating tasks the focus remains on that task being completed rather than

PRACTICE EXEMPLAR 2.2: ADVANCED PERIOPERATIVE PRACTICE SURGICAL CARE CO-ORDINATOR

Patients requiring elective surgical procedures often have complex physical and psychological needs that would benefit from experienced and specialist care pre-, intra-, and postoperatively. This approach can often be achieved with an APP who supports the patient during this period with specialist skills and experience such as counselling for consent and treatment, advanced health assessment and evaluation plus surgical skills to assist during surgery.

- Management of a specific patient group through the care process.
- APP of an interdisciplinary team of consultant surgeon, registrar, senior house officer and house officer.
- Acts as consultant on surgical care both internally and externally to the organisation.
- A team role of holistic patient care. An individual role of:

- Preoperative assessment and optimisation of condition for surgery and anaesthetic (advanced health assessment).
- Psychological and physical preparation for surgery.
- Involved in informed consent.
- Assist and perfom supervised surgery
- Initiate and interpret investigations where appropriate.
- Postoperative evaluation, follow-up, health promotion and patient education.
- Co-ordination with pre- and postoperative teams. An interface with medical and nursing teams such as pain, discharge, community and specialist nurses.
- Involvement in research and academia to advance colleagues, and perioperative nursing.

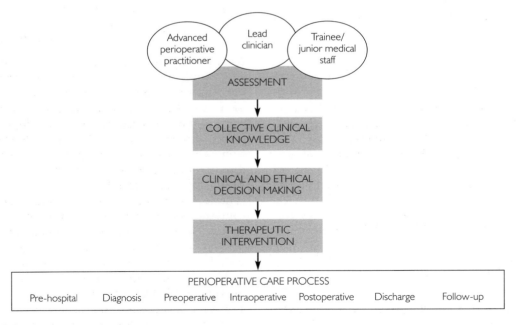

Figure 2.2 The perioperative care team

the care outcome of a holistic health assessment. Such task allocation has inevitably led to greater professional division i.e. 'that's a practitioner's/doctor's job' – creating a hiatus in the care process. Although care pathways have made an attempt to amalgamate the patient knowledge into a physical document this does not automatically manifest itself in better clinical decision making or care delivery.

There are two key features of this care model that are important to identify with. Firstly, that perioperative care begins before the patient enters the hospital, as they internalise and come to terms with their need for surgical intervention. Secondly, that the team consists of a range of practitioners who are able to assess and therapeutically intervene for the benefit of the patient. Such interventions may be physical in terms of investigations and clinical examination, but also spiritual and psychological support required during the care process.

It is important to emphasise that either of these interventions can be performed by any of the team members and therefore the roles of the practitioners may interchange, so the doctor can counsel and advise while the APP would examine, and vice versa depending on the situational context of care.

COLLABORATION IN PERIOPERATIVE ADVANCED PRACTICE

Collaboration is a key component and competency for any perioperative practitioner advanced or otherwise, a view that is reflected in the health science literature. In the past 20 years, a number of definitions have been developed. Baggs and Schmitt (1988) succinctly identify the following definition:

> *Nurses and physicians co-operatively working together, sharing responsibility for solving problems and making decisions to formulate and carry out plans for patient care.*
>
> Baggs and Schmitt (1988)

This definition highlights key elements of collaboration namely, co-operation, responsibility and decision making. It also suggests a dynamic and synergistic relationship between physician and nurse, with the emphasis on patient outcome. Central to many models of advanced practice is the concept of team and 'teamwork'. The terms 'teamwork' and 'collaboration' are used interchangeably; however the two meanings are subtly different. The implication of teamwork is that by joining a team one relinquishes identity and influence to achieve a common purpose, a laudable approach. However, as we have seen in care delivery using the holistic approach, professional identity and experience as a consultant are important values to bring to the bedside. This identity issue is well-explained by Jones (1994) who cites the American Nurses Association Policy statement on collaboration. This statement recognises the benefits that nursing has to add to collaboration with expert knowledge within a holistic framework; it suggests a mutuality and professional interdependence. It also identifies issues of power, identity and value that other definitions do not:

> *A true partnership, in which power on both sides is valued by both, with the acceptance of separate and combined practice spheres of activity and responsibilities, mutual safeguarding of the legitimate interest.*
>
> ANA (1980) p. 7

Most of the UK and US literature focuses upon the nurse–physician relationship; the concepts of power and partnership in relation to collaboration and advanced practice is a pivotal one.

Exploration of the historical developments of collaboration from the US and UK literature is helpful in relating this competency to perioperative practice. As we have seen, the specialisation *in* and *of* nursing coupled with the technological advances and rising expectations have been driving forces in modern health care. This changing landscape has also influenced collaborative relationships. The underlying theme suggests that collaboration is seen in terms of positive outcome, for patients, society and health-care professionals. These links have been established based upon very little empirical research, and are often suggested following analysis of data from nurse–physician relationship studies. Migueles and Brustowiscz (1997) linked improved patient care via collaboration in the perioperative setting, and found that this was achievable following greater professional understanding between nurses and physicians. They further suggest that the effects of collaboration in perioperative care can and will reduce the costs of health-care delivery. However this idea has been highlighted in other work. Woerth *et al.* (1997) support the cost-saving benefits of collaboration, with their work on coronary artery bypass grafting. Their examination of greater collaboration related to the learning curve in the developmental techniques in perioperative teams. This led to fewer complications, less time in the intensive care unit (ICU) and shorter hospital stay. Collaboration played an important role in these outcomes.

Professionally, some have seen collaboration as 'working with the enemy' and as having some pitfalls. Lorentzon (1998) views collaboration with uncertainty, reflecting that a collaborative programme could detract from the purity or 'unique identity' of professional knowledge. The implication is that collaboration is in some way a legitimising of intellectual professional practice.

Links between collaborative care and quality, cost and risk management have led to policy development in the UK. The Government White Paper *A First Class Service. Quality in the NHS* (DoH 1998c) unites these concepts with clinical governance. This suggests that with collaboration and greater professional understanding there would be a reduction of risk and its litigious consequences. In support the RCN (1998) guidance identifies collaboration and partnership as a basic principle within the framework of clinical governance. Much of the data for collaboration has focused on more qualitative issues surrounding decision making and ethical/moral implications of care between nurses and physicians. These are often concentrated in the traditional nurse–physician relationship, especially in specialist fields such as critical care (intensive care and anaesthesia). These ethical/moral decisions made as part of collabo-

rative working are important features of an APP's work. Baggs *et al.* (1997) looked extensively at the decision making process involved in patient care in intensive care. In a longitudinal descriptive correlation study, they found that collaboration is viewed more importantly by nurses than physicians, through the physician's belief that they are the primary decision makers. This is clearly evident in perioperative practice where surgeons still define the procedure and its timing. This hierarchical relationship is an area to be challenged by the APP. The surgeon's role is perceived to remain in authority and control, and as we have seen in this chapter, has a great deal to do with medical training and socialisation. Leadership within the team should be dynamic and shift, depending on what aspect of care is under discussion, but this may be a difficult concept to develop within teams headed by surgeons, as it may be seen as a threat to the traditional view of power and autonomy. This area of working relationship has been very seldom explored, although Stacey (1988) suggests that power and authority has shifted in health care, but boundaries are often redrawn without equalising the parties in favour of the medical staff.

As APPs gain greater knowledge and skills, the demarcation between disciplines in a traditional health-care structure are blurred, which may lead to conflict. Hanson and Spross (1996) suggest because of values held by physicians, plus the hierarchical structures of hospitals, medical staff will often see the relationship between themselves and the APP as one of total supervision. Challenging this boundary is important for perioperative practice, developing roles and professional status.

CONSULTANCY

Examination of the literature finds a wealth of information on the role of consultation in advanced practice. Definitions are prolific, as are descriptive and process models of consultancy.

Until recently the terms 'consultant or consulting' have been used synonymously with a medical practitioner. The role of consultancy in relation to advanced practice is not questioned, but investigation as to the most appropriate model is warranted. As APP redefines the boundaries of perioperative practice, contact in the form of consultation increases. Berragan (1998) charts the development of consultation linked with advanced practice. However influential advanced practice may have been in highlighting its role, the concept of consultancy is not new. Within the sphere of UK practice, the UKCC PREP (Post Registration Education and Practice Project) clearly identified the role of advanced practitioners as consultant practitioners and confirmed that they are crucial in the conceptual challenges and education of new clinical roles. Caplan (1970) and Caplan and Caplan's (1993) work is considered seminal in its conceptual development of consultation in health care. Caplan describes consultation in a process framework; in depth examination of his work reveals prerequisites of this. These are firstly, a request for consultation (therefore a consultee) and secondly a person with expert knowledge to gain from, encased in a problem-solving framework.

Schein (1988) develops the themes from Caplan's work to formulate a model of consultation that is more transferable to acute and critical care. Schein identified three models of consultation:

- Purchase of expertise
- Doctor–patient
- Process consultation.

Purchase consultancy and doctor–patient consultancy both mirror established relationships of the consultation framework developed by Caplan. Expertise can be purchased or requested, when the practitioner has amassed a level of knowledge that may be required by another organisation or for the purposes of professional education. Traditional doctor–patient consultation needs little explanation, other than this can be replaced by an advanced practitioner. Process consultation offers a new dynamic; it engenders elements of collaboration and consultation. The aim is to develop and teach other health professionals problem-solving skills rather than to solve the problem themselves, which is particularly useful in perioperative advanced practice where the diversity of consultation work can be extensive. The model of interdisciplinary perioperative care highlighted in Practice Exemplar 2.3 is a useful example of the diversity of collaboration and consultation. To encourage and enable an environment for problem-solving approaches to patient care, rather than adopting prescriptive authority would demonstrate the value of APP without devaluing or alienating other professional groups involved. Role conflict has already been established in this chapter regarding physicians; however conflict will arise from other healthcare professionals. Elcock (1996) provides evidence for this as he describes that 'consultant nurses' are often viewed as aloof, elitist and removed from patient care. This view is not consistent with those of others, and as 'process consultation' identifies, the role of the APP can improve care without direct 'hands on' action through leadership and teaching. Within perioperative practice a large base of experienced and skilled practitioners exists, and so consultancy for advanced practitioners would probably be a multimodel approach. Utilisation of other specialist practitioners would be paramount.

Additionally 'external' consultancy with the UK and NHS should also be taken on by the APP resulting in the dissemination of work such as publication and presentation, income generation through training and education and recognition for the organisation. However, Mills (1996) identifies that for both options, professional credibility and competence were essential. As a footnote, Manley (1997) in her action research of a nurse consultant's role in a critical care setting, found that consultancy cannot survive on its own as a job. It must be linked to collaboration to succeed in facilitating a quality patient-centred service.

PRACTICE EXEMPLAR 2.3:	ADVANCED PERIOPERATIVE PRACTICE EDUCATOR, CONSULTANT AND RESEARCHER

The technological advances in clinical work in the perioperative environment has seen an expansion in the role that training and education has to play in ensuring practitioners are able to meet the demands of theatre work. With the advances comes a responsibility to ensure that specialist skills are transferred to professional nursing members of the theatre team in a structured and cohesive manner. This educator role needs extensive researching to ensure that professional advancement is made for the individual nurse and the profession as a whole, and identifies with the global changes of the nursing role and the impact that they can have on future perioperative provision.

- The practitioner needs to have expert clinical knowledge to facilitate the educator role and is often combined with a teaching role within a higher education setting.
- Co-ordination of pre-registration student nurses and post-qualification professional nurses, development of education provision for advancing skills of the perioperative nurse.
- The practitioner must see the development of nursing as a linear progression from student to professional to specialist practitioner. This can be achieved by an educational individual performance review (IPR).

- As a consultant the practitioner acts as an interface between medical, nursing and managerial colleagues to adjust the boundaries of professional practice.
- It is important that research and audit is generated, not only in educational methods for perioperative nursing but also in clinical practice. This can be achieved in the following ways:
  - Development of own research projects and dissemination at national and international level.
  - Identify collaborative research and audit work between medical, nursing and paramedical roles.
  - Encouragement for professional and specialist nurses to research their clinical practice and work on methods for improving care.
  - Act as a research guide for perioperative nursing to identify areas of practice that would benefit from audit and research.

PROFESSIONAL LEADERSHIP AND CLINICAL CHANGE AGENT

Leadership has long been an important subject in health care, and in particular its relevance to advanced practice is an almost mandatory competency. Finding a useful definition is as fruitless as searching for a clear definition of advanced practice, and this section will not attempt to do so, but highlight what it may be and what it may mean to those in practice:

Leadership is not so much about technique and methods as it is about opening the heart. Leadership is about inspiration – of oneself and of others. Great leadership is about human experiences, not processes. Leadership is not a formula or a program, it is a human activity that comes from the heart and considers the hearts of others. It is an attitude, not a routine.

Lance Secretan (1998)

As McGee (1998) has identified, an ideal of an advanced practitioner should be through empowering to change the practice of others and serving in the best interests of the patients. This concept fits well with ideas of 'mastery' and excellence in clinical practice that has been demonstrated in the competencies of direct clinical care and consultancy. Campbell (1999) takes a refreshing view of leaders, drawing an important distinction between those positional leaders and those who are charismatic in being able to change practice, influencing group dynamics and truly becoming proactive to their clinical surroundings and shape, challenging the environment in which their patients are cared for. Campbell (1999) goes on to enhance her argument, identifying those characteristics including:

- Personal values
- Sensitivity
- Intelligence
- Interpersonal skills
- Enthusiasm
- Decisiveness.

However, these characteristics must be tempered with additional functions that transcend human traits. Leadership, as either a positive or negative, is perhaps the strongest variable in highlighting the role of the perioperative practitioner within the organisation or more globally in their profession. Kerfoot (2000) identifies that unity is an important paradigm that must be supported by every level of practitioner, and that unity comes from sharing a common vision.

Vision and visionary thinking are often key descriptors of leaders, but in many ways require a commitment of the individual to understand themselves in the context of their own strengths and weaknesses. Such personal awareness is often a vital prerequisite in the pursuit of a vision, and in many cases may be influenced by the organisation they work for, previous experience and influences on their career. Vision should be developed within the individual APP and may take many forms. Bower (2000) suggests that vision is also a strategic awareness of a preferred future and possible future level of practice. Alongside this, 'risk taking' has been recognised by many as an important step in controlling the vision and future direction of practice and demonstrates to others a confidence in stepping forward into the unknown and pushing back the boundaries of care delivery. Bower (2000) goes on to say that such 'risk taking' is always a calculated 'gamble' between proposed gains and losses, although visionary leaders may often have

a sense that there is a need to change that can be supported by their skills set. The natural assumption placed by McGee (1998) is that such skill/competencies are achieved through experience and education that are developed through advanced practice work. This may be true to an extent when the practitioner is considered expert in the field of practice, having a greater understanding of the system in which their patients are cared for. This also transcends practical work to include economic tasks, research and development, education and professional supervision.

Working as an APP often brings the individual into closer and enhanced level of working with professional colleagues, and is supported in terms of their credibility and developed value/belief system, often the cornerstone of their expert practice. Credibility is a characteristic which is further developed in the management chapter of this book. Such credibility may work at several levels with other health professionals, such as surgeons who value clinical skills, consistency, commitments, and loyalty for their service. Alternatively, they will use the same characteristics to support the professional perioperative practitioner as an interface of change with clinicians to their own working practices. Political agendas may also work to the advantage of the APP when working with the service development team who need a 'champion' to gain clinical 'buy in' where previous attempts may have failed (see Practice Exemplar 2.4).

Supporting or leading clinical change must be viewed as an integral role for the APP, and many models exist to support this process. Modern change management has altered dramatically, and it is not enough to assume that moving from A to B is sufficient. How the change was achieved and what sustainability it has should also be reflected upon. Managing clinical change must be supported by those with clinical expertise as this is central to the process of support and sustainability, i.e. getting the teams to own the change. The actual process of clinical project management can be achieved, and in many cases is better performed by a person who is unrelated to the area or is not a clinician.

PRACTICE EXEMPLAR 2.4: CREDIBILITY AND 'BUY IN' FOR CLINICAL CHANGE

A centrally funded health service redesign project was awarded to the district hospital, which had difficulties in managing its emergency workload. The perioperative advanced practitioner was identified to lead a redesign programme alongside their clinical work. The level of clinical 'buy in' and credibility to the person's role was seen as a significantly important leadership characteristic for both hospital management and clinicians. The project produced significant results, some of which were embedded into the organisational culture by the clinical team's ownership.

The text has so far concentrated upon the individual in support of leadership, but one must have people to lead. As is often the case the APP may be isolated from their peers due to the organisation structure or their role within the care team. This can often lead to assumptions that the individual is elitist which can have negative consequences on individual identity. Therefore the empowerment of others can often be an effective leadership strategy with which to counter some of the challenges posed by APP. Empowerment can take many forms including enhancement of patient care through education and development, which is described in Chapter 9. APP may mentor practitioners or provide supportive environment for personal and professional growth, utilising skills of guiding and coaching to both patients and staff (see Practice Exemplar 2.3).

COACHING AND GUIDING PATIENTS AND STAFF

There are many challenges faced by perioperative practitioners, as you are often involved in very complex care and unique care situations. These scenarios require the APP to coach and guide patients, their relatives and the staff caring for them, through complex systems. APP will develop complex strategies to shape and challenge the system to optimise care delivery. The author and former mentor, June Duesburry, had been working extensively with this concept, where:

a 'clinical navigator' is the link between the matrix of disciplines that make up the whole system of care, including primary and social care ... they are a promoter of integrated services who ensures the patient travels along the care pathway/trajectory in a smooth and timely fashion.

June Duesbury (2001) at Orthopaedic Collaborative Conference, London

Using such a holistic care approach that incorporates strategies of a 'navigator' will produce changes to the health of an individual and wider population. Perioperative practice must realign itself from the disease focus to a more societal one. Clarke and Spross (1996) state that such strategies must be a fundamental role where:

education provided by the ANP (APP) are best conceptualised as an interpersonal process of coaching through transition.

Clarke and Spross (1996) p. 140

In the perioperative setting, surgery is a transitional or significant life event and mode of facilitation must be viewed symbolically by the patient and APP. Clarke and Spross (1996) define the health goals in coaching and guiding as:

preventing future illness, decreasing chronicity, limiting relapse, alleviating suffering, responding to crisis.

Clarke and Spross (1996) p. 144

This philosophy is clearly important for all ANP, based in critical or acute care. Benner's (1984 and 1991) work is influential in the interventional role, and Benner extrapolates some fundamental skills for ANP including expert knowledge, ability to individualise illness, previous experience, and ability to create interpersonal competence with the patient. In its clinical application to the perioperative patient, it is useful to gain an understanding of the perception of health and illness and the perioperative patient. Turner (1995) articulates that:

An individual interprets their disorders ... upon the classification of illnesses which are available within a culture and by reference to general cultural values concerning appropriate behaviour.

Turner (1995) p. 207

The concept of the 'sick role' is well-documented and the 'Parsonian Model' (Parsons 1951) remains as applicable today in organisations. It is largely accepted that institutionalisation within the acute care system does take place. Therefore empowerment of the patient and greater involvement in care can be seen as a challenge for APP roles, and offers hope of reform in perioperative practice. Stacey (1988) remarks that health and illness need to be internalised as there are societal influences on health; certainly people feel responsible for their health and are largely defined by it. Stacey further states that:

with infectious diseases far less threatening in mass terms, chronic illnesses have assumed greater importance, and sickness has become a way of life, not a way of dying.

Stacey (1988) p. 143

In every-day perioperative care, two important factors must be taken into account when delivering such a care process. Firstly that during the preoperative assessment process, consideration must be given to what Leininger (1990) calls the emic (Insider) and etic (Outsider) perspective. This endogenous, exogenous framework mirrors the nurses' and patients' perceptions, experiences and expectations of surgery. Secondly this must be made in light of the cultural framework and family matrix, which play a distinct role in health.

The APP must therefore seek to understand all the social as well as physical interpretations of a patient's health and illness during the preoperative assessment process to ensure that they are supported along a positive health trajectory. However the etic perspective of patient care, concepts of control, powerlessness, and independence are important interpersonal dynamics for perioperative patients. The impact for APP is that unless patients are better informed, and motivated in relation to their health trajectory, then outcomes will be far worse in areas such as independence and powerlessness. Despite having to place a great deal of control of their health over to health-care professionals during hospitalisation, powerlessness is an important precursor to anxiety in the perioperative patient. As Bennett and Murphy (1997) identify, the empowerment approach, which also involves personal growth and development, is a particularly useful tool and is under-utilised in perioperative care. Although its foundations is in the humanist psychology movement (Maslow 1970; Rogers 1961) it is particularly apt for perioperative interventions.

The challenge posed by any perioperative health model is that there are many layers to the perioperative experience. This includes stress and anxiety related to powerlessness, surgery, disease and anaesthesia. Empowerment for perioperative patients can be seen as preparation and working through anxiety posed by surgery and disease. Janis (1958) and Salmon (1993) found this vital for patients to cope with the immediate threat to health (i.e. surgery) and long-term health trajectories associated with their disease process. As perioperative practitioners it is important to identify that surgery is just a small part of the patient's journey, and the impact as highlighted in Practice Exemplars 2.5 and 2.6 can be quite significant and must be managed with care and experience.

The overall aim and objective of a perioperative health model is to empower the patient within their disease and perioperative experience and reduce feelings of dependence. This can be achieved by utilising the perioperative experience

PRACTICE EXEMPLAR 2.5: COACHING AND GUIDING THROUGH CHANGE

A young female patient has been living with ulcerative colitis for many years, suffering pain and discomfort. She has had several admissions, including one bout when an emergency colectomy was performed, leaving her with an ileostomy. She spent several days on the high dependency unit and has had regular follow-ups since, including endoscopic examinations. This was a very stressful time for her and her family and it has been hard for her to adjust to the ileostomy. She believes her body image has suffered. As a result, she has ventured out less and less with her friends. During one of the follow-up visits to the hospital she is offered the chance for an ileo anal pouch procedure, the impact of which on her life will be great. The actual perioperative episode is an important defining moment and motivation will be high; the impact of carefully managed support pre-, intra- and post-surgery will be vital in supporting this transition. Can the long-term health impact be separated from the perioperative episode?

PRACTICE EXEMPLAR 2.6: SUPPORT FOR THE BREAST CANCER PATIENT

A female patient has been diagnosed with advanced breast cancer. This news has devastated her and she is having difficulties in coming to terms with the impact that this will have on her and her family life. The patient is counselled while further investigative work is done, and she is listed for a mastectomy with lymph node clearance. She is seen preoperatively by the APP who supports the information and counselling provided by the cancer nurses, and places the perioperative period in context of their disease, family matrix and cultural environment. The patient is on a trajectory that needs to be supported with consistent information from a range of professionals. Again, can the long-term health impact be separated from the perioperative episode?

as a symbolic life event for lifestyle change, and allowing the patient to 'let go' following discharge.

It is important to understand the impact of the perioperative experience and the implications this has on long-term trajectories of health described above. Salmon (1993) and Salmon *et al.* (1989) identify that medicine has defined the stress of surgery and hospital admission as an undesirable outcome that adversely affects postoperative recovery. Metabolic and endocrine changes are used as indicators of stress; however, they are normal physiological actions of tissue damage that aid recovery. The focus of perioperative research has been on the reduction of preoperative stress, through the use of psychological techniques. Janis (1958) and Salmon (1993) identify that anxiety preoperatively, in the psychological context, would help recovery. Salmon (1993) suggests that threats to health would allow patients to adjust more adequately to forthcoming events. Salmon (1993) describes this as:

realistic mental rehearsal for surgery
Salmon (1993) p. 324

This is a useful strategy to employ, particularly when acting as a facilitator in threat management, and promoting a process of 'working through' threats to health. The concept of 'working through threats' and empowerment are useful tools that can easily be implemented via emotional pre- and postoperative support, encouraging productive worry and reducing feelings of helplessness.

Therefore, understanding of the perioperative episode in relation to the disease process and the patient's life continuum is vital. Empowerment by the APP during this phase should also aim to create an environment of self-help and positive direction for the patient. This process can be utilised to lower trajectories of dependence and powerlessness later in life (see Figure 2.3).

The health trajectory gives a context framework to the perioperative health model. However within the actual perioperative experience it may cause a transitory increase in dependency and powerlessness caused by hospitalisation and surgical care (see Figure 2.4).

The use of life transition and events for behaviour change is an application that has its roots in developmental psychology, including Piaget, Freud and Erickson. Kimmel (1980) found that idiosyncratic transitions would allow change, reorientation and transition, changing a negative experience (i.e. hospitalisation and surgery) into a positive outcome (i.e. lifestyle change). The implications of this for the patient are important. Firstly in terms of the physical changes to health following surgery and altered body image after surgery. Secondly, in spiritual and emotional terms, relating to powerlessness and dependency, creating an awareness of the fallibility of self and their own individual health needs.

The process utilised to formulate change is based upon a 'stages of change' model developed by Prochaska and DiClemente (1984), as it allows flexibility to respond to individuals with different motivational needs. This 'stages of change' model is transposed upon the normal perioperative care continuum utilised by an APP (see Figure 2.4).

During the preoperative assessment, *precontemplation* is an initial step towards lifestyle changes and risk re-evaluation. It is an important time to explore previous attempts at change, exploring the emic and etic perspectives of health and broadly understand influences on the individual's lifestyle and health-related events.

Bennett and Murphy (1997) suggest that attempts at this stage to identify goals and change lifestyle may well lead to resistance. Informational needs should be addressed, aiming to personalise disease and prepare for the move from a steady psychological state to disequilibrium, and challenge beliefs via facilitation not argument. As Caplan (1964) suggests the experience can be used to benefit personal growth. At this point other agencies may be needed, to reinforce perception, including nurses, other APPs, doctors and psychologists as the credibility of the source of information and its trustworthiness have important influences on how the message is received, interpreted and acted upon.

The surgical episode should be in *contemplation*, the process of surgery acting as reinforcement as to the threat to health. The

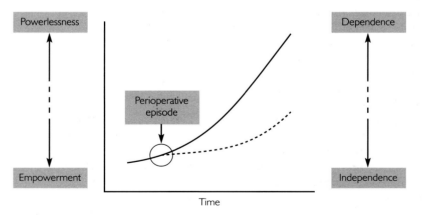

Figure 2.3 Perioperative health trajectories

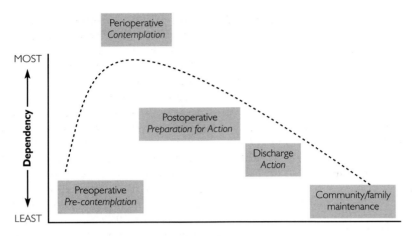

Figure 2.4 Stages of change model for perioperative health trajectory

process of anaesthetic and recovery is described as a symbolic awakening, a view that Moch (1998) identifies with her phenomenological examination of breast cancer and mastectomy patients, facilitating rebirth through illness.

Following immediate postoperative recovery, the patient needs to *prepare for action*; goal setting at this stage may lead to direct action from the patient in terms of lifestyle changes. The family must be involved so that outcomes are achievable within the home and community environment. Changes may include preparation for exercise, with the involvement of physiotherapy and occupational therapy, and identifying modes of exercise suitable for individual patients. Bennett and Murphy (1997) suggest that a focus is needed so that accommodation of new ideas can take place and this must be placed contextually in the hospital experience. The patient needs to identify that discharge is a reality and replace feelings of powerlessness with competence over situations that cause concern. The trajectory to be aimed for is lower than prior to admission. Fatalism must be replaced by hope and an improved emotional outlook.

Action and maintenance are inherently the difficult parts of any health model, and more often than not occur when the least support is avail-able. Lifestyle changes that are required to challenge sick roles must be made in the community and family environment. Support must be given to the patient so that hope does not turn to despair, and return the feelings of powerlessness. Backett (1990) identified that involvement of the family was vital in any lifestyle changing health model, making it clear that partners are not the only influences, and that children exert a significant effect on lifestyles within families. Johnson and Nicklas (1995) state that one approach taking into account these influences is to utilise the support of the family by improving the lifestyle of the family as a unit, leading to greater chances of a positive outcome.

This model of the 'navigated' surgical journey identifies several key features for the APP:

- Strong emphasis of holistic care integrated with advanced skills and competencies.
- Working across departmental and professional barriers to challenge variances in care delivery.
- Supporting and coaching perioperative practitioners in achieving effective outcomes for patients on their health trajectory.
- To reduce dependency and powerlessness for the patient.

APP coaches patients through the important and complex arena of the perioperative episode, and also supports staff in caring for these patients. The mastery of skills through technical expertise, clinical and professional development must be tempered with thoughtful self-reflection. There are often no precedents or protocols to support these processes and many may be developed through intuitive delivery and previous clinical scenarios. The APP must aim to see beyond the surgery to identify where their skills may challenge care delivery.

EVALUATING ADVANCED PERIOPERATIVE PRACTICE ROLES THROUGH RESEARCH AND AUDIT

The APP will use up-to-date research to support and direct practice; however, research utilisation and its application explains only part of its use in advanced perioperative practice. Despite a proliferation of advanced and specialist roles, evaluation through either research or audit is in its infancy. There is an important role for those in such positions to evaluate the impact of their role on individual patients as well as the organisation and perioperative practice generally. This assessment can be performed by the individual practitioner or through collaborative research within the perioperative setting.

Several fundamental evaluation questions are identifiable:

- Understanding the scope and role of advanced perioperative practitioners.
- Understanding the contextual issues of advanced perioperative practice.
- Identification of models of advanced perioperative practitioners and their future impact on health care.
- What barriers exist in fulfilling the true potential of advanced perioperative roles?
- What impact do advanced perioperative practitioners make in the health-care system?

The evaluation of these questions is a complex process that can be addressed though a variety of tools and techniques. The research techniques required by an advanced perioperative practitioner cannot be addressed within the framework of this chapter. This chapter will examine that process of evaluation and formulate a model of how this would influence current and future practice, rather than concentrate upon tools and techniques.

Several well-tested evaluation models exist when examining the impact of developing advanced practice roles, such as those made by Girouard (1996). What is useful from this work is the importance in understanding the structure, process and outcomes in assessing impact of changes in health-care delivery. The practical interpretation of these models is slightly more problematic and does not in many cases support the wider agendas in health care, in particular policy and the influence of the health-care organisation.

A continuum model that examines these points as the role develops from its early stages through to more complex long-term strategic goals is more helpful. It is during this continuum that audit and research must be directed by the practitioner to fulfill the knowledge and information requirements. Girouard's (1996) adapted evaluation model from Ventura *et al.* (1991) is a useful starting point, although contextually does require some work to identify its relevance to perioperative practice. The other deviation in our adapted model (see Figure 2.5) is the importance of linking the evolutionary development of the post to ongoing evaluation, as it is often the case such developments are tied to professional, organisational as well as economic goals, that have evolved through population and health community assessment. The initial focus for evaluation of advanced perioperative practice should try to understand what the role is attempting to do in relation to the population and/or the health community it serves.

To put it simply there are some broad questions that need addressing:

- What is the nature and scope of the problem faced by the population?
- What national targets are related to the population?

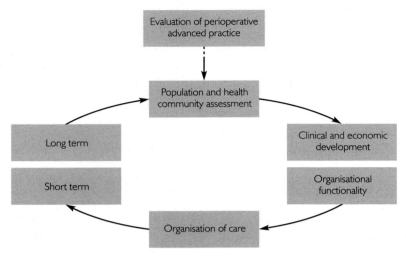

Figure 2.5 Evaluation model for advanced perioperative practice

- What internal organisation pressure or agenda does this fit?
- Is the proposed advanced practice role engaging with the population?
- What are the cost-effectiveness and the proposed benefits?
- What are the governance risks associated with its development?

These questions can be answered in many ways through user involvement/feedback, literature reviews, organisational and clinical audit, and existing research. In some cases this may have been identified through the practitioners' own clinical experience. For example, Practice Exemplar 1 on emergency surgery was originally identified through the practitioners' understanding of problems faced by emergency patients; this prompted a literature review which fed an audit of current practice that confirmed problems.

The clinical and organisational development stage is an important if often neglected area in advanced practice evaluation. Such clinical changes that may be proposed by the advanced practice role will involve significant cultural shift and in many cases challenge traditional boundaries of professional and departmental care. Such change should be structured to understand potential professional conflicts, including those that may exist between medical and perioperative boundaries that have been highlighted earlier in the chapter. Identification of the key stakeholders is vital for ongoing support and success and each stakeholder may require a different strategy to gain support (Figure 2.6).

• Surgeons and anaesthetists	• Perioperative audit
• Perioperative staff	• Research
• Nursing and quality directorate	• Morbidity and mortality meetings
• Finance department	• Directorate meetings
• Professional organisations	• Robust business case
• Clinical governance	• Publication and presentation
	• Risk assessment

Figure 2.6 Stakeholders and strategies for change in advanced perioperative practice development

The outcome from this clinical and organisational development stage will inform the key areas for change, scope the role and identify proposed areas for research and audit. Ultimately goal-setting by the organisation and professional bodies may determine those areas for examination that are detailed in the next stage.

Organisation functionality is often the first aspect of evaluative work undertaken by the APP and may examine those specific competencies that are important to the role's success such as expert practice, leadership, education, and service redesign. These are not in-depth analysis, but may be audited at a low level to assess actual workload compared to the proposed job plan. This may seem rather crude and rudimentary, but it is impossible to identify quickly, deviations from the proposed intervention strategy for the population concerned, and highlight tasks which may be added to the workload that are not valuable to the overall goal. Firstly, this initial foray must also start to formulate a proposed research and audit plan that will address some fundamental question of the role's quality, and the interactions that the role may have upon the perioperative team.

Secondly the questions may also start to address the impact on an individual patient and population. This period of role development is often described as 'bedding in', where formal analysis may not be targeted appropriately to ensure that research and audit is at the right level or direction for the advanced practitioner.

The short-term assessment goals are important milestones, and can be developed around the structure, process or outcome assessment, which is demonstrated in Figure 2.7.

Radford *et al.* (2001a, 2001b) demonstrate this short-term analysis in their evaluation of the APP in emergency surgery, when identifying impacts on admission to surgery time for a range of patients, plus organisation improvements to theatre utilisation and reduction in night-time operating. Longer term goals of assessment may involve a similar structure, as seen in Figure 2.8.

CONCLUSION

Central to this chapter has been the recognition that development of advanced perioperative practice must have patient care at the core. The aim

Assessment	Plan	Examples of projects
Administrative assessment	• Target setting improvements with organisation and professional body • Meeting key national goals for population or profession • Assessment of job plan	• Reports to organisation • Clinical diaries • Competency documents
Process assessment	• Impact on perioperative team • Impact on organisational care delivery • Service redesign and management of change	• Process mapping to identify how role has improved care • Audit examining department/hospital impact

Outcome assessment	• Patient pathway analysis
	• Care quality
	• Clinical effectiveness
		• Audit/research improving patient access and choice
		• Audit/research on care quality
		• Clinical effectiveness audit on:
		  – Utilisation of resources
		  – Cost per intervention
		  – Complications
		  – Service provision
		  – Choice and access

Figure 2.7 Short-term outcome assessment in advanced perioperative practice

Assessment	Plan	Examples of projects
Ongoing administrative assessment	• Target setting improvements with organisation and professional body • Meeting key national goals for population or profession • Re-assessment of job plan	• Reports to organisation • Clinical diaries • Competency documents
Process assessment	• Whole system redesign • Influencing wider health community • Influencing profession • Education and development • Research portfolio	• Process mapping • Audit • Research studies • Publications • Presentations
Outcome assessment	• Patient morbidity and mortality • Quality and resource utilisation • Effectiveness and cost	• Audit/research improving patient access and choice • Audit/research on care quality

Figure 2.8 Long term outcome assessment in advanced perioperative practice

has been to describe the various skills, competencies and responsibilities that are required to function at this level. There is a transition for every practitioner who moves from professional through specialist to advanced practice. Many practitioners may find it hard to separate perceived advanced practice roles that on the surface require them to be technical substitutes for anaesthetists or surgeons. This chapter has aimed to separate those technical skills, and examine how a different approach to care delivery can have significant impact for patients. However, the developing role does not stop there; new aspects of care delivery must be evaluated and managed to create a new frontier of perioperative practice. At the heart of this will be dynamic and assertive practitioners who are able to think critically and challenge the care delivery system to ensure the highest standards of care in the operating room. In the third millennium there have never been so many opportunities for the perioperative practitioner, which coincide with a time when pressures are at the peak to improve efficiency and productivity in health care. There still remains a credible threat to perioperative practice to be diluted into a task-based service that often negates its wider responsibilities to the health of an individual or community. Advanced perioperative practice offers real insight and challenge to existing views on perioperative practice and the impact it can make to holistic health improvement.

REFERENCES

American Nurse Association (1980) *Nursing: a social policy statement*. Washington DC: ANA.

Backett K (1990) Studying health in families: a qualitative approach. In: Cunningham A, Burley S and McKeganny (eds) *Readings in Medical Sociology*. London: Routledge.

Baggs IG and Schmitt M (1988) Collaboration between nurses and physicians. *Image* 20: 145–149.

Baggs I, Schmitt M, Mushlin A, Eldridge D, Oakes D and Hutson A (1997) Nurse physician collaboration and satisfaction with the decision making process in three critical care areas. *American Journal of Critical Care* 6(5): 393–399.

Barker M (1996) Should there be a theatre presence in the operating theatre? *British Journal of Nursing* 5(18): 1134–1137.

Benner P (1984) *From Novice to Expert: Excellence and Power in Clinical Nursing Practice*. Menlo Park: Addison Welsey.

Benner P (1991) The role of experience, narrative and community in skilled ethical compartment. *Advances in Nursing Science* 14(2): 1–21.

Bennett P and Murphy S (1997) *Psychology and Health Promotion*. Buckingham: OUP.

Berragan L (1998) Consultancy in nursing: roles and opportunities. *Journal of Clinical Nursing* 7: 139–143.

Bigbee J (1996) History and evolution of advanced nursing practice. In: Hamric A, Spross J and Hanson C (eds) *Advanced Nursing Practice: An Integrative Approach*. Philadelphia: WB Saunders.

Bower F (ed) (2000) *Nurses Taking the Lead: Personal Qualities of Effective Leadership*. London: WB Saunders.

Brennan B (1999) The challenge of tomorrow. In: Nightingale K (ed) *Understanding Perioperative Nursing*. London: Arnold.

Campbell L (1999) Leadership for theatre managers. In: Nightingale K (ed) *Understanding Perioperative Nursing*. London: Arnold.

Caplan G (1964) *Principles of Preventative Psychiatry*. New York: Basic Books.

Caplan G (1970) *The Theory and Practice of Mental Health Consultation*. London: Tavistock.

Caplan G and Caplan R (1993) Mental Health Consultation and Collaboration. San Francisco: Waveland.

Castledine G (1995) Defining specialist. *British Journal of Nursing* 4(5): 264–5.

Castledine G (1998) Clinical specialists in nursing in the UK: the early years. In: Castledine G and McGee P (eds) *Advanced and Specialist Nursing Practice*. Oxford: Blackwell Scientific.

Clarke E and Spross J (1996) Expert coaching and guidance. In: Hamric A, Spross JD and Hanson C (eds) *Advanced Nursing Practice: An Integrative Approach*. Philadelphia: WB Saunders.

Denny E (1999) *The Emergence of the Occupation of District Nursing in 19th Century England*. PhD Thesis, University of Nottingham.

Department of Health (1993) *Hospital doctors: training for the future: the report on the working group on specialist medical training*. London: HMSO.

Department of Health. (1998a) *Nurse consultants*. Health Service Circular 98/161. London: HMSO.

Department of Health. (1998b) *Making a difference*. London: HMSO.

Department of Health (1998c) *A first class service: quality in the new NHS*. London: HMSO.

DHSS (1970) *Lewin Report – The organisation and staffing of operating departments*. London: HMSO.

DHSS (1972) *Report of the committee on nursing*. Chair: Professor Asa Briggs. CMNB 5115. London: HMSO.

DHSS (1977) *The extending role of the clinical nurse*. HC (77) 22 June 1977. London: HMSO.

Dunn L (1997) A literature review of advanced clinical nursing practice in the United States of America. *Journal of Advanced Nursing* 25(4): 814–819.

Elcock K (1996) Consultant nurse: an appropriate title for advanced practitioner? *British Journal of Nursing* 5(22): 1376–1381.

Girouard S (1996) Evaluating advanced nursing practice. In: Hamric A, Spross JD and Hanson C (eds) *Advanced Nursing Practice: An Integrative Approach*. Philadelphia: WB Saunders.

Ham C, Smith J and Temple J (1998) *Hubs, Spokes and Policy Cycles*. London: Kings Fund.

Hamric A, Spross JD and Hanson C (1996) *Advanced Nursing Practice: An Integrative Approach*. Philadelphia: WB Saunders.

Hanson C and Spross JD (1996) Collaboration. In: Hamric A, Spross JD and Hanson C (eds) *Advanced Nursing Practice: An Integrative Approach*. Philadelphia: WB Saunders.

Hay R (1994) A nurse's place is at the bedside. *Nursing Standard* 30(8): 42.

Holmes S (1994) Development of the cardiac surgeon's assistant. *British Journal of Nursing* 3(5): 204–209.

Hughes E (1951) Studying the nurse's work. *American Journal of Nursing* 10(1): 1–22.

Janis I (1958) *Psychological Stress*. New York: Wiley.

Johnson C and Nicklas T (1995) Health ahead – the heart smart family approaches to prevention of cardiovascular disease. *American Journal of Medical Sciences* 310: 127–132.

Jones RA (1994) Nurse physician collaboration: a descriptive study. *Holistic Nursing Practice* 8(3): 38–53.

Kerfoot K (2000) Nursing in the new world of healthcare. In: Chaska N (ed) *The Nursing Profession: Tomorrow and Beyond*. London: Sage.

Kimmel D (1980) *Adulthood and Ageing*. New York: Wiley.

Leininger M (1990) Importance and uses of ethnomeds, ethnography and ethno nursing research. In: Cahon M (ed) *Recent Advances in Nursing: Research Methodology*. Edinburgh: Churchill Livingstone.

Lorentzon M (1998) The way forward: nursing research or collaborative health care research. *Journal of Advanced Nursing* 27(4): 675–676.

Manley K (1997) A conceptual framework for advanced practice: an action research project operationalizing an advanced practitioner/consultant nurse role. *Journal of Clinical Nursing* 6(3): 179–190.

Maslow A (1970) *Motivation and Personality*. New York: Harper Row.

McGee P (1998) Advanced practice in the UK. In: Castledine G and McGee P (eds) *Advanced and Specialist Nursing Practice*. Oxford: Blackwell Scientific.

Migueles E and Brustowicz R (1997) Interdisciplinary quality improvement in the perioperative program: a collaborative model. *Nursing Clinics of North America* 32(1): 215–230.

Millington C (1976) Clinical nurse consultant in anaesthetics. *Nursing Mirror* 142(20): 49–50.

Mills C (1996) The consultant nurse: a model for advanced practice. *Nursing Times* 14(92): 33–34.

Moch S (1998) Health with illness: concept development through research practice. *Journal of Advanced Nursing* 28(2): 305–310.

National Association of Theatre Nurses (1993) *The role of the nurse as first assistant*. Harrogate: NATN.

National Association of Theatre Nurses (1994) *The nurse as surgeon's assistant*. Harrogate: NATN.

NHSME (1989) Bevan Report – *Management and utilisation of operating departments*. London: HMSO.

NHSME (1991) *Junior doctors – the new deal*. London: HMSO.

Parsons T (1951) *The Social System*. Glencoe, IL: Free Press.

Prochaska J and DiClemente C (1984) *The Transtheoretical Approach: Crossing Traditional Boundaries of Change*. Homewood: Irwin.

Radford M (2000) A framework for perioperative advanced practice. *British Journal of Perioperative Nursing* 10(1): 50–54.

Radford M, Johnston P, Williamson A and Jewkes A (2001a) Management of the minor surgical emergency workload by specialist nurse pre-assessment and co-ordination. *British Journal of Surgery* 88(s1): 27.

Radford M, Johnston P, Williamson A and Jewkes A (2001b) Co-ordination of the emergency surgical workload by specialist nurse pre-assessment: the effect on emergency theatre operating patterns. *British Journal of Surgery* 88(s1): 27.

Reilly C, Challands A, Barrett A and Read S (1996) *Professional Roles in Anaesthetics: A Scoping Study*. Leeds: NHS Executive.

Rogers C (1961) *On Becoming a Person*. Boston: Houghton Mifflin.

Royal College of Nursing (1998) *Guidance for nurses on clinical governance*. London: RCN.

Salmon P, Pearce S, Smith C, Heys A, Manyande A, Peters N and Rashid J (1989) The relationship of preoperative distress to endocrine responses to subjective responses to surgery: support for Janis's Theory. *Journal of Behavioural Medicine* 11: 599–613.

Salmon P (1993) The reduction of anxiety in surgical patients: An important nursing task or the medicalisation of preparatory worry? *International Journal of Nursing Studies* 30(4): 323–330.

Schein EH (1988) *Process Consultation (Vol 11): Lessons for Managers and Consultants*. Reading, MA: Addison Welsey.

Secretan L (1998) Industry Week. www.industryweek.com

Stacey M (1988) *The Sociology of Health and Healing: A Textbook*. London: Unwin.

Thibodeau J and Hawkins J (1994) Moving towards a nursing model in advanced practice. *Western Journal of Nursing Research* 16: 205–218.

Turner B (1995) *Medical Power and Social Knowledge*, 2nd edn. London: Sage Publications.

UKCC (1994) *The future of professional practice: the council's Standards for Education and Practice Following Registration*. London: UKCC, p. 20.

UKCC (1992a) *Code of professional conduct*. London: UKCC.

UKCC (1992b) *Scope of professional practice*. London: UKCC.

Ventura M, Crosby F and Feldman M (1991) An information synthesis to evaluate nurse practitioner effectiveness. *Military Medicine* 156 (6): 286–291.

Wicker P and Strachan R (2001) Education focus – advancing perioperative care. *British Journal of Perioperative Nursing* 11(1): 28–33.

Woerth S, Cranfill I and Neal JM (1997) A collaborative approach to minimal invasive direct coronary artery bypass. *Association of Operating Room Nurses Journal* 66(6): 994–1001.

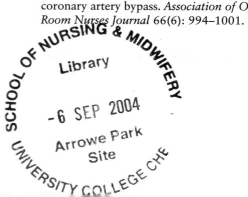

3 PRINCIPLES OF INFECTION CONTROL

Pat A Hutchinson

CHAPTER AIMS

- **To explain the chain of infection**
- **To describe host-specific defence mechanisms against infection**
- **To examine blood-borne viruses and the perioperative environment including health clearance**
- **To discuss infection control in the pre- and perioperative phases including standard (universal) precautions**
- **To provide an overview of infection control in hospitals.**

INTRODUCTION

Application of the principles of infection control is a fundamental part of effective health care. In order to manage infection control effectively, all practitioners need knowledge, in relation to key micro-organisms, their mode of transmission, methods of control and how to apply these in practice. The general principles of infection control are based on the use of practices and procedures that prevent or reduce the likelihood of infection being transmitted from a source (e.g. person, contaminated fluids, equipment) to a susceptible individual. This is commonly referred to as the chain of infection.

The chain of infection

The chain of infection is often described as having six links that represent the chain of events leading to the transmission of infection:

1 **A source of infectious agents** (bacteria, viruses, fungi).

2 **Reservoirs** in which the organisms may survive to multiply (e.g. people, animals, food, water, equipment). The most common reservoir and source of micro-organisms in clinical areas are the patients themselves, particularly their excretions (such as blood, urine, faeces, and vomit), secretions (such as pus, wound exudates) and skin lesions. Since it is impossible to eliminate exposure to all body fluids it is important that all practitioners should follow Standard (Universal) Precautions at all times and hence remove one or more of the other links in the chain of infection.

3 **Portals of exit** are where these micro-organisms leave the body of the infected or colonised individual (e.g. droplets, excreta, secretions, skin).

4 **Methods of transmitting** these micro-organisms from person to person by the following routes:
   - *Direct contact:* with body surfaces or fluids of an infected person
   - *Indirect contact:* involves the transfer of micro-organisms indirectly from one person to another (or endogenously from one body site to another) via contaminated hands, equipment (e.g. urine measuring jugs, laryngoscope blade), surfaces, animals, food or water
   - *Airborne spread:* contaminated skin scales, aerosols of contaminated droplets from patient sneezing and coughing
   - *Vectors:* such as flies, fleas, cockroaches, mosquitoes and other insects that harbour infectious agents
   - *Ingestion:* Micro-organisms enter the gastrointestinal tract with contaminated food and water (e.g. salmonella)
   - *Inoculation:* Micro-organisms may be introduced via skin and mucous membranes by accidental injury, injection, bites or during surgical incision.

5 **Portals of entry** are ways through which the micro-organisms are able to enter the body of another individual. This can be via the genito-urinary tract, the alimentary tract through the ingestion of contaminated food, the skin, mucous membranes and the respiratory tract via inhalation of organism such as tuberculosis.

6 **Susceptible individuals** have variable resistance to infection depending on their age, underlying disease and other factors that may compromise their immune status such as medical treatment with immunosuppressive drugs or irradiation. The risk of transmission of infection is higher for patients undergoing invasive procedures, and for patients who stay in hospital for a long time. Indwelling devices like catheters may also increase the risk of infection, particularly when used over long periods. Glynn *et al.* (1997) found that invasive devices increase a patient's risk of infection sevenfold.

An infection will not be able to develop if one of the links in the chain is removed or controlled. However, it would be impossible to eradicate the second and sixth links, namely the **reservoirs** of infection and the **susceptible individuals**. For that reason, infection control practice tries to eliminate the third and fourth links, i.e. the **means of transmission** so as to prevent pathogenic organisms from gaining access via the **portals of entry**. The single most effective means of achieving this is through effective handwashing.

HOST-SPECIFIC DEFENCE MECHANISMS AGAINST INFECTION

All infections need a route of some sort by which to gain access to the body and the body in turn has developed defence mechanisms to reduce its vulnerability.

First lines of defence

- **Skin** – The first line of defence that an invading micro-organism meets is the physical barrier provided by intact skin. Skin has a low pH and pathogenic bacteria fail to survive for long in this acid environment, but it allows the growth of harmless bacteria such as *Staphylococcus epidermidis*, micrococci and diptheroids (normal skin flora organisms). However this balance is easily disrupted by the use of broad-spectrum antibiotics. These wipe out the normal flora which is replaced by potentially more harmful organisms, particularly if the individual is hospitalised. When the integrity of the skin is broken, for example, by a surgical incision or inflammation, it provides an obvious portal of entry for infection.

- **Respiratory tract** – The majority of micro-organisms are prevented from entering the bronchial tree by hairs in the nose, which filter particles, and the cough reflex, which prevents their aspiration. However procedures such as intubations and tracheotomy bypass the normal respiratory defence mechanism.

- **Conjunctiva** – The surface of the eyeball is constantly irrigated with tears from the lachrymal glands. Tears remove micro-organisms by mechanical action (with eyelids). The enzyme lysozyme in tears has antibacterial properties that form an effective barrier against infection.

- **Genitourinary tract** – The constant downward flow of urine through the ureter and bladder helps avoid ascending infections. However this is bypassed when a urinary catheter is inserted.

- **Gastrointestinal tract** – Gastric juices are highly acidic and a pH of between 2 and 3 destroys most ingested bacteria.

Second lines of defence

If invading micro-organisms get through the first line of defence and enter the tissues, further non-specific host responses are stimulated. These include the inflammatory response, phagocytic cells, eosinophils, complement proteins, interferon and natural killer cells.

BLOOD-BORNE VIRUSES AND THE PERIOPERATIVE ENVIRONMENT

Theatre practitioners on a daily basis are exposed to blood and body fluids, aerosols from power tools, splashes and risks of percutaneous injury from instruments, blades and needles. For this reason alone it is essential that practitioners working in the high-risk environment of an operating theatre are aware of the potential risks and incorporate safe systems of practice to avoid occupational exposure to blood-borne pathogens.

Conversely, patients can be at risk of acquiring blood-borne viruses from health-care workers (HCWs). The three most important blood-borne viruses from an occupational exposure point of view are hepatitis B, hepatitis C and HIV.

HEPATITIS

Hepatitis is a general term used to describe inflammation and enlargement of the liver. Toxins and some drugs can cause the condition but it is most commonly caused by a viral infection. Hepatitis can be divided into two groups based on their mode of transmission, namely, the faecal–oral route and the blood-borne route.

Faecal–oral route

Hepatitis A virus (HAV)

Hepatitis A is a picornavirus that is excreted in large amounts in faeces and spreads from person-to-person by hand contact or by contamination of food or water. HAV does not result in chronic infection or long-term liver disease. A vaccine against HAV is available and is recommended for travellers where there is a risk of contracting infection.

Hepatitis E virus (HEV)

Hepatitis E is caused by a calicivirus but is similar to hepatitis A in that it is spread by water contaminated with faeces and from person-to-person via the faecal–oral route. HEV is rare in developed countries, but is endemic in parts of India, Pakistan, Africa and South America (Ayliffe *et al.* 2000).

Blood-borne route

Hepatitis B virus (HBV)

Hepatitis B is a viral infection of the blood that causes inflammation and enlargement of the liver. Severity can range from subclinical infection that is only detected by the presence of serological markers or impaired liver function tests, to a ful-

minating, fatal case of hepatitis. HBV is spread predominately though exposure to blood by inoculation through the skin; this is known as the parenteral route. It can also be passed from an infected mother to her unborn baby (the transplacental route) or via sexual contact.

A common mode of transmission of HBV to health-care workers is occupational exposure via accidental needlestick or other contaminated sharp injuries.

Diagnosis of HBV

Serological markers are viral proteins found in the blood that can indicate the presence of infection or its stage of resolution. There are three different components of the virus that may be detected in the serum of an infected person:

1   **Hepatitis B surface antigen (HBsAg)** is found on the outer protein coat of the virus. It is the earliest indicator of acute infection and is also indicative of chronic infection if its presence persists for more than 6 months. Anti-HBs is the specific antibody to hepatitis B surface antigen. Its appearance 1–4 months after onset of symptoms indicates clinical recovery and subsequent immunity to HBV.
2   **Hepatitis B core antigen (HBcAg)** is derived from the protein envelope that encloses the viral DNA, and it is not detectable in the bloodstream. If infected by HBV, an antibody to the core of the virus (antiHBc) develops. To differentiate between natural immunity and vaccine acquired immunity, a special test for antiHBc IgG is carried out. When positive, this indicates naturally acquired immunity (vaccine-induced immunity would only be anti-HBs positive).
3   **Hepatitis B 'e' antigen (HbeAg)** is generally detectable in patients with acute infection. The presence of HbeAg in serum correlates with higher titres of HBV and greater infectivity.

A diagnosis of acute HBV infection can be made on the basis of the detection of IgM anti-HBc. This is generally detected at the time of clinical onset and declines to sub-detectable levels within

6 months. IgG anti-HBc persists indefinitely as a marker of past infection.

Hepatitis C virus (HCV)

Hepatitis C (HCV) was first isolated in 1989 and has been identified as one of the major causes of chronic liver disease throughout the world (Choo *et al*. 1989). There are six major genetic types of the HCV with varying virulence; at least 40% are genotype 1; of the remainder the majority is types 2 and 3. Infections with genotypes 4, 5 and 6 are relatively rare in Britain (NICE 2000).

HCV rarely causes symptoms in either the initial exposure or during the disease's progression. This means many people are not aware that they have the virus or how or when they were infected, but up to 75–80% of those infected with HCV develop chronic infection (Villano *et al*. 1999). It may take 10–30 years before clinical symptoms manifest themselves and by this stage any damage to the liver will be irreparable. In developed countries, it is estimated that 90% of persons with chronic HCV infection are current and former injecting drug users and those with a history of transfusion of unscreened blood or blood products (WHO 2000).

The predominant route of transmission is parenteral via blood products and contaminated needles. Historically, blood transfusion and use of non-inactivated blood products such as clotting factors were a frequent cause of HCV. After the introduction of blood products treated with heat in 1988, and the screening of blood in 1991, injecting drug abusers have become the most significant route for transmission of HCV in the UK. Other routes of transmission are exposure to infected blood from tattooing, skin piercing, sharing toothbrushes and razors, and to a lesser degree, sex and perinatal transmission. Similar to HBV, HCV is not spread by sneezing, hugging, coughing, food or water, sharing eating utensils, or casual contact.

Diagnosis of HCV

A commonly used test is called an enzyme immunoassay (ELISA) for hepatitis C virus antibody. These tests look for the antibodies, or chemicals, in the blood that the body produces in response to the HCV. A positive antibody test is evidence of previous exposure to HCV, but gives no indication whether the virus is still present.

Any antibody-positive specimens should be confirmed by the polymerase chain reaction (PCR) assay for HCV RNA, which is a direct indicator of ongoing infection. HCV RNA can be detected in serum 10 days after exposure and will persist in those who become chronic carriers. Detection of the RNA viral genome in blood confirms the diagnosis of current HCV infection.

Treatment for HCV

A recent study suggested that early treatment of acute hepatitis C infection might prevent chronic infection (Jaeckel *et al*. 2001). The National Institute for Clinical Excellence (NICE) issued guidance on the use of ribavirin and interferon

Table 3.1   Interpretation of hepatitis B serology results

Tests	Results	Interpretation
HBsAg	Negative	Susceptible
anti-HBc	Negative	
anti-HBs	Negative	
HBsAg	Negative	Immune due to natural infection
anti-HBc	Positive	
anti-HBs	Positive	
HBsAg	Negative	Immune due to hepatitis B vaccination
anti-HBc	Negative	
anti-HBs	Positive	
HBsAg	Positive	Acutely infected
anti-HBc	Positive	
IgM anti-HBc	Positive	
anti-HBs	Negative	
HBsAg	Positive	Chronically infected
anti-HBc	Positive	
IgM anti-HBc	Negative	
anti-HBs	Negative	
HBsAg	Negative	Four interpretations possible*
anti-HBc	Positive	
anti-HBs	Negative	

*1. May be recovering from acute HBV infection.
2. May be distantly immune and test not sensitive enough to detect very low level of anti-HBs in serum.
3. May be susceptible with a false positive anti-HBc.
4. May be undetectable level of HBsAg present in the serum and the person is actually a carrier.

Source: Center for Disease Control (CDC) www.cdc.gov/ncidod/diseases/hepatitis/b/Bserology.htm

Table 3.2   Test for the detection of HCV

Type of test	Description of test
Enzyme-linked immunosorbent assay (ELISA)	This tests for antibodies to HCV and confirms contact with HCV, but does not show whether the virus is still replicating or is actively present.
Recombinant immunoblot assay (RIBA)	This is similar to the ELISA test and is used as a confirmation. It may indicate chronic liver damage.
Polymerase chain reaction (PCR)	This test indicates whether the virus is in the blood. It shows replication and active infection.

alpha for the treatment of moderate to severe hepatitis C (NICE 2000). Patients are given interferon taken alone or in combination with ribavirin in attempts to clear the virus and reduce the risk or slow the development of liver disease. The primary aims of the treatment are to achieve normal liver function tests and sustained clearance of hepatitis C virus, i.e. negative PCR test, both of which need to be sustained for at least 6 months after treatment has stopped.

Occupational exposure to HCV

The risk of transmission following a single percutaneous exposure from a hepatitis C antibody positive source is probably between 1.2 and 3.0%. In an Italian study between 1992 and 1993, 331 (51%) hollow-bore needlestick, 105 (16.5%) suture needles or sharp object injuries, 85 (13%) mucous membrane contaminations and 125 (19.5%) skin contaminations were reported. Out of these exposures, four HCV seroconversions were observed after hollow-bore needlestick injuries and no seroconversion occurred from the other routes mentioned (Puro *et al.* 1995). Sulkowksi *et al.* (2002) also report there has been no transmission of HCV via intact skin.

Box 3.1   Treatment for HCV

Interferon alpha is usually administered subcutaneously, three times a week for six months.

Ribavirin is a nucleoside analogue with a broad spectrum of antiviral activity against RNA viruses that is administered orally.

Six months of combination therapy costs £4800 (this excludes monitoring, counselling etc.)

Source: NICE (2000)

Conversely, to date there have been five incidents in the UK in which hepatitis C-infected health-care workers have transmitted infection to 15 patients, which has led to further recommendations from the Advisory Group on Hepatitis (AGH) to protect patients (DOH 2002a). (See later section on the guidelines for health clearance for blood-borne viruses for more detail.)

Hepatitis D virus (HDV)

Hepatitis D virus, also known as the '*delta agent*', is found only in people who are also infected with hepatitis B virus. HDV cannot cause infection in the absence of HBV and the HBV vaccine prevents both types of infection.

Hepatitis G virus (HGV)

Hepatitis G virus (HGV) is also referred to as GBV-C agent. The full clinical significance of the infection with this virus, whether it is a true hepatrophic virus, and its natural history are yet unknown. It has been transmitted by blood transfusions and transmission to HCWs via needlestick injuries has also been reported (Shibuya *et al.* 1998).

Human immunodeficiency virus (HIV)

The human immunodeficiency virus (HIV) is a blood-borne virus, first recognised in 1981. HIV is a RNA retrovirus. This means that the genetic information of the virus consists of RNA, but it also has an enzyme, *reverse transcriptase*, that converts the RNA to DNA and then incorporates it into the DNA of the host cell.

By the beginning of the 21st century it was estimated that there had been 22 million HIV-related deaths worldwide, and that there were 36 million people living with HIV infection. In the

UK it is estimated that there have been nearly 15,000 deaths and that the number of people living with diagnosed infection is currently around 25,000. This number is rising around 12% per annum (DOH 1998a).

Diagnosis of HIV

Detection of infection is normally by serological tests for anti-HIV antibodies in the blood. These are usually detected after 3 months when the individual has seroconverted.

Transmission of HIV

HIV is present in the blood and other body fluids of infected individuals. Transmission of the virus can occur though sexual intercourse, receipt of infected blood or blood products, donated organs and semen. Vertical transmission from mother to child can also occur. Finally it can be transmitted through the sharing or reuse of contaminated needles.

Occupational exposure to HIV

As of 1998, there have been 95 definite cases of occupational HIV infection and a further 191 cases of possible occupationally acquired HIV infection. Out of these figures, 12 cases were reported in the UK, of which four were definitely acquired occupationally (Evans and Abiteboul 1999). Percutaneous exposure to HIV-infected blood is the major route of transmission in occupational exposure and the risk is estimated at 0.3%. That is approximately one infection in 300 exposures compared with a 2–40% risk for hepatitis C virus (one in 30) and a 3–10% (one in three) risk for hepatitis B virus (Riddell and Sherrard 2000) (see Table 3.3 for summary). A case–control study identified four factors associated with increased risk of occupationally acquired HIV infection (Cardo *et al.* 1997):

1 Visible blood on the device, which caused the injury (e.g. hollow-bore needle)
2 Injury with a needle which had been placed in the source patient's artery or vein
3 A deep injury
4 The source patient had a terminal HIV-related illness.

Table 3.3 A summary of transmission rates, available vaccines and post-exposure prophylaxis (PEP) for HIV, HBV and HCV

Virus	Transmission rate following injury	Vaccine available	Post-exposure prophylaxis
HIV	1 in 300	NONE	Combination antiretroviral therapy
Hepatitis B	1 in 3 If source is 'e' antigen positive	YES	Vaccine and/or immunoglobulin
Hepatitis C	1 in 30	NONE	

The study concluded that in situations where there was larger volumes of blood, and a source patient with a high viral load, the risk of HIV transmission after percutaneous exposure would exceed the average risk of 1:300 (Cardo *et al.* 1997).

The risk of transmission from a mucocutaneous exposure (via broken skin and mucous membrane) has an estimated risk of 0.03%. One incident that highlights the risks of acquiring blood-borne viruses from blood splashes was reported in the *Nursing Standard* in 1995. An Italian auxiliary nurse was diagnosed as HIV positive, two months after a test tube containing patient's blood shattered and a drop entered her eye (Anon 1995).

Treatment for HIV

Currently there is no cure for HIV infection or any vaccine that can protect against it. However, treatment with anti-HIV drugs is allowing people with HIV infection to live longer.

Post-exposure prophylaxis (PEP) for HIV

A designated consultant such as an occupational health consultant, consultant in genito-urinary medicine or in A&E departments will only prescribe PEP after a risk assessment is carried out. This will determine whether the exposure to blood or body tissue was known to be, or strongly suspected to be, infected with HIV. PEP will not be offered following contact with low-risk materials (e.g. urine, vomit, saliva and faeces) unless they are visibly blood-stained (DOH 2000a).

Box 3.2 Post-exposure prophylaxis (PEP)

> Are you aware of the post-exposure prophylaxis policy in your local work area?
>
> Do you know whom to contact in the event of possible HIV exposure?
>
> Do you know who can prescribe PEP in your workplace?
>
> Where can the emergency starter packs be located at weekends, nights and Bank Holidays?
>
> Do you know when chemoprophylaxis should be initiated following an exposure?

The PEP regime uses a combination of drugs with activity at different stages in the viral replication. A **reverse transcriptase inhibitor** blocks the action of the reverse transcriptase process so that virus replication is prevented and a **protease inhibitor** prevents the virus from forming.

The UK guidelines for the use of PEP recommend that a combination of three antiretroviral drugs is used. These are **zidovudine, lamivudine and indinavir** (see Table 3.4). Chemoprophylaxis should be initiated within one hour of exposure or at least within 24–36 hours (National AIDS Manual 2001) for a period of four weeks. These antiretroviral drugs are all licensed for the treatment of HIV infection but not for its prevention.

Table 3.4 Post-exposure prophylaxis guidelines (DOH 2000a)

Name	Type of drug	Dose	Side effects
Zidovudine plus	Reverse transcriptase inhibitor	200 mg t.d.s. or 250 mg b.d	Nausea, vomiting, diarrhoea, abdominal pain, cough, headache, insomnia.
Lamivudine plus	Reverse transcriptase inhibitor	150 mg b.d	
*Indinavir or	Protease inhibitor	800 mg t.d.s	Malaise, muscle disorders
Nelfinavir	Protease inhibitor	750 mg t.d.s or 1250 mg b.d.	

*This was the original drug in the PEP starter packs in 1997.

For this reason they may still only be prescribed on 'a named basis' only for PEP.

Guidelines for health clearance for blood-borne viruses

The Department of Health set up an expert group in 2001 to assess the potential health risks posed to patients from health-care workers new to the NHS infected with serious communicable diseases. This assessment was to refer particularly to HIV, hepatitis B, hepatitis C and tuberculosis and to identify what measures were required to minimise these risks (DOH 2003).

Health clearance for blood-borne viruses is proof that the individual is not infectious for hepatitis B and C and that they are HIV negative. This clearance will be required for posts or careers involving exposure-prone procedures (EPPs). These new proposals are not intended to prevent those infected with blood-borne viruses from working in the NHS but to restrict them from working in those clinical areas where their infection may pose a risk to patients in their care.

Procedures considered *not to be exposure prone* are where the hands and fingertips of the worker are visible and outside the patient's body at all times and internal examinations or procedures that do not involve possible injury to the worker's gloved hands from sharp instruments and/or tissues. Provided routine infection control procedures are adhered to at all times, examples include:

Box 3.3 Definition of exposure-prone procedures

> Exposure-prone procedures are those in which there is a risk that injury to the worker may result in exposure of the patient's open tissues to the blood of the worker (bleed-back) These procedures include those where the worker's gloved hands may be in contact with sharp instruments, needle tips or sharp tissues (spicules of bone or teeth) inside a patient's open cavity, wound or confined anatomical space where the hands or fingertips may not be completely visible at all times (DOH 2002a).

- Taking blood (venepuncture)
- Setting up and maintaining IV lines or central lines (providing any skin tunnelling procedure used for the latter is performed in a non-exposure manner, i.e. without the operator's fingers being at any time concealed in the patient tissues in the presence of a sharp instruments)
- Minor surface suturing
- The incision of external abscesses
- Routine vaginal or rectal examinations
- Simple endoscopic procedures.

Health-care workers moving into training or a post involving EPPs *for the first time* should be treated as 'new' and will require additional health clearance for serious communicable diseases unless there is already a record of testing for BBVs. This will include for instance junior doctors entering

surgical specialties and post-registration nurses in operating theatres (see Table 3.5).

The National Minimum Standards for Independent Care (DOH 2002c) require all HCWs in the independent health-care sector to comply with DOH guidelines about infection with blood-borne viruses including hepatitis C. HCWs who apply for a post or training which may involve EPPs *and who decline* to be tested for HIV, hepatitis B and C should not be cleared to perform EPPs.

STANDARD (UNIVERSAL) PRECAUTIONS IN THE PERIOPERATIVE ENVIRONMENT

Universal Precautions, now more commonly referred to as Standard Precautions, were introduced nearly two decades ago, largely in response to the HIV/AIDS epidemic and an

Table 3.5 The standard health checks required for serious communicable diseases for HCWs new to the NHS and additional health checks required to perform exposure prone procedures (EPPs)

	Standard health checks for HCWs new to the NHS	Additional health checks for HCWs new to the NHS who will perform EPPs	
Hepatitis B	Immunisation • 3 doses are given at 0, 1 and 6 months after the first. • After a further 2–3 months a blood sample is given to test for antibodies.	Tested for hepatitis B surface antigen (HBsAg), which indicates current hepatitis B infection (DOH 2000b)	
		If negative for HBsAg should be immunized and response to vaccine checked (anti-HBs)	**If positive** for HBsAg, to be tested for hepatitis B e-markers
			If e-antigen (HBeAg)-positive not allowed to perform EPPs **If e-antigen negative** the hepatitis B viral load (HBV DNA) is tested. **If the viral load is greater than 10^3 genome equivalents per ml, not allowed to perform EPPs**. This test is repeated on annual basis.
Hepatitis C	Offered a hepatitis C antibody test and if positive a hepatitis C RNA test.	Tested for hepatitis C antibody. If positive should be tested for hepatitis C RNA to detect the presence of current infection. **If hepatitis C RNA-positive** not allowed to perform EPPs (DOH 2000a)	
		Hepatitis C-infected HCWs who have been treated with antiviral therapy and who remain **hepatitis C virus RNA negative** for at least 6 months after cessation of treatment **should be permitted to return to EPPs**. Further checks to show that the HCW is still HCV RNA negative to be repeated 6 months later.	
HIV	Offered an HIV antibody test	Tested for HIV antibody. **If HIV antibody-positive** not allowed to perform EPPs (UK Health Departments 1998a)*	

*Revised guidance to be issued in 2003 (DOH 2002b)

urgent need to protect hospital personnel from blood-borne infections (CDC 1987). The Department of Health first endorsed similar UK recommendations in 1990, to protect HCWs against infection with blood-borne viruses (UK Health Departments 1990).

Standard Precautions are recommended for the treatment and care of all patients, regardless of their perceived infectious status and should incorporate safe systems for handling blood (including dried blood), other body fluids, secretions and excretions (excluding sweat), non-intact skin and mucous membranes (see Box 3.4). *All practitioners should assess the task or activity that is to be completed and not the individual who is to receive the care* (NATN 1998).

In situations when Standard Precautions may be insufficient to prevent transmission of infection **Additional Precautions** should be applied for patients known or suspected to be infected or colonised with epidemiological important or highly transmissible pathogens that may not be contained with standard precautions alone, for example:

- Airborne transmission (*Mycobacterium tuberculosis*, measles virus, chickenpox virus)
- Droplet transmission (mumps, rubella, pertussis, influenza)
- Direct or indirect contact with dry skin (colonisation with methicillin-resistant *Staphylococcus aureus* (MRSA) or with contaminated surfaces)
- Any combination of these routes.

In the ward setting this may mean allocation of the patient into a single room with en-suite facilities. Also the use of personal protective equipment may be indicated such as a particulate filter mask for tuberculosis. Rostering of immune HCWs to care for a patient with, for example, chickenpox is also beneficial. However in the operating theatre the risk of transfer of infection from one patient to the next in a general surgical operation list is small. In a plenum ventilated operating theatre there is no reason for it to lie empty for more than 15 minutes following a dirty operation before a clean procedure is per-

Box 3.4 Standard (Universal) Precautions to be taken for the care of all patients include:

> - Handwashing
> - Skin care
> - Wearing appropriate personal protective equipment for the task or activity in hand: gloves, apron, gown, masks, eye protection
> - Safe use and disposal of sharps
> - Refer to local policies for the safe disposal of: clinical waste, linen, management of spillages, decontamination procedures for instruments, equipment and environment and management of needlestick injuries
>
> It is important that all practitioners incorporate these principles into their everyday practice because the patient's infectious status may not have been determined if undergoing emergency surgery or the laboratory tests are incomplete.

formed providing the theatre is thoroughly cleaned (Ayliffe *et al.* 2000; HIS 2001). Surfaces that do not have direct contact with the patient such as the floor, wall and light become no more contaminated after a dirty operation than after a clean one (Hambraeus *et al.* 1978). However the operating table and all equipment and instruments that come into contact with more than one patient have a greater potential for transmission of infection between dirty and subsequent cases than air. A vertical laminar flow theatre needs only 5 minutes to replace the full volume of air in the theatre (HIS 2002).

RECENT EVIDENCE-BASED GUIDELINES

The epic Project: Developing National Evidence-Based Guidelines for Preventing Health-Care Associated Infections (2001)

In 1998, the Department of Health (England) commissioned the first phase of national evidence-based recommendations for preventing health-care associated infections. These guidelines issued in 2001 are for all health-care practitioners, to incorporate into their practice and local protocols, when caring for all hospital inpatients all the time. The standard principles of good practice are divided into four areas:

1 Hospital environmental hygiene
2 Hand hygiene
3 The use of protective equipment (PPE)
4 The use and disposal of sharps.

However they do not address the additional infection control requirements of specialist settings, such as the operating department (Pratt et al. 2001).

The Hospital Infection Society (HIS) Working Party on Infection Control in Operating Theatres (2002)

In 1999 this group was established in order to provide clear and practical guidelines for infection control and theatre practitioners. Three subgroups were formed to look at:

1 Behaviours and rituals in the operating theatre.
2 Guidelines for the environmental monitoring (including bacteriological air sampling) of operating theatre facilities.
3 To consider optimal theatre facilities whether ultra clean or conventional operating (theatre) ventilation is required. This work is still in progress (HIS 2002).

In both of the above projects the same grading system was used to describe the strength, quality and direction of evidence that supports a guideline recommendation. These are:

- **Category 1**: generally consistent findings in a range of evidence derived from a majority of acceptable studies.
- **Category 2**: evidence based on a single acceptable study, or a weak or inconsistent finding in multiple acceptable studies.
- **Category 3**: limited scientific evidence that does not meet all the criteria of 'acceptable studies', or an absence of directly applicable studies of good quality. This includes published expert opinion derived from systematically retrieved and appraised professional, national and international publications.

The next part of the chapter is divided into two phases – pre- and perioperative. Each phase reviews the key infection control procedures that all practitioners should use in the care of all patients undergoing a surgical procedure to minimise the transmission of infection to staff and between patients. Each phase is underpinned by the recommendations from the *epic* Guidelines (Pratt *et al.* 2001) and the HIS Working Party Guidelines on Infection Control in Operating Theatres (HIS 2002).

PREOPERATIVE PHASE

Admission

Pre-admission assessment and an increase in day-case surgery have reduced the length of time patients have to be in hospital prior to surgery. Cruse and Foord (1980) demonstrated that shorter stays are associated with lower infection rates. The relationship between the numbers of preoperative days and the likelihood of infection are: after 1 day, the wound infection rate is 1.2%; after 7 days this increases to 2.1%; and after 14 days or more the wound infection rate increases to 3.4% (Cruse 1992). There are two possible explanations for this: one is that patients requiring extended preoperative stay are likely to be debilitated or present with a coexisting illness that might predispose them to wound infection (Ayliffe *et al.* 2000). The other is that the length of preoperative stay results in lowering patient resistance or increased pathogenic skin contamination (Mishriki *et al.* 1992).

Preoperative preparation of the patients
Showering
The benefit of preoperative bathing, with or without antiseptic soaps to reduce skin flora, remains unclear. A number of studies demonstrated that showering using an antimicrobial product reduced the bacterial load on the skin (Garibaldi 1988; Kaiser *et al.* 1988; Hayek 1987). One study by Byrne *et al.* (1990) identified that the greatest fall in bacterial skin flora was achieved by the first and second showers and that there was

no further significant fall with subsequent showers. From this study they recommended that each patient undergo three preoperative showers with 4% chlorhexidine detergent. Other studies, some of which were large-scale controlled trials, showed no such beneficial effect of one to three showers (Lynch *et al.* 1992; Rotter *et al.* 1988; Ayliffe *et al.* 1983). The HIS working party concluded that there was no evidence that chlorhexidine showers reduce the incidence of postoperative infection and graded it a **Category 1 recommendation** (HIS 2002).

Shaving

A number of studies have demonstrated that shaving the skin before an operation increases the risk of wound infections (Cruse and Foord 1973; Alexander *et al.* 1983; Cruse 1986). The criteria to shave should be based on the need to view or access the surgical site and should be carried out close to the time of surgery. This avoids the risk of traumatising the skin and providing an opportunity for the skin to become heavily colonised with bacteria at the surgical site.

The HIS working party graded it a **Category 1 recommendation** stating that 'Only the area to be incised needs to be shaved and, if this cannot be done by depilatory cream the day before operation, it should be done in the anaesthetic room immediately preoperatively, using clippers rather than a razor. Shaving brushes should not be used' (HIS 2002, p. 8).

Patients' clothing

The routine removal of patients' underwear was first introduced when nylon underwear could potentially cause static electricity. Today the removal of the patient's underwear should only occur if it is going to interfere with the operation site or there is a risk of the patient's own underwear being soiled by the use of skin preparations in theatres. In both cases disposable underwear should be made available in order to maintain the patient's dignity. Brown (1993) described this ritual of removing patients' underwear as the 'most illogical of rituals'. The HIS Working Party (2002) recommend that this practice be stopped for the good reason that it causes embarrassment to the patient and serves no useful purpose. However in respect of removing all other items of the patient's own clothing prior to some surgery e.g. cataract surgery, the HIS working party conclude that further work is required to confirm whether this is necessary (HIS 2002).

Transport of the patient to theatre

Prior to the patient going to theatre they should be dressed in a freshly laundered theatre gown. If being transported on a bed then it should be made up with fresh bed linen to minimise the shedding of particles into the air when the bedding is disturbed (Litsky and Litsky 1971). Moreover the patient can be transferred to the anaesthetic room or to the operating theatre on their bed, without additional risk of infection, providing the bed linen pack (i.e. the upper layers rather than under sheet) is not brought into the operating theatre itself (Ayliffe *et al.* 2000).

The practice of a two trolley system and the provision of a trolley transfer area are no longer required as there is no evidence that transferring of the patient to a clean trolley reduces the likelihood of contamination of the theatre and has little significance in increasing wound infection rates (Ayliffe *et al.* 1969; Lewis *et al.* 1990). The HIS Working Party (2002) concurred with this, also in the use of clean bed linen prior to the patient being transferred to the theatre, and graded it a **Category 2 recommendation**.

Provision of overshoes

Humphreys *et al.* (1991) carried out a study of floor bacterial counts that involved shoes with and without covers. They demonstrated that there was no significant reduction to the bacterial floor counts in the theatre if shoe covers were worn, concluding that it was an unnecessary and costly practice, and did not benefit the patients. In addition the issue of hand contamination by donning and removal of overshoes was highlighted as a potential risk to patients (Carter 1990; Caunt 1991; Weightman and Banfield 1994).

Mathias (2000) suggested that overshoes could be worn to avoid shoes being overly contaminated by blood and body fluids. The Guidelines for Prevention of Surgical Site Infection (Mangram *et al.* 1999) also support this view. In addition, the UK Health Department (1998b) guidelines for protecting health-care workers against infection with blood-borne viruses advise that Wellingtons or calf-length boots should be available. These offer more protection than shoes and further reduce the risk of blood–skin contact. The HIS Working Party recommended that the practice of wearing overshoes should cease. This is a **Category 3 recommendation** (HIS 2002).

Visitors to theatres
There is no evidence to support the practice of visitors wearing overgowns and overshoes in the anaesthetic room. If the visitor is to enter the operating theatre itself then they should change into theatre suits. The HIS Working Party concurred and graded it a **Category 3 recommendation** (HIS 2002).

PERIOPERATIVE PHASE

Theatre personnel clothing

Scrub attire
The National Association for Theatre Nurses (NATN) recommends that all personnel who enter semi-restricted and restricted areas of the perioperative environment should be in clean, freshly laundered theatre attire which should be changed when soiled or wet. Trouser suits, as opposed to dresses, should be worn. These should be of a closely woven material, easily washed at high temperatures. The material should also be lint free, cool and comfortable to wear. Maintained in good repair these will give a professional appearance (NATN 1998).

The HIS Working Party concluded that when leaving the theatre temporarily, there was insufficient evidence to support the wearing of cover gowns over surgical attire. However, it is recommended that local policy reflect aesthetic and discipline requirements. This is a **Category 3 recommendation** (HIS 2002).

Theatre footwear
Well-fitting footwear with impervious soles should be worn. These need to be cleaned after every use to remove splashes of blood and body fluid. Procedures need to be in place to ensure that this is undertaken at the end of every session. This is a **Category 3 recommendation** (HIS 2002). However, the problems in achieving this safely were highlighted in a study by Agarwal *et al.* (2002). They revealed that 44% of all operating boots tested were contaminated with blood and bacteria. In light of the fact that HIV, hepatitis B and C can survive in dry blood for up to 5 weeks and longer (Cattaneo *et al.* 1996), they concluded that the present practice of manual cleaning of boots is unsatisfactory and recommended that boots be washed in automatic washing machines (Agarwal *et al.* 2002). A similar study by Thomas *et al.* (1993) found that 36%, 40% and 57% of boots examined in three different hospitals were contaminated with blood.

Whatever method is used to clean theatre footwear, a risk assessment should be carried out and if manual cleaning is the chosen method then appropriate training and personal protective equipment must be provided and worn.

Removal of jewellery
Both the NATN (1998) and the Association of Operating Room Nurses (AORN 2000a) recommend that jewellery (i.e. necklaces, ear-rings and rings with stones) be removed. This was also the recommendation of the HIS working party who graded it a **Category 3 recommendation**. However on the issue of wedding rings the HIS Working Party concluded that theatre practitioners ('scrub and non-scrub') may continue to wear these. But in the case of surgeons they may be advised to remove a wedding ring when working with metal prostheses. They cite one piece of research from Nicolai *et al.* (1997) who found multiple glove perforations at the base of the ring finger in surgeons who wore a wedding ring during major joint replacement operations.

Finger nails

Finger nails should be kept short, clean and free of artificial nails (NATN 1998; AORN 2000a). Studies by Hedderwick *et al.* (2000) and McNeil (2000) demonstrated that artificial nails harbour more pathogens such as Gram-negative bacilli and yeast bacteria, even after handwashing, than nurses with natural nails. Another study by Moolenar *et al.* (2000) suggested that nurses' long and artificial fingernails might have had a role in *Pseudomonas aeruginosa* transmission in a neonatal intensive care unit, which led to 16 infant deaths.

However the recommendation in the use of nail polish differs between the NATN and AORN recommendations. NATN recommend that nails should be free of nail polish (NATN 1998). AORN have modified its recommendation to allow the surgical conscience of each practitioner to decide whether to wear nail polish in the operating theatre (AORN 2000a). This decision was based on a study by Wynd *et al.* (1994) who found no increase in microbial growth related to wearing *freshly applied nail polish*. However, the study further suggested that nail polish worn longer than four days or chipped any time during that four-day period had a tendency to harbour greater numbers of bacteria. Theatre practitioners will need to consult their own local uniform and theatre policies.

Theatre caps

Theatre caps are principally worn to reduce the dispersal of hair and skin scales and protect the wearer from contamination such as blood and body fluids (ICNA 2002a). In a study by Humphreys *et al.* (1991) the effect of surgical theatre headgear on air bacterial counts was explored. They concluded there was little evidence that the wearing of headgear reduces bacterial contamination in the theatre and therefore caps should only be worn by the scrub team given their proximity to the operative field, particularly in a laminar flow field. The NATN (1998) recommend that all theatre staff keep their hair covered as a matter of routine at all times. The HIS Working Party recommend that there is no need for non-scrubbed staff members

of the operating team to wear disposable headgear; however common sense dictates that hair should be kept clean and out of the way. Hats must be worn in laminar flow theatre during prosthetic implant operations. This is a **Category 3 recommendation** (HIS 2002).

THE USE OF STANDARD (UNIVERSAL) PRECAUTIONS IN THE PERIOPERATIVE ENVIRONMENT

Hand hygiene

The single most important factor in prevention of infection in hospitals is hand hygiene. Historically, a Hungarian obstetrician, Ignaz Philip Semmelweis, was accredited for highlighting this in 1847. He believed that 'cadaveric particles' were responsible for high rates of puerperal fever and death. After Semmelweis introduced a simple handwashing policy for all physicians and medical students to use chlorinated lime after performing postmortems and before coming into contact with women in labour, the death rate fell from 22% to 3%.

Since 1847, a plethora of research on hand hygiene has been published, but compliance remains poor. One recent study cites several reasons for low compliance (Pittet *et al.* 2000):

- Skin irritation
- Inaccessible hand washing supplies
- Wearing gloves
- Being too busy
- Not thinking about it.

The Committee of Public Accounts viewed this poor compliance with guidance on hand hygiene as inexcusable (Taylor *et al.* 2001). In response to this, the Department of Health highlighted that through the Control Assurance Standards on Infection Control NHS Trusts were required to have a policy on hand hygiene and provide education and training in this area. They also pointed out that the recent national evidence-based guidelines included seven recommendations on hand hygiene (Pratt *et al.* 2001).

In 2001, The NHS Purchasing and Supply Agency (PASA) in collaboration with the ICNA and the Hand Hygiene Liaison Group set out to develop an improved range of paper hand towels that were more absorbent and softer to use. The low quality paper hand towels that were currently available was another reason cited for poor hand hygiene. This phase of the project was completed in 2002 and the new, improved ranges of paper hand towels are available from NHS Supplies. The next phase is due to look at soap systems and in conjunction with the National Patient Safety Agency (NPSA), PASA have already commenced a separate trial of alcohol-based hand cleansers, to develop a national standard for the gel. This work will also explore wall-mounted and individual dispensers.

NPSA is a special health authority created to co-ordinate the efforts of all those involved in health care, and more importantly to learn from patient safety incidents occurring in the NHS. One of NPSA's projects is an integrated hand hygiene campaign. This is the first initiative of its kind to involve patients in improving hand hygiene. The NPSA plan is to test whether, by using a combination of communication methods and practical steps such as making hand cleaning gel easily accessible on the wards, lasting changes in behaviour can be achieved. This is initially only occurring in six NHS Trusts who have been provided with a hand hygiene improvement toolkit, the contents of which include staff badges inviting patients to remind them to clean their hands, patient leaflets, posters aimed at staff and supplies of disinfectant hand gel. It is the intention of the NSPA that the campaign will go nationwide in 2004.

The aims of hand decontamination

The aim of hand decontamination is to significantly reduce the carriage of potential pathogens on the hands (Larson 1995). Gould (2002) suggests that the terminology surrounding hand washing should be changed to hand 'decontamination' so that all health-care staff view hand hygiene as a priority when they have direct patient contact.

All theatre practitioners are well aware of the importance of a diligent scrub technique, but may fail to remember to wash their hands when carrying out other activities in the operating department. One of the seven recommendations on hand hygiene is that all health-care workers' hands *must* be decontaminated immediately before *each* and *every* episode of direct patient contact or care and after any activity or contact that potentially results in hands becoming contaminated. This is a **Category 3 recommendation** (Pratt *et al.* 2001).

Choice of cleansing agents commonly found in operating departments

- **Liquid soap and water** – is used to remove transient micro-organisms acquired on the hands before they can be transferred, commonly referred to as a 'social' hand wash. Unlike antiseptics they do not kill micro-organisms or inhibit their growth, so their effectiveness is limited. In the operating department it can be used in areas such as changing facilities, toilet areas and all other areas where a higher level of skin disinfection is not required.
- **Chlorhexidine, iodophors (e.g. povidone-iodine) and triclosan** – these are products used either for hygienic hand disinfection where the transient micro-organisms are largely destroyed or for a surgical scrub where the transient micro-organisms and readily detachable residents are removed or destroyed.
- **Alcohol-based products** can be used for both hygiene hand disinfection and surgical scrub. However it is important to highlight that alcohol-based products *do not remove micro-organisms* but rapidly destroy them on skin surfaces, so they are therefore only suitable to be used for clean hands. All visible contaminates must be first removed with soap and water or a detergent-based solution. Ethyl alcohol and isopropanyl or n-propyl alcohol are the two main alcohols that are combined with other antimicrobials, e.g. chlorhexidine or triclosan, plus the addition of an emollient to reduce the drying effect on skin. They have a rapid broad-spectrum antimicrobial activity but have limited effect on spores (ICNA 2002b).

Box 3.5 How do you choose which surgical scrub preparation to use? Is it by performance or preference?

- **Chlorhexidine** is more effective against Gram-positive than Gram-negative bacteria. In vitro studies have demonstrated activity against viruses including HIV, herpes simplex and influenza virus, as well as some activity against fungi. Organic matter minimally affects it. One of the main advantages is its residual activity (up to 6 hours) and it is less irritating than iodophors.
- **Iodophors (povidone-iodine)** has a rapid broad-spectrum antimicrobial activity. It is neutralised in the presence of organic matter and can cause skin irritation.
- **Triclosan** is effective against Gram-positive and most Gram-negative bacteria and fungi. It has variable activity against Pseudomonas species. It is minimally affected by organic matter and is commonly used in commercial hygiene products. Triclosan has proven useful for theatre practitioners who have developed hypersensitivity to other surgical scrub products.

Source: ICNA 2002b.

Skin care

Skin damage is generally associated with the detergent base of the preparation and possibly poor handwashing technique. Common errors seem to be: not wetting the hands before applying soap or antiseptic detergent; not rinsing thoroughly to remove residual soap; and not drying the hands carefully. The *epic* Guidelines recommend that a hand cream should be applied regularly to the hands to protect the skin from the drying effects of regular hand decontamination. Also, should a particular product currently used in the workplace cause skin irritation, occupational health advice should be sought. This is a **Category 3 recommendation** (Pratt *et al.* 2001).

PERSONAL PROTECTIVE EQUIPMENT (PPE)

The *epic* Guidelines' overall recommendation for the use of personal protective equipment is a **Category 3 recommendation**:

Select protective equipment on the basis of an assessment of the risk of transmission of micro-organisms to the patient, and the risk of contamination of health-care practitioners' clothing and skin by the patient' blood, body fluids, secretions and excretions.

Pratt *et al.* (2001) p. 29

Studies have shown that there is no consistent approach towards the use of PPE and confusion as to which item to wear and when (McCoy *et al.* 2001). The Protective Clothing: Principles and Guidelines (ICNA 2002a) emphasise the importance of protective clothing as an essential component in reducing cross-infection, whilst challenging the ritualistic use of protective clothing by promoting evidence-based practice.

Plastic aprons

Single use fluid repellent aprons will protect the practitioner from contamination with blood, body fluids and micro-organisms and must be discarded after each task or episode of care. This is a **Category 3 recommendation** (Pratt *et al.* 2001).

Examples of use are:

- Prior to handling contaminated swabs and specimens
- Cleaning in between cases and at the end of theatre lists
- Dealing with spillages
- When cleaning contaminated equipment
- Whenever there is a risk of contamination to theatre attire.

A full-body, fluid-repellent gown should be worn where there is a risk of extensive splashing of blood, body fluids, secretions and excretions, with the exception of sweat, on to the skin of health care practitioners. This is a **Category 3 recommendation** (Pratt *et al.* 2001).

Theatre gowns and drapes

Traditionally the sole purpose of theatre gowns and drapes was to reduce wound infections by providing a barrier to prevent the transfer of micro-organisms from the patient's own skin flora and the skin of operating staff, into the surgical wound. However, the polycotton fabrics still in use today in the NHS provide little or no resistance to microbial penetration, especially when wet. Nor do they protect health-care practitioners from being contaminated by the patient's blood or bodily fluids. These findings were confirmed by Werner *et al.* (2001) who investigated the quality of the surgical gowns and drapes used in England, Wales and France. The findings of the study revealed that cotton and polyester materials were still widely used; of the 199 reusable items examined, over half failed the initial visual inspection, due to holes impairing functionality. A total of 88% showed a lower liquid resistance than required in the critical area (see Box 3.6) compared with 2% in the single-use drapes examined. Furthermore up to 92% of the reusable drapes and gowns allowed bacterial penetration in critical areas under wet conditions. The study concluded that the percentage of conspicuous faults, mainly associated with reusable products, reflect the 'random risk' posed to both patients and operating personnel when using these products (Werner *et al.* 2001). Even earlier than this, Moylan *et al.* (1987) carried out a comprehensive study following up postoperative infection rates in 2000 general surgical operations. They concluded that the risks of infection are 2.5 times greater with traditional textiles than with single-use products.

Box 3.6 Definition of the critical area of a drape or a gown

This is the area with a greater probability of being compromised by the transfer of infective agents in and out of the wound. These are fronts and sleeves of surgical gowns, and the fenestrations and openings of drapes.

Source: Report from an *Independent Multidisciplinary Working Group* (2003).

The continued use of these traditional materials will not be a future option in the UK, as reusable or disposable gowns and drapes are now classified as medical devices. As such, they must be CE marked to meet the European Directive on device safety known as 93/42/EEC, which since 1998 has been mandatory in the European Union (EU) countries. In addition, the first part of a new EU Standard EN 13795–1 will require both single-use and reusable drapes and gowns to be resistant to liquid penetration, and resistant to microbial penetration with a minimal release of particles (i.e. lint). The further use of cotton and polyester cotton-blended drapes and surgical gowns is not recommended.

The debate as to whether individual trusts opt for single use or reusable drapes and gowns may carry on for now, but what is for certain is that the continued use of the traditional cotton material has no place in the modern operating theatre.

Masks and eye protection

The national evidence-based guidelines state that facemasks and eye protection should be worn where there is a risk of blood, body fluids, secretions and excretions splashing into the face and eyes'. Respiratory protective equipment should be used when clinically indicated. Both of these are **Category 3 recommendations** (Pratt *et al.* 2001).

Masks

Since the introduction by von Mikulicz in 1897 the surgical mask has become an integral part of theatre clothing. Historically the principle function of a mask was to protect patients from the potential shedding of micro-organisms from staff and protect the health-care worker from potential exposure to micro-organisms (ICNA 2002a). Although still used in the operating theatres for this purpose, there is little evidence that they reduce the risk of surgical wound infection (Hubble *et al.* 1996). However, health-care workers require protection from splashes of potentially infected blood and bodily fluids onto the mucous membranes of the eyes and mouth.

The HIS Working Party (2002) concluded there is insufficient evidence to continue the use of masks to prevent wound infection. They did accept that it would be prudent for the 'scrub' team to wear a facemask for prosthetic implant operations. This is a **Category 2 recommendation** (HIS 2002). Patients undergoing procedures involving prosthetic implants are at a higher risk of acquiring a surgical site infection because only a low level of inoculum of low pathogenicity organisms (e.g. *Staphylococcus epidermidis*) is needed because of the presence of a foreign body.

In contrast, the AORN recommendations on wearing masks in the operating theatre are that all persons entering restricted areas of the surgical suite should wear a mask when there are open sterile items and equipment present (AORN 2002b). AORN acknowledges that there is a difference of opinion in the literature regarding wearing masks in the operating theatre. Mitchell and Hunt (1991) suggested that the wearing of facemasks by non-scrubbed staff working in an operating room with forced ventilation appears to be unnecessary. However AORN suggest that the risk of contamination is dependent on the airflow in the area, the amount of traffic, personnel practices, and other factors that would be impossible to consistently monitor. Until further research provides more definitive answers they will continue wearing masks.

Type of masks and tuberculosis

The interdepartmental working group for TB (DOH 1998b) recommends that all persons should wear particulate filtration masks during high-risk procedures such as cough-inducing or aerosol-generating procedures. Particulate filtration masks must filter particles down to 1 micron in diameter and it is suggested that they provide a greater than 95% (i.e. filter leakage of 5%) filtration efficiency for particles with a median diameter of 1.0 μm at a rate of 50 litres per minute (CDC 1994).

Box 3.7 Guide to selection, wearing and disposal of facemasks

Always ensure masks are:

- Appropriate for their purpose. The following need to be determined to ensure selection of the appropriate mask: What is it to be used for? Is it to protect the patient, the healthcare worker or both? What is the hazard? What is the particle size of the hazard and how is it transmitted?
- A fresh mask should be worn for each operation and should be replaced when it becomes damp (HIS 2002; Romney 2001; European Standard 2001).
- Worn and fitted according to the manufacturers' instructions. If not fitted correctly the efficiency of the mask is reduced (European Standard 2001; Curran and Ahmed 2001 and DOH 1998c).
- The mask should not be touched by hands while being worn. It should be handled as little as possible.
- Removed by touching the strings and loops only.
- Not worn loosely around the neck but removed and discarded as soon as practicable after use.
- Never reused once removed.

Box 3.8 A dust/mist respirator or particulate filtration mask *must* be worn by all staff entering a room for:

- Suspected or known tuberculosis (TB): for cough inducing, aerosol generating procedures e.g. bronchoscopy and sputum induction.
- Known or suspected drug resistant TB or multidrug resistant TB.
- Known or suspected TB: when entering body cavities or dissecting viscera or organs in which Mycobacterium tuberculosis is a possibility e.g. theatre, mortuary.

These approved masks can retain their efficiency for up to 8 hours but they are **single-use items and once removed they must never be reused.**

Source: ICNA 2002a.

Masks and surgical smoke and laser plumes

During surgical procedures using a laser or electrosurgery units (ESU), the thermal destruction of tissue creates a smoke by-product (NIOSH 1999). Research studies have shown that this smoke plume can contain toxic gases and vapours such as benzene, carbon monoxide, hydrogen cyanide, formaldehyde, methane, phenol, styrene, toluene, particulate matter, gases, mutagens, carcinogens, DNA, blood and blood-borne pathogens (Giordano 1996). In fact, there have been over 80 chemicals identified so far in surgical smoke (Kokosa and Eugene 1989).

General global consensus is that surgical smoke, regardless of the device used to create the airborne contaminants, is an occupational health hazard and must be properly evacuated (Smalley 1997). However, general room ventilation is not sufficient by itself to capture contaminants generated at the source of the surgical site; nor is the practice of using ordinary suction tubing with a Yankauer sucker attached to a wall or portable suction unit, which was intended to capture liquids, not particulates or gas. The two major local exhaust ventilation approaches recommended for health-care personnel to use in order to reduce surgical smoke levels are portable smoke evacuators and room suction systems (NIOSH/CDC 1996). In respect of facemasks, NIOSH recommend that these should be used as a secondary means of personal protection because no mask will filter out all airborne contaminants (NIOSH 1999). Some masks filter particles to approximately 5 microns in size; masks used in laser procedures filter particles to about 0.1 microns. However, particles can be much smaller than 0.1 and therefore additional measures are necessary.

Eye protection

Eye protection should be worn to protect the mucous membrane of the eye (conjunctivae) during all procedures where the risk of splash (including lateral splashes) or aerosol spray is likely (UK Health Departments 1998b). The common types available in health-care settings are goggles, visors and face shields (single-use items that incorporate a mask with a plastic shield). Whichever type is used they should all be comfortable to wear, fit correctly and allow for clear uncompromised vision (ICNAb 2002a). In a study by Quebbemen et al. (1991) they concluded that facial contamination from blood and body fluids was more likely during orthopaedic, cardiothoracic and vascular surgery compared with gynaecology and general surgery.

Gloves

Gloves play a dual role, as a barrier for personal protection against blood-borne pathogens, other micro-organisms and hazardous substances (e.g. chemicals) and the prevention of infection.

Gloves must be worn for invasive procedures, contact with sterile sites and non-intact skin, mucous membranes, and all activities that have been assessed as carrying a risk of exposure to blood, body fluids, secretions and excretions; and when handling sharp or contaminated instruments. This is a **Category 3 recommendation** (Pratt et al. 2001). All glove types commonly used in the NHS need to conform to the BS-EN455 parts 1, 2, and 3 (British Standards Institution 1994a and b and 2000) and since 1998, all devices which include examination and surgeon gloves must comply with European law (DOH 1998c).

Natural rubber latex

Gloves manufactured from natural rubber latex (NRL) are still considered to give the best protection against blood-borne viruses, as well as maintaining dexterity. Due to this NRL remains the material of choice for gloves when dealing with blood and bodily fluids (ICNA 2002c; Pratt et al. 2001; Russell-Fell 2000).

In 1996 guidance was issued to health-care workers highlighting the potential problems caused by NRL sensitivity (Medical Devices Agency [MDA] 1996). Then in 1998 the MDA issued further guidance regarding the use of cornstarch powder in medical gloves linked with sensitisation (MDA 1998). Haglund and Junghanns (1997) reported that cornstarch powder, which was traditionally used to make donning gloves easier, has been proven to be harmful and is associated with adhesions, latex allergy and increasing risks of infection associated with invasive devices contaminated with cornstarch powder.

A number of studies in operating theatres have demonstrated that wearing two pairs of latex gloves (double-gloving) significantly reduces the risk of exposure to blood and should be considered when undertaking an exposure prone procedure (EPP) or when glove punctures are likely e.g. orthopaedics, obstetric, cardiothoracic and gynaecology procedures (UK Departments 1998b). The HIS Working Party concluded that wearing double gloves at surgical procedures helps to protect the wearer from viral transmission. There is no evidence that perforated gloves increase the incidence of infection and needle-puncture of a glove is not an indication to change gloves. If any action is taken it is preferable to don a second pair of gloves to protect the operating surgeon or individual undertaking the procedure. This is a **Category 1 recommendation** (HIS 2002).

Safe management of sharps

Sharp injuries and contamination incidents are important risks for the transmission of blood-borne pathogens to health workers, particularly in the operating theatre. Most cases of occupational transmission of viruses occur from (i) percutaneous exposure when the skin is cut or penetrated by a needle or other sharp object, for example scalpel blade, trocar, teeth and bone spicules; or (ii) from contamination of mucous membranes of eyes, mouth and broken skin which is referred to as mucutaneous exposure.

Causes of needlestick injuries

Eistenstein and Smith (1992) cited several reasons for causes of needlestick injuries. These were recapping of needles, transfer of used sharps to point of disposal, sharps not discarded after use, or overfilled sharp containers. Resheathing of needles has been proven to be by and large a dangerous practice, because if the needle misses the sheath, it will puncture the

hand holding it. Houang and Hurley (1997) found that knowledge of risk was not sufficient to encourage correct procedures as highlighted by Heydon (1995), who reported an incident concerning a 33-year-old occupational health worker in New Zealand who pricked a blister on the palm of the hand of an employee with a history of acute hepatitis C. The OH worker sustained a needlestick injury when she resheathed the needle and was diagnosed with hepatitis C two months later. In an attempt to reduce the incidence of needlestick injuries to the minimum, the UK Departments of Health have recommended a reduction in the use of sharp devices wherever possible and to consider introducing needle protective devices (UK Departments 1998b).

Preventing needlestick injuries

In order to reduce the risk of percutaneous exposure at the operating table the following actions were recommended by the UK Departments (1998b):

- Avoid hand to hand passing of sharp instruments during an operation.
- Establish a 'neutral zone'; this can be a tray, kidney basin or an identified area in the operative field, which ensures the safe passage of sharps.
- Ensure scalpels and sharp needles are placed in the designated neutral zone and removed promptly away from the operative field when not in use.

If however a theatre practitioner sustains a needlestick injury, they should immediately follow the actions outlined in Box 3.9. If the needlestick injury was from a high-risk source of blood-borne viruses, see Table 3.4 for further information on post-exposure prophylaxis (PEP).

Sharps must be discarded into a sharps container conforming to European and British Standards (BS 7320, 1990) and United Nations recommendations (UN 3291, 1999) at the point of use.

Box 3.9   First aid treatment for needlestick injuries

- The injured area should be encouraged to bleed and washed with soap and water
- Contamination of mucous membranes (eyes, mouth) should be flushed with water
- Wounds should be cleaned, sutured and dressed as appropriate
- Report incident to occupational health department and line manager
- Complete an accident form.

Safe management of spillages

All blood and body fluid spillages should be removed promptly, using 1% hypochlorite solution (10,000 parts per million [p.p.m.] of available chlorine) or chlorine-releasing granules; this is necessary to neutralise and make safe the spillage prior to disposal. In situations where there are minor contaminations of surfaces a dilution of 0.1% hypochlorite (1000 p.p.m. available chlorine) can be used. If chlorine disinfectants cannot be used then spills should be removed using detergent and hot water. It should be noted that in the case of urine spillages, chlorine-based products should not be used as they may react with urine to produce a chlorine vapour (DOH 1990). Consult local infection control policy for further information on the products used and the procedure for dealing with body fluids spills in your workplace.

Safe management of linen

Linen should be separated into used linen (soiled or fouled) and infected linen and then re-processed according to HSG (95)18 Hospital Laundry Arrangements for Used and Infected Linen (DOH 1995). Consult local infection control policy in your workplace for further information.

Safe disposal of waste

All waste must be properly segregated, labelled, stored, transported and disposed of in accordance with expert guidance (Health Service Advisory Committee 1999). Consult the local infection control policies in your work area for further information.

Environmental cleaning in the theatre suite

Floors of the operating room should be disinfected at the end of each session and scrubbed daily. Wall washing is recommended twice yearly. Specific spillages of blood or body fluids should be dealt with immediately. Mop buckets for spillage should be emptied after each use and kept dry until the next occasion when they are required. Lint-free cloth is recommended for all operating theatre cleaning. This is a **Category 3 recommendation** (HIS 2002).

AN OVERVIEW OF INFECTION CONTROL IN HOSPITALS

The Government has given infection control a high political priority. The 1997 White Paper, 'The New NHS: Modern, Dependable' proposed shifting the focus of management in the NHS from finance to quality of care with excellence guaranteed to all patients. In 1998 a Consultation document 'A First Service: Quality in the New NHS' described how quality standards would be delivered locally through a system of *clinical governance* (DOH 1998d).

1998 saw the publication of the House of Lords Science and Technology Select Committee Enquiry into Antibiotic Resistance that recommended that infection control and basic hygiene should be at the heart of good management and clinical practice, with resources being re-directed accordingly (House of Lords 1998). Both the Government's response and the issuing of Health Service Circular Resistance to Antibiotic and other Antimicrobial agents (HSC 1999/049) support this view in raising the profile of hospital-acquired infection. Furthermore the National Planning and Priority Guidance for 1999/2000 highlighted the prevention of HAI, communicable disease and antimicrobial resistance as key issues in public health (HSC 1999/242).

Since then the following guidance from the Department of Health was issued to the NHS

Trusts which either gave specific guidance on the management and control of HAI or made reference to this issue:

- Control Assurance Guidelines supplementing HSC 1999 123 (DOH 1999b).
- Modernising Health and Social Services: National Priorities Guidance 2000–01 and 2002–03 (DOH 1999b).
- HSC2000/002 The Management and Control of Hospital Infection (DOH 2000c).

Hospital-acquired infection

A nosocomial or hospital-acquired infection (HAI) is any infection that develops as a result of hospital treatment from which the patient was not suffering or incubating at the time of admission to hospital. About 9% of inpatients have a HAI at any one time (Emmerson *et al.* 1996; DOH/PHLS 1995) and a further 20–70% of surgical wound infections present after discharge from hospital (Holtz and Wenzel 1992). In 1995 it was stated that 30% of HAI could be prevented by better application of existing knowledge and implementation of realistic infection control policies (DOH/PHLS 1995). However following the National Audit Office

Box 3.10 Five facts about HAIs

- There are at least 300,000 hospital infections a year.
- They are estimated to cost the NHS around £1 billion a year.
- They can mean 11 extra days in hospital – but some infections only present after patient discharge.
- Hospital infections may kill: a crude estimate suggests as many as 5000 patients may die annually as result of HAI and a further 15,000 HAI is a significant contributing factor (DOH/PHLS 1995).
- Not all HAI are preventable, but ICTs believe that they could be reduced by 15% avoiding costs totalling £150 million.

Source: National Audit Office (2000).

Report (2000) infection control teams (ICTs) now believe that 15% of HAI is now a more realistic preventable figure.

The cost of hospital-acquired infection

In 1997, The Department of Health commissioned the Central Public Health Laboratory and the London School of Hygiene and Tropical Medicine to assess the burden of HAI in terms of the costs to the public sector, patients, informal carers and society as a whole. The key findings of this 13-month study in one NHS trust were extrapolated to provide results for all NHS trusts throughout England. This information then determined the overall costs to the National Health Service (NHS) to be around £1 billion (Plowman *et al.* 2000).

It was noted by Plowman *et al.* (2000) that although a shorter hospital stay will reduce the risk of acquiring an infection for surgical patients the risks are likely to be highest on the day of surgery and the days immediately following.

Surveillance of hospital-acquired infection

Surveillance is defined as the collection and analysis of data on infections occurring in patients and staff, and dissemination of the results to the relevant personnel so that appropriate actions can be taken.

The SENIC Report (Study in the Efficacy of Nosocomial Infection Control) demonstrated the

Box 3.11 Key findings from the socioeconomic burden of HAI study

- Hospital costs for patients who develop an HAI are 2.8 times greater than for those who do not.
- HAIs add £2917 per case to the cost of a hospital stay.
- Patients with a HAI remain in the hospital, on average, 2.5 times longer (equivalent to 11 extra days).
- HAIs are estimated to cost the hospital sector £930.6 million a year in inpatient costs.

Source: (Plowman *et al.* 2000).

value of well-organised surveillance and infection control programmes in the USA. Through reporting the rates of infection to individual surgeons, a reduction of 32% was achieved. In contrast, hospitals that had no effective programmes saw infection rates increase by 18% (Haley *et al*. 1985). This reduction in wound infection rates in conjunction with surveillance and feedback programmes was reproduced in other studies (Cruse 1986; Olsen *et al*. 1990).

The SENIC study identified several factors that increased the likelihood of developing a surgical wound infection. These included the type of surgery (clean or contaminated), the duration of the operation and the site of surgery (Haley *et al*. 1985). The CDC term for infections associated with surgical procedures was changed from surgical wound infection to surgical site infection (SSI) in 1992 (Horan *et al*. 1992). These infections are now classified into three categories: (i) superficial incisional SSI (skin and subcutaneous); (ii) deep incisional SSI (deep soft tissue-muscle and fascia); and (iii) organ/space SSI, and they are used by all USA hospitals who participate in the Centers for Disease Control (CDC) National Nosocomial Infections Surveillance System (NNIS) (Garner *et al*. 1988; Horan *et al*. 1992).

In 1996, the Department of Heath in England and the Public Health Laboratory Service (PHLS) established a similar scheme for England. This was based on the USA version that has been in use for several decades. The English scheme was known as the Nosocomial Infection National Surveillance Scheme (NINSS). Its purpose was to improve the quality of patient care by reducing infection rates. Participation in the NINSS scheme was voluntary and enabled hospitals to compare their data against aggregated anonymised data from other participating hospitals.

In 2000, the Department of Health established a new NHS Healthcare Associated Infection Surveillance Steering Group (HAISSG) to review the 5-year old NINSS project and make recommendations to expand and develop the scheme further to meet the needs of local NHS Trusts and overall surveillance needs. Also in 2000 the Minister of State for Health, John Denham,

announced that surveillance of hospital-acquired infection should be made compulsory for all NHS Acute Trusts.

In April 2001, compulsory reporting of bacteraemia caused by methicillin-resistant *Staphylococcus aureus* (MRSA) was introduced. The first year's report featuring the results of the MRSA bacteraemia rates from the 187 acute NHS Trusts in England was published in 2002 (PHLS 2002). Since July 2003, these results are to be used as a performance management indicator. The indicator will then form part of the balanced scorecard that will contribute to the star ratings for acute hospital trusts. The next tranche of HCAI surveillance to be rolled out will be the mandatory reporting of bacteraemia due to glycopeptide resistant enterococci (GRE) in October 2003 and *Clostridium difficile*-associated diarrhoea in January 2004. In respect of the surgical site infections it is believed the mandatory reporting will focus initially on orthopaedic surgery in April 2004 (DOH 2003).

Post-discharge surveillance

Studies in the US and UK confirm that between 50 and 70% of surgical wound infections occur post-discharge (Holtz and Wenzel 1992; Plowman *et al*. 2000). The Department of Health, recognising the need for effective post-discharge surveillance, funded the PHLS to evaluate post-discharge surveillance methods for surgical wound infections and determine an acceptable methodology to collect comprehensive reliable data. The NAO Report (2000) recommended that NHS Trusts should carry out some form of post-discharge surveillance in order to obtain a more accurate picture of their performance in relation to hospital-acquired infection.

CONCLUSION

Hospital-acquired infection remains a serious issue for health professionals and patients. Surgery is changing rapidly: where it is carried out, the increasing technology, the length of time patients remain in hospital, and the practitioners who undertake it. Therefore in order for infection control to be effective, all theatre practitioners must observe the principles of infection control practice. These principles are based on national evidence-based guidelines, and should be followed in your daily practice towards all patients, at all times, to help minimise the transmission of infection between patients and staff and to reduce perioperative hospital-acquired infections.

REFERENCES

Agarwal M, Hamilton-Stewart P and Dixon RA (2002) Contaminated operating room boots: the potential for infection. *American Journal of Infection Control* 30: 179–183.

Alexander JW, Fischer JE, Boyajian M *et al.* (1983) The influence of hair-removal methods on wound infections *Archives of Surgery* 118: 347–352.

Anon (1995) Italian nurse in AIDS compensation test case. *Nursing Standard* 9(46): 12.

AORN (2000a) Recommended practices for environmental cleaning in the surgical practice setting. In: *Standards, Recommended Practices and Guidelines.* Denver: AORN, pp. 255–260.

AORN (2000b) Recommended practices for surgical attire. In: *Standards, Recommended Practices and Guidelines.* Denver: AORN, 183–188.

Ayliffe GAJ, Babb JR, Collins BJ and Lowbury EJL (1969) Transfer areas and clean zones in operating suites. *Journal of Hygiene* 67(3): 417–425.

Ayliffe GAJ, Noy MF, Babb JR, Davies JG and Jackson J (1983) A comparison of pre-operative bathing with chlorhexidine-detergent and non medicated soap in the prevention of wound infection. *Journal of Hospital Infection* 4(3): 237–244.

Ayliffe GAJ, Fraise AP, Geddes AM and Mitchell K (2000) *Control of Hospital Infection: A Practical Handbook*, 4th edn. London: Arnold.

British Standards Institution (1990) BS 7320 *British Standards specification for sharps containers.* London: BSI.

British Standards Institution (1994a). *Medical gloves single use, Part 1: specification for freedom from holes.* BS-EN 455-1. London: BSI.

British Standards Institution (1994b) *Medical gloves single use, Part 2: specification for physical properties.* BS-EN 455-2. London: BSI.

British Standards Institution (2000) *Medical gloves single use, Part 3: requirements and testing for biological evaluations.* BS-EN 455-3. London: BSI.

Brown GH (1993) The sacred cow contest. *Canadian Nurse* 89: 31–33.

Byrne DJ, Napier A and Cuschieri A (1990) Rationalizing whole body disinfection. *Journal of Hospital Infection* 15(2): 183–187.

Cardo DM, Culver DH, Ciesielski CA *et al.* (1997) A case–control study of HIV seroconversion in healthcare workers after percutaneous exposure. Centers for Disease Control and Prevention Needlestick Surveillance Group. *New England Journal of Medicine* 337(21): 1485–1490.

Carter R (1990) Plastic overshoes – an unacceptable risk? *Nursing Times* 86(13): 63–64.

Cattaneo C, Nuttall PA and Sokol RJ (1996) Detection of HIV, hepatitis B and hepatitis C markers in discarded syringes and bloodstains. *Science and Justice* 36(27): 1–4.

Caunt H (1991) The evolution of theatre dress. *Nursing* 4(42): 23–24.

Centers for Disease Control and Prevention (1987) Recommendations for prevention of HIV transmission in health-care settings. *Morbidity and Mortality Weekly Report* 36 (No 2 suppl): 001.

Centers for Disease Control and Prevention (1994) Guidelines for preventing the transmission of Mycobacterium tuberculosis in health care facilities. *Morbidity and Mortality Weekly Report* 43 (No RR-13): 1–132.

Choo QL, Kuo G, Weiner AJ, Overby LR, Bradley DW, Houghton M (1989) Isolation of a cDNA clone derived from a blood-borne non-A, non-B viral hepatitis genome. *Science* 244: 359–362.

Considering the consequences: an evaluation of infection risk when choosing surgical gowns and drapes in today's NHS. *Report from an Independent Multi-disciplinary Working Group.* February 2003.

Cruse PJE and Foord R (1973) A 5-year prospective study of 23,649 surgical wounds. *Archives of Surgery* 107: 206–210.

Cruse PJE and Foord R (1980) The epidemiology of wound infection: a 10-year prospective study of 62939 wounds. *Surgical Clinics of North America* 60(1): 27–40.

Cruse PJE (1986) Surgical infection: incision wounds. In: Bennett JV and Brachman PS (eds) *Hospital Infections*, 2nd edn. Boston: Little Brown, pp. 423–436.

Cruse PJE (1992) Classification of operations and audit of infection In: Taylor EW (ed) *Infection Control in Surgical Practice.* Oxford: Oxford University Press.

Curran E and Ahmed S (2001) Do healthcare workers need to wear masks when caring for patients with pulmonary tuberculosis? *Communicable Disease and Public Health* 3(4): 240–243.

Department of Health (1990) Spills of urine: potential risk of misuse of chlorine-releasing disinfecting agents. *Safety Action Bulletin* 59(90): 41.

Department of Health (1995) *Hospital laundry arrangements for used and infected linen*. Heath Safety Guidance (HSG) (95)18. London: DoH.

Department of Health/Public Health Laboratory Service (1995) *Hospital infection control. Guidance on the control of infection in hospitals*. HSG (95)10. London: DoH.

Department of Health (1998a) *Prevalence of HIV in England and Wales 1997*. Summary Report from the Unlinked Anonymous Surveys Screening Group. London: DoH.

Department of Health Interdepartmental Working Group on Tuberculosis (1998b) *The prevention and control of tuberculosis in the United Kingdom: UK guidance on the prevention and control of 1. HIV-related tuberculosis and 2. Drug-resistant, including multiple drug-resistant, tuberculosis*. London: The Stationery Office.

Department of Health (1998c) *Medical devices directive – CE marking*. EL(98)5. London: The Stationery Office.

Department of Health (1998d) *A first class service: quality in the new NHS*. London: DoH.

Department of Health (1999b) HSC 1999/123 *Governance in the new NHS. Control assurance statement 1999/2000: Risk management and organization controls*. HSC 1999/123. London: DoH.

Department of Health (2000a) *HIV – post exposure prophylaxis*. Guidance from UK Chief Medical Officer's Expert Advisory Group on AIDS. London: The Stationery Office.

Department of Health (2000b) *Hepatitis B infected healthcare workers*. HSC 2000/020. London: DoH. http://www.doh.gov.uk/nhsexec/hepatitisb.htm

Department of Health (2000c) *The management and control of hospital acquired infection*. HSC 2000/002. London: DoH.

Department of Health (2001) *National strategy for sexual health and HIV*. London: DoH. Website: http://www.doh.gov.uk/nshs/index.htm

Department of Health (2002a) *Hepatitis C infected health care workers* (HSC 2002/010). London: DoH. http://www.doh.gov.uk/hepatitisc

Department of Health (2002b) *HIV infected healthcare workers: a consultation paper on management and patient notification*. London: DoH. http://www.doh.gov.uk/aids.htm

Department of Health (2002c) *Independent health care: national minimum standards regulations*. London: DoH.http://www.doh.gov.uk/ncsc/ independenthealthcare.pdf

Department of Health (2003) *Consultation on graft guidance on health clearance for serious communicable disease: new health care workers*. London: DoH.http://www.doh.gov.uk/healthclear/index.htm

Eisenstein HC and Smith DA (1992) Epidemiology of reported sharp injuries in tertiary care hospital. *Journal of Hospital Infection* 20(4): 271–280.

Emmerson AM, Enstone JE, Griffin M, Kelsey MC and Smyth ET (1996) The Second National Prevalence Survey of Infection in Hospitals – overview of the results. *Journal of Hospital Infection* 32(3): 175–90.

European Standard (2001) *Performance requirements and test methods for surgical masks intended to be used as medical devices*. Brussels: European Committee for Standardisation, Central Secretariat.

European Standard EN 13795-1 (2002) *Surgical drapes, gowns and clean air suits, used as medical devices, for patients, clinical staff and equipment – Part 1: General requirements for manufacturers, processors and products*. European Committee for Standardisation.

Evans BG and Abiteboul D (1999) A summary of occupationally acquired HIV infections described in published reports to December 1997. *Eurosurveillance* 4(3): 29–32.

Garibaldi RA, Skolnick D, Lerer T, Poirot A, Graham J, Krisuinas E and Lyons R. (1988). The impact of preoperative skin disinfection on preventing intraoperative wound contamination. *Epidemiology* 9(3): 109–113.

Garner JS, Jarvis WR, Emori TG, Horan TC and Hughes JM (1988) CDC definitions for nosocomial infections 1988. *American Journal of Infection Control* 16(3): 128–140.

Giordano BP (1996) 'Don't be a victim of surgical smoke' (Editorial) *AORN Journal* 63: 520–522.

Glynn AA, Ward V, Wilson J, Charlett A, Cookson B, Taylor L and Cole N (1997) *Hospital Acquired Infection: Surveillance, Policies and Practice*. London: Public Health Laboratory Service.

Gould D (2002) Hand decontamination. *Nursing Times* 98(46): 48–49.

Haglund U and Junghanns K (eds) (1997) Glove powder – The hazards which demand a ban. Proceedings of a meeting. London, United Kingdom, May 1996. *European Journal of Surgery* (Suppl) 579: 4–55.

Haley RW, Culver DH, White JW, Morgan WM, Emori TG, Munn VP and Hooton TM (1985) The efficacy of infection surveillance and control programs in preventing nosocomial infections in the US hospital. *American Journal of Epidemiology* 121(2): 182–205.

Hambraeus A, Bengtsson S and Laurell G (1978) Bacterial contamination in a modern operating theatre. Importance of floor contamination as a source of airborne bacteria. *Journal of Hygiene* 80: 57–67.

Hayek LJ, Emerson JM and Gardner AM (1987) A placebo-controlled trial of the effect of two preoperative baths or showers with chlorhexidine detergent on postoperative wound infection rates. *Journal of Hospital Infection* 10(2): 165–72.

Health Service Advisory Committee (1999) *Safe disposal of clinical waste.* London: HMSO.

Health Service Circular (1999) *Resistance to antibiotics and other antimicrobial agents: action for the NHS following the Government's response to the House of Lords, Science and Technology Select Committee report 'Resistance to antibiotics and other antimicrobial agents'.* HSC 1999/049. London: DoH.

Hedderwick SA, McNeill SA, Lyons MJ and Kauffman CA (2000) Pathogenic organisms associated with artificial fingernails worn by healthcare workers. *Infection Control and Hospital Epidemiology* 21(8): 505–509.

Heydon J (1995) Hepatitis C from needlestick injury. *New Zealand Medical Journal* 108(992): 21.

Holtz TH and Wenzel RP (1992) Post discharge surveillance for nosocomial wound infections: A brief review and commentary. *American Journal of Infection Control* 20(4): 206–213.

Horan TC, Gaynes RP, Martone WJ, Jarvis WR and Emori TG (1992) CDC definitions of nosocomial surgical site infections, 1992: A modification of CDC definitions of surgical wound infections. *American Journal of Infection Control* 20(5): 271–274.

Hospital Infection Society Working Party (2002) *Behaviour and rituals in the operating theatre.* http://www.his.org.uk

Houang E and Hurley R (1997) Anonymous questionnaire survey on the knowledge and practice of hospital staff in infection control. *Journal of Hospital Infection* 35(4): 301–306.

House of Lords Select Committee on Science and Technology (1998) *Resistance to antibiotics and other antimicrobials.* Seventh report. London: The Stationery Office.

HSC 1999/242 (1999) *Modernising health and social services: national priorities guidance for 1999/00–2001/02.* London: DoH.

Hubble MJ, Weale AE, Perez JV, Bowker KE, MacGowan AP and Bannister GC (1996) Clothing in laminar flow operating theatres. *Journal of Hospital Infection* 32: 1–7.

Humphreys H, Russell AJ, Marshall RJ, Ricketts VE and Reeves DS (1991) The effect of surgical theatre head-gear on air bacterial counts. *Journal of Hospital Infection* 19(3): 175–180.

Humphreys H, Marshall RJ, Ricketts VE, Russell AJ and Reeves DS (1991) Theatre over-shoes do not reduce operating theatre floor bacterial counts. *Journal of Hospital Infection* 17(2): 117–123.

Infection Control Nurses Association (2002a) *Protective clothing: principles and guidance.* London: ICNA.

Infection Control Nurses Association (2002b) *Hand decontamination guidelines.* London: ICNA.

Infection Control Nurses Association (2002c) *A comprehensive glove choice.* London: ICNA.

Jaeckel E, Cornberg M, Wedemeyer H *et al.*, German Acute Hepatitis C Therapy Group (2001) Treatment of acute hepatitis C with interferon alfa-2b. *New England Journal of Medicine* 345(20): 1452–1457.

Kaiser AB, Kernodle DS, Barg NL and Petracek MR (1988) Influence of preoperative showers on staphylococcal skin colonization: a comparative trial of antiseptic skin cleansers. *Annals of Thoracic Surgery* 45(1): 35–38.

Kokosa J and Eugene J (1989) Chemical composition of laser tissue interaction of smoke plume. *Journal of Laser Applications* 59–63.

Larson E (1995) APIC Guidelines for handwashing and hand antisepsis in health care settings. *American Journal of Infection Control* 23(4): 251–69.

Lewis DA, Weymont G, Noakes CM *et al.* (1990) A bacteriological study of the effect on the environment of using a one or two trolley system in theatre. *Journal of Hospital Infection* 15(35): 35–53.

Litsky BY and Litsky W (1971) Bacterial shedding during bed stripping of reusable and disposable linens as detected by the high volume air sampler. *Health Laboratory Scientist* 8(1): 29–34.

Lynch W, Davey PG, Malek M, Byrne DJ and Napier A (1992) Cost-effectiveness analysis of the use of chlorhexidine detergent in preoperative whole-body disinfection in wound infection prophylaxis. *Journal of Hospital Infection* 21(3): 179–191.

Mangram AJ, Horan TC, Pearson ML, Silver LC and Jarvis WR (1999) Guideline for Prevention of Surgical Site Infection, 1999. Centers for Disease Control and Prevention (CDC) Hospital Infection Control Practices Advisory Committee. *American Journal of Infection Control* 27(2): 97–132.

Mathias JM (2000) Sacred cow survey. Use of cover gowns, shoe covers falls to new low. *OR Manager* 16(9): 1, 9–11, 13–14.

Medical Devices Agency (1996) *Latex sensitisation in the healthcare setting. Use of latex gloves.* (DB (96)01). London: The Stationery Office.

Medical Devices Agency (1998) *Medical Devices Directive (MDD). Latex medical gloves (surgeons and examination). Powdered latex medical gloves (surgeons and examinations).* MDA SN9825 (June). London: MDA.

McCoy KD, Beekman SE, Ferguson KJ, Vaughn TE, Torner JC, Woolson RF and Doebbeling BN (2001) Monitoring adherence to Standard Precautions. *American Journal of Infection Control* 29(1): 24–31.

McNeil SA, Foster CL. Hedderwick SA and Kaufman CA (2000) Effect of hand cleansing with antimicrobial soap or alcohol-based gel on microbial colonization of artificial fingernails by healthcare workers. *Clinical Infectious Diseases* 32(3): 367–372.

Mishriki SF, Jeffery PJ and Law DJW (1992) Wound Infection: the surgeon's responsibility. *Journal of Wound Care* 1(2): 32–36.

Mitchell NJ and Hunt S (1991) Surgical face mask in modern operating rooms – a costly and unnecessary ritual? *Journal of Hospital Infection* 18: 239–42.

Moolenaar RL, Crutcher JM, San Joaquin VH *et al.* (2000) A prolonged outbreak of *Pseudomonas aeruginosa* in a neonatal intensive care unit: did staff fingernails play a role in disease transmission? *Infection Control Hospital and Epidemiology* 21(2): 80–85.

Moylan JA, Fitzpatrick KT and Davenport KE (1987) Reducing wound infections – improved gown and drape barrier performance. *Archives of Surgery* 122: 152–157.

National AIDS Manual (2001) *AIDS Reference Manual.* London: National AIDS Manual. Website: www.aidsmap.com

National Association of Theatre Nurses (1998) Preparation of personnel. In: *Principles of Safe Practice in the Perioperative Environment.* Harrogate: NATN, pp. 65–67.

National Audit Office (2000) *The management and control of hospital acquired infection in acute trusts in England.* HC 230 Session 1999-00. London: National Audit Office. http://www.nao.gov.uk

National Institute for Clinical Excellence (2000) *Guidance on the use of ribavirin and interferon alpha for hepatitis C.* London: NICE.

National Institute for Occupational Safety and Health (1996) *Control of smoke from laser/electric surgical procedures.* Publ no 96–128. Cincinnati: OSHA (NIOSH), pp. 1–2.

NHS Executive (1998) *National priorities guidance for 1999/00–2001/02: modernising health and social services.* London: NHS Executive.

Nicolai P, Aldam CH and Allen PW (1997) Increased awareness of glove perforation in major joint replacement. A prospective, randomised study of Regent Biogel Reveal gloves. *Journal of Bone and Joint Surgery* (Br) 79(3): 371–373.

NIOSH (1999) Control of smoke form lasers/electric surgical procedures. *Applied Occupational and Environmental Hygiene* 14(2): 71.

Olsen MM and Lee JT Jr (1990) Continuous 10-year wound infection surveillance. Results, advantages and unanswered questions. *Archives of Surgery* 125: 794–803.

Pittet D, Hugonnet S, Harbarth S, Mourouga P, Sauvan V, Touveneau S and Perneger T (2000) Effectiveness of a hospital-wide programme to improve compliance with hand hygiene Infection Control Programme. *Lancet* 356(9238): 1307–1312.

Plowman R, Craves N, Griffin M, Roberts J, Swan A, Cookson B and Taylor L (2000) *The socio-economic burden of hospital acquired infection.* London: Public Health Laboratory Service.

Pratt RJ, Pellowe C, Loveday HP and Robinson N (2001) The *epic* Project: Developing National Evidence-based Guidelines for Preventing

Healthcare Associated Infections. *Journal of Hospital Infection* 47 (Suppl): S1–S82.

Public Health Laboratory Service (2002) The first year of the Department of Health's mandatory MRSA bacteraemia surveillance scheme in acute NHS Trusts in England: April 2001–March 2002. *CDR Weekly* 12(25): 1–17.

Puro V, Petrosillo N and Ippolito G (1995) Risk of hepatitis C seroconversion after occupational exposures in health care workers. Italian Study Group on Occupational Risk of HIV and Other Blood-borne Infections. *American Journal of Infection Control* 23(5): 273–277.

Quebbemen EJ, Telford GL, Hubbard S, Wadsworth K, Hardman B, Goodman H and Gottlieb MS (1991) Risk of blood contamination and injury to operating room personnel. *Annals of Surgery* 214(5): 614–620.

Riddell LA and Sherrard J (2000) Blood-borne virus infection: the occupational risks. *International Journal of STD and AIDS* 11(10): 632–639.

Romney MG (2001) Surgical face masks in the operating theatre; re-examining the evidence. *Journal of Hospital Infection* 47: 251–256.

Rotter ML, Olesen Larsen S, Cooke EM *et al.* (1988) A comparison of the effect of pre-operative body bathing with detergent alone and with detergent containing chlorhexidine gluconate on the frequency of wound infections after clean surgery. The European Working Party on Control of Infection. *Journal of Hospital Infection* 11(4): 310–320.

Russell-Fell FW (2000) Avoiding problems: evidence based selection of medical gloves. *British Journal of Nursing* 9(3): 125–184.

Shibuya A, Takeuchi A, Sakurai K and Saigerji K (1998) Hepatitis G virus infection from needlestick injuries in hospital employees. *Journal of Hospital Infection* 40(4): 287–290.

Smalley PJ (1997) Update on regulation on surgical smoke and its management. *Surgical Services Management* 3(3): 31–35.

Sulkowski MS, Ray SC and Thomas DI (2002) Needlestick transmission of hepatitis C. *Journal of the American Medical Association* 287(18): 2406–2413.

Taylor K, Plowman R and Roberts JA (2001) *The challenge of hospital acquired infection*. London: National Audit Office, The Stationery Office.

Thomas JA, Fligelstone LJ, Kerwood TE and Rees RW (1993) Theatre footwear: a health hazard? *British Journal of Theatre Nursing* 3(7): 5–9.

UK Health Departments (1990) *Guidance for clinical health care workers: protection against infection with blood-borne viruses*. Recommendations of the Expert Advisory Group on AIDS and the Advisory Group on Hepatitis. London: The Stationery Office.

UK Health Departments (1998a) AIDS/HIV infected health care workers: guidance on the management of infected healthcare workers and patient notification HSC 1998/226. http://www.doh.gov.uk/aids.htm

UK Health Departments (1998b) *Guidance for clinical health care workers: protection against infection with blood-borne viruses*. Recommendations of the Expert Advisory Group on AIDS and the Advisory Group on Hepatitis. London: The Stationery Office. http://www.doh.gov.uk/aids.htm

United Nations (1999) UN 3291 *Recommendations on the transport of dangerous goods, model regulations*, 11th edn. Geneva: UN.

Villano SA, Vlahov D, Nelson KE, Cohn S and Thomas DL (1999) Persistence of viremia and the importance of long-term follow-up after acute hepatitis C infection. *Hepatology* 29(3): 908–914.

Weightman NC and Banfield KR (1994) Protective over-shoes are unnecessary in a day surgery unit. *Journal of Hospital Infection* 28(1): 1–3.

Werner HP, Feltgen M and Schmitt O (2001) Quality of surgical drapes and gowns – investigation in England, Wales and France. *Hygiene of Medicine* 26: 62–75.

World Health Organization (2000) Hepatitis C Act. Sheet No 194 http://www.who.int/inf-fs/en/fact164.html

Wynd CA, Samstag DE and Lapp AM (1994) Bacterial carriage on the fingernails of OR nurses. *AORN Journal* 60: 796, 799–805.

4 PRINCIPLES OF ANAESTHETIC PRACTICE

Melanie Oakley and Christine Spiers

CHAPTER AIMS

- To explore the anaesthetic practitioner's role in terms of airway management, haemodynamic assessment and induction and maintenance of anaesthesia
- To expand the practitioner's knowledge of anaesthetic pharmacology
- To consider the potential hazards associated with anaesthesia and the practitioner's role in supporting the patient when complications occur
- To briefly review emergency situations in anaesthetic practice.

Anaesthesia is derived from the Greek word meaning 'not or without sensation'; this definition is still applicable to modern day anaesthesia. It allows surgery to take place without the patient feeling any sensation of pain. Anaesthesia can be general, where the patient is rendered unconscious, or local where a block is employed to produce a lack of pain and sensation. This can be carried out with or without sedation, or a combination of general and local anaesthesia can be used. Good and safe anaesthesia will maintain homeostasis and ensure a patent airway. The patient will be cardiovascularly stable with the circulating volume replaced as necessary. The body will be protected in terms of thermoregulation and injury. This will be done in the presence of pre-existing conditions, and serious life threatening injury. The technique employed will be chosen by the anaesthetist as a result of assessment of the patient prior to anaesthesia.

THE ANAESTHETIC PRACTITIONER'S ROLE IN ANAESTHESIA

The patient undergoing anaesthesia will be apprehensive about the procedure. The anaesthetic practitioner is there to ensure continuity of care during their time in the operating department. In order to do this the practitioner must have knowledge of the anaesthetic technique to be used, the pharmacological agents and the type of surgery. In addition the anaesthetic practitioner must be aware of pre-existing medical conditions which will impact on the care given to the patient, as well as providing psychological support.

Two grades of staff work within the anaesthetic area in the UK. Firstly, there are practitioners who have undergone a three-year general training. In order to work in anaesthetics, practitioners must obtain the ENB 182 Anaesthetic Nursing certificate or equivalent. With the demise of the National Boards this will be in the form of diploma or degree modules in specialist anaesthetic practice. Following the course practitioners will consolidate the skills learnt while on the course for at least six months.

In the UK practitioners can only work in the anaesthetic area if they have an anaesthetic qualification (Association of Anaesthetists 1989). This means that prior to embarking on an anaesthetic qualification, no prior experience will have been gained, although the individual may have worked in recovery.

The other grade of staff is the operating department practitioner (ODP). They will have completed a two-year course in operating department practice. This was originally a City and Guilds qualification, which subsequently became NVQ level 3 and now is a diploma level course. This qualification enables ODPs to work in all areas of the operating department.

The role of the anaesthetic practitioner will vary in each country around the world. For example in North America the role is that of the practitioner anaesthetist assessing patients and administering anaesthesia. Whereas in the UK the anaesthetic practitioner works with the anaesthetist ensuring continuity of patient care, they do not administer anaesthesia, although this is open to continuing discussion, particularly with the predicted shortfall in consultant anaesthetists (Bailey 1995). The NHS Management Executive carried out a scoping study in 1996, which concluded that practitioner anaesthetists would not enhance anaesthetic patient care in this country. Added to this, the Royal College of Anaesthetists was fast-tracking senior anaesthetic registrars and it was predicted that the shortfall would be filled within two years. However more recently the Changing Workforce Programme, part of the Modernisation Agency, is examining the possibility of setting up non-physician anaesthetist programmes (NHS Modernisation Agency 2002).

The role of the anaesthetic practitioner is varied, but there should be a move away from using the term 'assistant to the anaesthetist'. Primarily anaesthetic practitioners are there to ensure that patients are anaesthetised safely with the least amount of anxiety possible on the patient's part. They are not there to assist the anaesthetist as appears to be the common misconception (MacRae 1996; Association of Anaesthetists 1989). The dictionary defines assistant as a 'helper' or 'subordinate worker' (Sykes 1982). This description demeans the role of the anaesthetic practitioner and does not respect them as a professional with specialist knowledge and skills (Oakley 1999).

The role can incorporate the following, although this may vary in different institutions:

- Preassessment of the patient, particularly in day surgery.
- Checking the anaesthetic machine, monitors and ancillary equipment, tailoring it to the patients on the list.
- Welcoming the patient into the operating department and making all the necessary safety checks.

- Assessing the patient for anxiety and altering the care given accordingly.
- Caring for the patient during induction, maintenance and reversal of anaesthesia, advocating for them where necessary.
- Maintaining all documentation.
- Communicating with the recovery/ITU/HDU where applicable and transferring the patient to the appropriate area safely.

AIRWAY MANAGEMENT IN ANAESTHESIA

The management of the patient's airway during anaesthesia is central to the whole anaesthetic. Whether maintaining an airway during anaesthesia or post-anaesthesia the aims are the same:

- Safeguard the patency of the airway
- Ensure adequate oxygenation and ventilation
- Prevention and protection from aspiration.

To enable the aims of airway maintenance to be fulfilled, the patient's airway must be assessed. As a result of this a plan for the management of the airway can be derived. This will be based on a number of factors: the results of the airway assessment; the type of surgery; previous anaesthesia; and past and present medical history. These factors will be combined, enabling an individualised plan of how to manage the patient's airway. In anaesthesia there are many methods of maintaining an airway and the anaesthetic practitioner must be familiar with them and the indications for their use.

Safeguard the patency of the airway

Assessment of the airway

It is essential to assess the patient's airway prior to anaesthesia, as a potential difficult intubation has to be excluded. Assessment will take the form of external examination of the neck, face and mandible. The patient will be asked to open their mouth as wide as they can and neck, flexion will be assessed. Internal examination of the teeth and oropharynx will be made. The results of this assessment will be amalgamated with recent chest and neck X-rays and past anaesthetic history. Tests can be used to indicate the degree of difficult intubation. The most commonly used one is the Mallampati test as shown in Figure 4.1. This is a predictive test based on the pharyngeal view as to the likely view on laryngoscopy. On laryngoscopy further grading can be carried out on a I–IV scale, grade I being the vocal cords visible through to grade IV where the epiglottis is not visible (Hobbs 2001). If a difficult intubation is predicted the anaesthetic practitioner must prepare for this.

Broadly there are three ways to maintain an airway during anaesthesia:

1. Bag and facemask
2. Laryngeal mask airway (LMA)
3. Endotracheal tube.

Bag and facemask

Currently the bag and facemask has limited use during anaesthetic maintenance. Before the advent of the laryngeal mask airway it was the main method of maintaining an airway during anaesthesia in a spontaneously breathing patient. Currently its main area of use is preceding intubation while waiting for the muscle relaxant to take effect.

Advantages
- Enables maintenance of a patent airway while ventilating the patient with the other hand (a skill rapidly being lost with the advent of the laryngeal mask airway).

Disadvantages
- It requires practice to maintain an airway with a facemask and ventilate the patient at the same time.
- Potential risk of aspiration (does not protect against regurgitation).
- When using a black facemask the anaesthetist is unable to see if the patient has vomited or breaths clouding the mask; for this reason clear facemasks are safer.
- Can cause damage to the face when excessive pressure is used keeping the airway patent with a facemask.

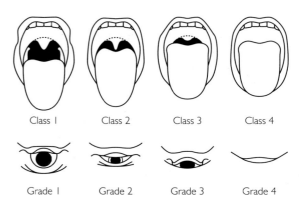

Figure 4.1 Mallampati classification for predicting difficult intubation

- Should only be used for short procedures.
- When used with a clausen harness there is a risk of the airway becoming obstructed.

Laryngeal mask airway

Dr Brain designed the laryngeal mask airway as an alternative to the bag and facemask system of ventilation. It came into clinical use in the late 1980s (Brimacombe 1993) and has revolutionised airway management during anaesthesia and postoperatively.

The design is simple. The shape was derived from taking plaster casts of the cadaveric larynx. Initially an adaptation of the Goldmann dental mask was used and from this evolved the shape that is now commonly used today. As the use of the laryngeal mask airway has increased, so have the types available. Initially sizes 3 and 4 were available for women and men respectively. Now paediatric sizes have been added plus armoured versions for use in surgery where there is a risk of damage to the tube or in positions where there is a risk of tube kinkage. More recently a disposable variety has become available together with the LMA PRO-SEAL™. The latter has a double tube for gastric secretions and allows for the passage of a nasogatric tube. It is thought that it prevents gastric insufflation (Simpson and Popat 2002; Soliz *et al.* 2002). Added to this the intubating laryngeal mask (ILMA) has evolved (Erickson *et al.* 2002). This has a high intubating success rate, particularly in patients who are potentially difficult to intubate in the conventional manner. However it is expensive and this precludes its routine use.

The cuff of the LMA is described as elliptical with a tube coming from the upper end. The tip of the mask rests on the upper oesophageal sphincter with the sides facing the pyriform fossae and upper border under the tongue (see Figure 4.2). Insertion of the LMA is simple and easy to learn with good retention of the skill (Stone *et al.* 1994) and more recently its use as a form of airway management during cardiopulmonary resuscitation has been reviewed (Hand 1999).

Advantages
- Non-invasive form of airway management.
- Can be put down immediately following induction of anaesthesia; propofol has been found to be the most suitable induction agent (Brown *et al.* 1991).
- One airway from induction to recovery.
- Negates the need for laryngoscopy – less trauma to mucosa of the mouth.
- Reduced incidence of sore throat (Millar *et al.* 1997).
- Tolerated at lighter planes of anaesthesia.
- Insertion and removal have minimal effects on the cardiovascular response.
- Can be used to ventilate patients.

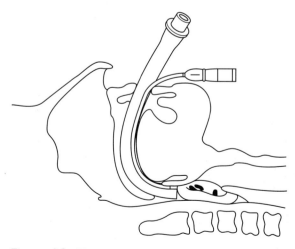

Figure 4.2 The laryngeal mask airway

Disadvantages
- This a diminution in the skills needed to maintain an airway with a facemask.
- Contraindicated in patients who are at risk of aspiration.
- Owens *et al.* (1995) suggested an increased incidence of reflux to the level of mid to upper oesophagus, although they had no incidence of aspiration.
- Higher risk of laryngospasm due to increased secretions.

Endotracheal tube

This remains the gold standard of airway management. The endotracheal tube is introduced into the larynx with the aid of a laryngoscope and gently pushed through the vocal cords; if pushed further there is danger of the tube being advanced into the right main bronchus resulting in only one lung being ventilated.

The endotracheal tube provides a patent and secure airway throughout anaesthesia. Numerous types are available, such as oral, nasal, south facing, double lumen and armoured, which can be utilised in a variety of surgical procedures.

Advantages
- Secure airway with minimal risk of aspiration
- A variety of tubes are available
- Fulfills all the aims of airway management
- Gives perfect control of the airway.

Disadvantages
- Invasive, can cause damage to the vocal cords
- Laryngoscopy stimulates the vagus nerve and can cause bradycardia; it can also damage the mucosa of the mouth and teeth
- Skill is required to intubate and retention of these skills is poor
- With the advent of the LMA there is less opportunity to develop and practice intubation.

Ensure adequate oxygenation and ventilation

The anaesthetic machine

The anaesthetic machine enables the delivery of anaesthetic gases and vapours. In its simplest form it would be devoid of monitoring equipment and ventilators. In the new electronic models usually all the monitoring is built in. It is the anaesthetic practitioner's responsibility to check the machine prior to use. The checklist usually followed is the one produced by the Association of Anaesthetists (1997). The newer machines are self-diagnostic. However the anaesthetic practitioner should demonstrate knowledge of these machines and how to check them prior to use. These machines have many more safety features than the generation prior to them.

Anaesthetic breathing circuits

Breathing circuits consist of tubes of varying degrees, which deliver fresh gas and vapours to the patient. Some of the expired gases are rebreathed and thus breathing circuits are classified as rebreathing systems (Shields and Werder 2002). Breathing circuits are normally described using the Mapleson classification ranging from A–F. Efficiency of these circuits are measured in terms of the amount of fresh gas required to prevent rebreathing during ventilation.

Principles of anaesthetic breathing circuits

- They should deliver adequate inspired oxygen concentration
- There should be efficient elimination of carbon dioxide
- Dead space must not be significantly increased
- There should be very little resistance to inspiration or expiration
- The breathing circuit should enable spontaneous and assisted ventilation
- It should protect the patient from barotrauma
- It should be safe, reliable, lightweight and inexpensive
- Scavenging of waste gases should be simple (Simpson and Popat 2002).

VENTILATION IN ANAESTHESIA

Ventilation is used in anaesthesia to maintain gas exchange when a muscle relaxant is used. In normal respiration the expansion of the rib cage and lowering of the diaphragm create a negative pressure in the thoracic cavity and air is sucked into the lungs. The negative pressure also draws blood into the heart from the inferior and superior venae cavae. Expiration occurs as a result of elastic recoil of the respiratory muscles and the alveoli. Compliance is the term used for the ability of the lungs to expand under pressure. Secreted by cells lining the alveoli is a substance called surfactant; this allows the surface of the alveoli to expand, reducing the surface tension and thus lessening the work of breathing and aiding lung compliance.

Artificial ventilation has the opposite effect to normal ventilation by causing a positive pressure within the thoracic cavity (intermittent positive pressure ventilation [IPPV]). This causes a rise in central venous pressure readings and lowers the cardiac output and blood pressure. Artificial ventilation also reduces the oxygen consumption required for normal respiratory effort and decreases lung compliance.

The most important terminology in ventilation is minute volume (MV), tidal volume (TV) and rate (R). Minute volume is the volume of gas delivered by the ventilator in one minute. Tidal volume is the volume of each breath and the rate is the number of ventilations per minute. Pulmonary ventilation is calculated by TV × R = MV.

Ventilators used in anaesthesia can broadly fit into two categories (see Figure 4.3).

Some ventilators may be used to compress bellows in a separate system which contains an anaesthetic gases-bag in a bottle ventilator. Compressed air is used as the driving gas and this forces the bellows down. The fresh gas flow in the bellows is delivered to the patient. The fresh gas flow and the driving gas are kept separate.

Prevention and protection from aspiration

In any airway situation where the patient is rendered unconscious there is the risk of vomiting or regurgitation. Vomiting is an active process, which will usually happen as the swallowing reflexes are abolished, or when they return. In the anaesthetic situation this is upon induction and emergence from anaesthesia. Regurgitation is a passive process and during anaesthesia is

PRESSURE GENERATORS
Compression of the bellows – inspiration

Weight of the bellows has to be altered if the lungs are difficult
to ventilate (low compliance)

Not an ideal ventilator for patients with 'stiff' lungs or high
airways resistance

If resistance is too high bellows will hardly compress and the tidal
volume will be inadequate

FLOW GENERATORS
Powerful enough to overcome low compliance or high
airways resistance

↓

Divided into two groups:
1. Those using high gas pressure
2. Those using a powerful motor

Figure 4.3   Ventilators used in anaesthesia

silent. It is thought to occur in up to 25% of patients undergoing anaesthesia (Davies and Warwick 2001). If unnoticed the patient can aspirate the stomach contents leading to aspiration pneumonitis. The incidence of aspiration is 1–6/10,000 with a mortality rate of 5% and in the obstetric population this is doubled (Davies and Warwick 2001).

In the non-emergency population aspiration is avoided by assessment of the patient to identify at risk groups, and fasting the patient. Fasting is a controversial issue. It was established in the early 1990s that having clear fluids up to 2–3 hours prior to surgery does not alter the stomach pH or increase gastric volume significantly and solid food is acceptable 6 hours prior to surgery (Kallar and Everett 1993). However anecdotally patients are still fasting from midnight and from six in the morning when on an afternoon list.

If a patient has aspirated they will demonstrate symptoms of breathlessness and will cough. Stomach contents will be seen in the oropharynx

---

GUIDELINES FOR PREOPERATIVE FASTING

These guidelines are for any patient over the age of one-year undergoing either elective or emergency surgery.

ELECTIVE SURGERY:

- Patients should fast for *six hours* from food or milk drinks.
- Clear fluids may be taken up to *two hours* before the scheduled start time of the list.
- It is recommended that all elective patients should be encouraged to drink a glass of water *two hours* before the scheduled start of the list (i.e. 07.00 h for a morning list and 12.00 h for an afternoon list).
- The routine use of pharmacological agents* to reduce the risk of pulmonary aspiration is not indicated in all patients.

EMERGENCY SURGERY:

- All patients undergoing emergency surgery *should be fasted of solids and fluids for at least six hours preoperatively*, except in the event of life or limb threatening situations when the surgical imperative overrides the risk of aspiration – the anaesthetist will treat this patient as for a 'full stomach'.
- Intravenous fluids should be instituted to cover maintenance and expected fluid deficits.
- A nasogastric tube should be inserted for patients with suspected bowel obstruction.
- Patients with gastrointestinal disease, following trauma and/or the administration of opioids or other drugs, alcohol ingestion or pregnancy have longer gastric emptying times. The administration of pharmacological agents* to reduce the risk of gastric aspiration may be indicated after discussion with the anaesthetist.

PLEASE NOTE:

If you are in doubt about any particular patient then please contact the relevant anaesthetist or the on-call anaesthetic team for advice.

*These include drugs such as gastrointestinal stimulants (metoclopramide), gastric secretion blockers (ranitidine, omeprazole, lansoprazole), antacids (sodium citrate), antiemetics (ondansetron, prochlorperazine) or anticholinergics (atropine, scopolamine).

Reproduced with kind permission of Dr ADB Williamson FRCA, Consultant Anaesthetist, Good Hope Hospital NHS Trust.

on extubation, and there may also be increased airway pressure. Other signs include tachypnoea, and a wheeze and crackles may be heard on chest auscultation. The patient will become cyanosed, tachycardic, pulmonary oedema will develop and there will be radiographic changes.

Management of aspiration

If aspiration has occurred or is even suspected the patient should be placed on their side in the head down position. Stomach contents should be suctioned from the oropharynx and 100% oxygen administered. The patient should be intubated if inadequate oxygenation and ventilation or if tracheobronchial suction is required, or if the patient is unable to protect their own airway. If established aspiration, the treatment takes the form of oxygen therapy, ventilatory support, removal of the aspirate, bronchodilators, antibiotics, fluid balance and corticosteroid therapy (Davies and Warwick 2001).

In summary, management of the patient's airway during anaesthesia is of the utmost importance and the anaesthetic practitioner must be well-versed in the airway adjuncts available and the principles of airway management.

HAEMODYNAMIC ASSESSMENT

The safety of the patient during intubation and anaesthesia is of paramount concern to all practitioners and there are a burgeoning number of assessment tools available to assist the practitioner in assessing and maintaining the patient's haemodynamic status during the anaesthetic period.

A comprehensive haemodynamic assessment may be achieved by using both invasive and non-invasive methods, and it is essential that anaesthetic practitioners are confident with the equipment available, and that they are able to evaluate and act upon the data yielded from these assessments to the benefits of their patients.

It is valid to note some important points with regard to monitoring devices. Both invasive and non-invasive monitoring is a useful adjunct to care, but it is imperative that all practitioners remember that there is a patient at the end of this equipment. Increasingly complex monitoring equipment, while clinically invaluable, may be very frightening for patients (and their carers if present) and reassurance, explanation and support is always needed.

Secondly the range of values derived from various techniques may be very wide and it is essential to consider the results in the context of the patient's clinical status. For example a patient with chronic obstructive pulmonary disease (COPD) may have a consistently low SpO_2 (88%), or a patient with chronic cardiac disease may have a consistently raised central venous pressure (CVP) of >12 mmHg, but these values may be 'normal' for these individuals.

Thirdly, there is the need to take measurements at regular intervals in order to be able to observe trend patterns. A single value in isolation may be of little value, whereas a trend in an abnormal direction will be far more helpful.

Lastly, the importance of regularly serviced and calibrated equipment is imperative to ensure that measurements taken are accurate and equipment is safe to use. The use of the mercury sphygmomanometer is slowly being phased out due to the known hazards of this substance. The anaesthetic practitioner has a duty to ensure that they possess adequate technical skills and understanding of data retrieved in order to obtain the best possible outcome for their patients. The ability to act as the patient's advocate is fundamental in the anaesthetic room, especially once the patient is rendered mute by the anaesthetic agents and the insertion of an artificial airway.

TYPES OF MONITORING

The nature of monitoring is frequently referred to as invasive, or non-invasive and the use of each will vary according to the clinical situation, although generally the more serious the patient's clinical situation, the more complex and intensive the monitoring assessment needed. Non-invasive monitoring involves no breach in the body surface, whereas invasive monitoring involves the use of probes or catheters inserted into the body in order to derive measurements.

- Assessment of heart rate and rhythm
- Assessment of blood pressure
- Assessment of skin perfusion
- Assessment of oxygen saturation (SpO$_2$)

Figure 4.4 Non-invasive assessments

- Central venous pressure (CVP) monitoring
- Arterial blood pressure monitoring

Figure 4.5 Invasive assessments

The range of non-invasive and invasive methods to be considered in this chapter are listed in Figures 4.4 and 4.5.

In this chapter an overview of the method of employing the techniques and a discussion of limitations and uses of the methods will be given. The evaluation of data derived and the application of the methods to clinical scenarios will be considered elsewhere (Chapter 6).

Assessment of heart rate and rhythm

The arterial pulse

Arterial pulses should be assessed for:

- Rate
- Rhythm
- Volume.

Although the radial pulse is frequently used, palpation of an artery closer to the heart is usually better for appreciating the character or volume of the pulse waveform. In clinical practice, radial, brachial, carotid and femoral pulses are frequently palpated to gain the following information.

Rate

The pulse should be counted for 30 seconds, unless it is irregular, when it should be assessed for at least 1 minute. In a healthy adult the normal heart rate ranges from 60–100 beats per minute. A heart rate less than 60 per minute is termed a bradycardia and is often seen in individuals taking beta-adrenergic blockers (such as atenolol); a heart rate greater than 100 beats per minute is called a tachycardia and is often associated with anxiety, pain or hypovolaemia.

Rhythm

The normal pulse is regular, or very slightly irregular. If the pulse is irregular there are many benign and malignant reasons for this, which are explained in Chapter 6. An occasional irregularity may be caused by ectopic beats, whereas an irregularly irregular pulse may indicate atrial fibrillation. Many individuals have a slightly irregular pulse, whereby the rate quickens on inspiration and slows on expiration – this is called sinus arrhythmia and is considered a normal variant (Spiers 2002). An assessment of the apical and peripheral pulse rate may be helpful in situations where atrial fibrillation is suspected.

Volume

The volume of the pulse is dependent upon the difference between the systolic and diastolic blood pressure – the pulse pressure. A low volume pulse is often seen in patients with chronic heart disease and suggests myocardial insufficiency; a high volume pulse is often seen in patients with anaemia. *Pulsus paradoxus* is a diminished volume of the pulse during inspiration and occurs in conditions which limit venous return to the heart such as constrictive pericarditis, right ventricular infarction and pericardial tamponade.

ECG monitoring

The best non-invasive method for evaluating the heart rate and rhythm is the ECG. Electrocardiography has been described as the most valuable diagnostic tool in modern medicine as it gives a continuous picture of the heart's electrical activity in real time (Jevon and Ewens 2002). Cardiac monitoring is a minimum requirement during the anaesthetic phase of patient care (Association of Anaesthetists 2000) and therefore rhythm interpretation is a core skill for perioperative practitioners to acquire (Simpson and Popat 2002).

Technological advances have led to sophisticated monitoring systems which incorporate a variety of alarms, computerised rhythm analysis and assessment of haemodynamic parameters. Many coronary care units utilise continuous 12-lead recording, although for the perioperative settings the use of a three-electrode placement will suffice. All personnel in operating theatres should be familiar with monitor operation and electrode placement as well as being able to recognise commonly presenting arrhythmias (Spiers and Stinchcombe 2002).

The ECG is a graphic representation of the electrical activity generated by the heart during the cardiac cycle (Moriarty 1999). Electrical events arise from the activity of the conduction system of the heart and in the majority of cases, the electrical events precede mechanical contraction of the heart.

Cardiac conduction system

The heart can essentially be considered as a four-chambered double-sided muscle pump which generates effective cardiac output to the body. In a healthy heart, the cardiac chambers contract in synchrony, atria followed by ventricles, to optimise the cardiac output. The cardiac contraction is stimulated by the rapid transmission of an elec-trical signal which spreads across the heart in an orderly manner in order to enable this synchrony (Spiers and Stinchcombe 2002). The electrical impulse starts in the sinoatrial node, which is the primary pacemaker of the heart, and then spreads via the atrioventricular node into the intraventricular conduction system, which comprises of the bundle branches and Purkinje fibres (Figure 4.6).

ECG waveforms

There is a direct relationship between the electrical events which occur in the conduction system and the ECG waveforms which are displayed on the cardiac monitor or ECG recording paper. These ECG waveforms are labelled alphabetically and begin at the P wave. This labelling system began over nine decades ago and is attributed to a Dutch physiologist Willem Einthoven who arbitrarily designated the waveforms as P, QRS and T waves.

The P wave represents the initiation of the electrical signal by the sinoatrial node and the spread of the excitation wave across the atria resulting in atrial depolarisation. The QRS complex represents transmission of the excitation

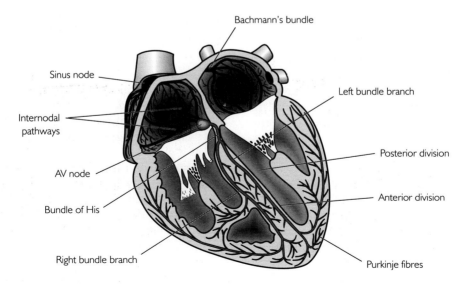

Figure 4.6 Cardiac conduction system

wave into the intraventricular conduction pathways and the resultant ventricular depolarisation. The ST segment, T wave (and U wave if present) represent ventricular repolarisation. The relationship of these waveforms to the electrical events and to the cardiac cycle is represented in Figure 4.7.

Monitoring leads

Monitoring electrodes placed on the body's surface detect this electrical activity and this is transmitted via the monitoring leads to the cardiac monitor where the waveforms are amplified and displayed. The placement of the electrodes on the body surface is arranged in such a way as to create an effective 'view' of the electrical activity in the conduction system. In a standard three-lead system, the red lead is placed on the right arm, the yellow lead is located on the left

arm and the black or green lead is placed on the left leg. Increasingly, these electrode placements are being placed on the body torso rather than on the limbs and a variety of other placements may be encountered. For example, electrode placement on the posterior aspect of the shoulder is also acceptable and is clearly useful when the anterior placement would interfere with the surgical field (Jacobson 1998). A useful mnemonic for remembering the lead placement is **Ride Your Bike – R** (RA), **Y** (LA), **B** (LL). Wherever the electrodes are placed, some simple rules apply:

- The electrodes should be placed equidistant from and in a triangle around the heart (Huszar 2002). If the electrodes are placed on the torso, the red (RA) and yellow (LA) electrodes should be positioned on the shoulders and the black (LL) placed just above the right

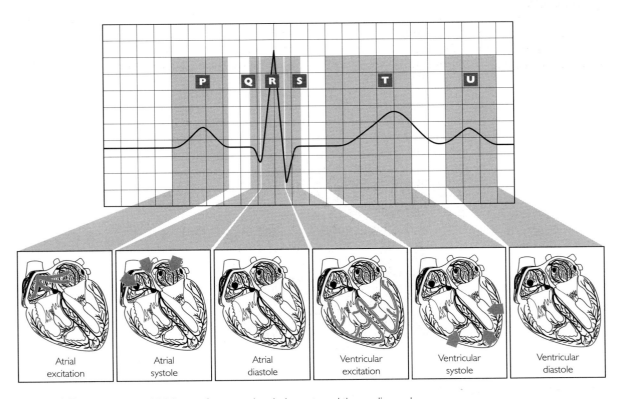

Figure 4.7 Relationship of ECG waveforms to electrical events and the cardiac cycle

hip. However, if the wrists are used for the red and yellow electrodes, then the left ankle is the appropriate placement for the LL lead.

- The electrodes should be equidistant from each other, but should not be placed too close together. If electrodes are placed too far away from the heart, the resulting ECG trace may be too small.
- The electrodes should be placed over soft tissue areas as this will facilitate the detection of the electrical impulses. McConnell (2001) suggests avoiding areas of dense fat or bony prominences, and avoidance of the recommended position for defibrillation pads is strongly advised.

Creating effective contact between the electrode and the skin surface is imperative in order to gain high quality monitor traces. Electrodes are impregnated with gel, which facilitates conduction across the skin; however, this contact can be impeded if the skin is not clean, is particularly sweaty or is very hairy. Wash the skin with a simple soap and water solution and dry it thoroughly before electrode placement. If the skin is very hairy it may be necessary to trim the hairs, but do not shave as this may irritate or damage the skin.

Occasionally, despite effective skin preparation, a good trace is still not visible on the monitor screen and this is referred to as *artifact* or *'electrical noise'*. This may be due to additional internal or external electrical activity interfering with the recording of cardiac electrical activity. External activity may be caused by interference from alternating current (AC) equipment such as infusion pumps or mobile phones and internal activity is due to muscle tremor such as seen when a patient is shivering with cold or fright. Reducing the amount of interference may occasionally be achieved by moving essential equipment further away from the patient and by replacing electrodes and monitoring leads if possible. It is imperative that an interpretable trace is gained in order to maintain patient safety during anaesthesia (Spiers and Stinchcombe 2002).

When the electrodes are placed in the positions described above a discernible trace should

appear on the monitor which resembles the P, QRS and T waves previously described. This is Lead 11 and it is the most frequently used lead for monitoring the heart rhythm, as in this lead the P wave is easily seen, and the QRS and T wave are tallest in amplitude. When this trace is observed in a regular rhythm across the monitor screen at a rate between 60 and 100 beats per minute it is referred to as a *sinus* rhythm (originating from the sinoatrial or sinus node) (Figure 4.8). Further discussion of rhythm interpretation is included in Chapter 6.

Assessment of blood pressure

Arterial blood pressure is the force exerted by the volume of blood on the arterial walls. It is a dynamic and changing pressure, which gives valuable information about the haemodynamic status of a patient. Blood pressure is a function of cardiac output and systemic peripheral resistance and it can therefore be influenced by a number of different factors. Blood pressure varies considerably throughout the day and is affected by emotion, pain, time of day and circadian rhythm. It is important to note that anxiety alone can raise the blood pressure by 30 mmHg and this should be taken into account when the patient first arrives in the anaesthetic room.

Non-invasive measurement of blood pressure depends upon occlusion of an artery with a cuff and either detection of Korotkoff sounds (auscultatory method) or oscillometry. The oscillometric method (Dynamap) uses an automated machine and cuff to compress the artery and measures blood pressure by sensing arterial pulsations or oscillations (Clinton 2003). The auscultatory method employs a sphygmomanometer and cuff to occlude the artery and a stethoscope to detect

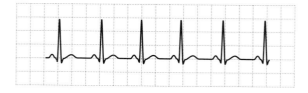

Figure 4.8 Rhythm strip – sinus rhythm

sounds of turbulent blood flow within the artery following release of the arterial compression (Jowett and Thompson 2003). The sounds are known as Korotkoff sounds after the Russian army surgeon who first identified them in 1905.

The first method (oscillometry) is more commonly employed in operating departments partly due to its ease of use and also due to the aforementioned problems associated with the mercury sphygmomanometer. Aneroid gauges and mercury devices must be regularly calibrated and checked by medical engineering departments to ensure accuracy. A number of sources of error exist with non-invasive blood pressure measurement and guidelines on accurate BP measurement have been published by the British Hypertension Society (British Hypertension Society and the Practitioners Hypertension Association 1997). Many of the problems associated with inaccurate recordings are related to inappropriate cuff sizes or incorrect positioning of the arm in relation to the patient's heart. Table 4.1 gives guidance on good practice to achieve accurate recordings and to avoid the commonly encountered pitfalls.

There are many advantages to using the auscultatory method of blood pressure measurement. The equipment needed is minimal, readily available and relatively simple to use. There is no risk to patients and it is a relatively painless procedure to perform. There are also many disadvantages to the method as have been highlighted in Table 4.1. Numerous studies over many decades have highlighted the potential

Table 4.1 Problems and recommended practices for measuring auscultatory blood pressure. Adapted from Jowett and Thompson 2003 and Darovic 2002.

Problem	Possible causes	Rationale and changes to practice
False high blood pressure	Cuff is too small	A small cuff does not disperse the pressure adequately across the arterial surface. *Use appropriate cuff size – see Table 4.2*
	Cuff is not centred over the artery	Higher external pressure is needed to compress the artery. *Reposition cuff with the bladder overlying antecubital fossa*
	Arm is located below heart level	Hydrostatic pressure influences the arterial pressure. *Reposition the arm to heart level.*
	Very obese arm	A cuff which is too small for a large arm will result in too little compression of the artery at the suitable pressure level. *Use appropriate cuff size – see Table 4.2*
	Unsupported arm	The isometric muscle contraction needed to hold the arm up against gravity will raise the blood pressure. *Support the arm horizontally with pillows.*
False low reading	Cuff too large	The pressure is spread over too large a surface area and it produces a damping effect on the Korotkoff sounds. *Use appropriate cuff size – see Table 4.2*
	Arm located above heart level	Hydrostatic pressure influences the arterial pressure. *Reposition arm to heart level*
	Difficulty with determining the onset of the first Korotkoff sound and distinguishing last sound	If mercury column is allowed to fall too quickly, sounds will be missed. *Allow column of mercury to drop at 2 mm/s and measure systolic and diastolic pressure to nearest 2 mmHg*
Falsely variable readings	Difficulty with hearing Korotkoff sounds	Shocked patients and patients with bradycardia. *Use stethoscope with total length not exceeding 16 inches and examiners should have normal hearing acuity with background noise kept to a minimum*
	Differences in recordings between arms	There is always slight variation in pressure between arms due to haemodynamic variability. A 15 mm Hg systolic pressure difference may indicate subclavian artery stenosis or aortic dissection. *Initial blood pressure should be recorded in both arms. For continuous comparative readings use one arm only and record which arm is being used on observation charts.*

pitfalls and limitations of the method and the issue of using the correct cuff size is frequently cited as an important source of error (Maskrey 1999; O'Brien *et al.* 1995; Croft and Cruikshank 1990). The bladder size needs to be at least 80% of the arm's circumference. A variety of cuff sizes are now available for width and length. Table 4.2 summarises the recommendations for cuff sizes in a variety of child and adult sizes.

Automated blood pressure monitoring (oscillometric method)

Automated blood pressure monitoring has become increasingly popular in perioperative areas as it is able to provide regular measurements of systolic, diastolic and mean arterial pressures without the use of a stethoscope, without manual inflation and deflation of the sphygmomanometer cuff and without patient contact. This therefore frees up the health-care practitioner from frequent, routine blood pressure measurements, while the alarm systems enable the practitioners to be alerted to haemodynamic changes. The oscillometric (Dynamap) method detects blood pressure by sensing the arterial pulsations caused by cyclic pressure changes due to pulsatile blood flow (Darovic 2002).

This method of blood pressure is relatively reliable in haemodynamically stable individuals and will be accurate to ±10 mmHg in such healthy individuals. However, reliability and accuracy has been questioned in critically ill patients who are haemodynamically unstable, particularly if they are hypotensive and shocked (Darovic 2002; O'Brien *et al.* 1995). Ironically, it is these patients who are frequently monitored using automated monitoring.

Table 4.2 Recommended cuff sizes for non-invasive blood pressure monitoring. Adapted from Jowett and Thompson 2003 and Hatchett 2002

	Cuff width (cm)	Cuff length (cm)	Arm circumference (cm)
Child	8.0–10.0	20–23	Up to 25
Adult	12.0–13.0	23	Up to 33
Large adult	13.0–15.0	35	Up to 38
Obese adult	15.0–18.0	35	Up to 42

Overall automated blood pressure devices have a role in monitoring trends in blood pressure and in tracking patients who require regular measurements during operative and diagnostic procedures, but their use in critically ill patients is debatable. Conscious patients may express distress at the cyclic tourniquet and arm cuffs may abrade the skin if wrinkles and ridges are present in the cuff. This may result in pressure injuries and occasionally bruising to sensitive or elderly skin.

Assessment of skin perfusion

Assessment of skin perfusion, colour and temperature augment the other haemodynamic measurements. Vasoconstriction and loss of circulatory volume may result in decreased skin perfusion which is characterised by pallor, cool peripheries, mottled skin, and a delayed capillary refill (>2 seconds) as blood is shunted away from the skin and skeletal muscle to the central organs (Clinton 2003). In operating theatres, changes in external temperatures and exposure of large surface areas to temperature change may result in a compensatory vasoconstriction and this does not necessarily herald circulatory shock. Assessment of these factors needs to be considered in the context of all the other haemodynamic values measured.

Assessment of oxygen saturation (SpO$_2$)

Pulse oximetry is probably the most significant advance in patient monitoring since the advent of electrocardiography. It is a simple non-invasive device, which monitors the percentage of haemoglobin, which is saturated with oxygen (SaO$_2$%).

How oximetry works

Oximetry works on the simple principle that oxygenated and deoxygenated blood differ in colour; arterial blood appears red and venous blood appears blue. Oximetry detects the amount of saturated versus desaturated haemoglobin in arterial blood by measuring the amount of light absorbed at two different wavelengths. The system works by alternately emitting two light sources, which emit intense red and infrared light. Saturated haemoglobin (oxyhaemoglobin) absorbs more infrared light, whereas desaturated haemoglobin absorbs more red light. The light sources shine through the pulsatile capillary beds to a light-sensitive photodiode positioned on the opposite side of the capillary bed and the resulting signal registers the percentage of arterial haemoglobin that is saturated with oxygen from the blood pulsating in the capillaries (hence 'pulse' oximetry) (Jowett and Thompson 2003).

The pulse oximeter consists of a probe attached to the patient's finger, ear lobe or occasionally bridge of the nose and connects to either a portable unit or to the cardiac monitor. The advantage of pulse oximetry is that it is easy to apply, entirely non-invasive and well-tolerated by patients. The monitor unit will display the oxygen saturation as a percentage value, the pulse rate and a plethysmographic waveform of the pulse.

Oxygen saturation

Oxygen saturation tells us how much of the arterial oxygen is combined with haemoglobin; this is referred to as oxygen saturation and is expressed as a percentage. Hence:

$$\text{Oxygen saturation } (\text{SaO}_2\%) = \frac{\text{Amount of oxygen carried by the haemoglobin}}{\text{Amount of oxygen that can be carried by haemoglobin}}$$

When oxygen combines with haemoglobin it is called oxyhaemoglobin and this amount is closely related to the PaO_2 of the blood. The oxyhaemoglobin dissociation curve is 'S'-shaped rather than linear, hence the relationship between arterial oxygen and oxygen saturation is not linear (Figure 4.9). Essentially one can see that when the PaO_2 remains between 10 and 13 kPa on the flat part of the curve oxygen saturation remain high (>95%). However a comparatively small fall in oxygen saturation to 90% actually equates to a fall in PaO_2 to 8 kPa, due to the rapid decline in the curve at the end of the plateau. Other factors that may cause the curve to shift either to the right or the left are temperature, increased $PaCO_2$ and raised pH and therefore it

can be seen that oxygen saturation values are not always reflective of arterial oxygen levels, particularly at lower values. Similarly the device does not give information on the PaO_2 or $PaCO_2$ levels within the blood or the acid–base balance system. The normal value for oxygen saturation is greater than 95% in healthy adults, although patients with chronic obstructive pulmonary disease (COPD) may have a normal level of less than 90% (Fox 2002). It is important to remember that the oximeter does not give an indication of the oxygen content of the blood nor of the haemoglobin level. Therefore if a patient is anaemic, the oxygen saturation may record as 100%, but the oxygen content of the blood may be low (Clinton 2003).

Problems with pulse oximetry

Pulse oximetry offers an accuracy of ±2% in the range of 70–100% saturation (Hill and Summers 1994). It is a useful means of ensuring that the patient's oxygen saturation is satisfactory, obviating the need for arterial blood gas analysis, but a number of factors may reduce the accuracy in SpO_2 monitoring, and clinicians should be aware of these factors.

- **Poor tissue perfusion.** The probe can only function if enough pulsatile blood passes between the light source and detector. Situations which result in poor perfusion or vasoconstriction will therefore result in inaccurate or even no recorded readings. Many arrhythmias, particularly the tachyarrhythmias

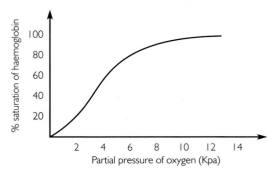

Figure 4.9 The oxygen dissociation curve

may cause inadequate and irregular perfusion (Woodrow 1999); the peripheral vasoconstriction seen in hypotension, hypovolaemia, cardiac failure and peripheral vascular disease may also cause unreliable measurements (Moyes 1998).

- **Motion artefact.** Shivering, seizures and persistent limb tremor (Parkinson's disease) may all result in an inadequate signal. Most movement artefact occurs from the probe slipping across the patient's skin. Ensuring that the probe is adequately secured and that the cable is sufficiently long to permit the patient some movement will diminish this problem (Jowett and Thompson 2003).

- **Excessive ambient light.** Excessive ambient light from sunlight, surgical lamps or flickering fluorescent lights may saturate the detector and cause erroneous readings. In one particularly disturbing incident Poets *et al.* (1993) reported how an oximeter probe became detached from a premature baby, but still recorded an oxygen saturation of 98–99%. It became evident that the readings disappeared when the room lights were switched off!

- **Abnormal haemoglobins.** Conditions which alter haemoglobins, such as carboxyhaemoglobin (carbon monoxide poisoning) and drugs which cause methaemoglobinaemia (lignocaine and nitrates) may produce unreliable saturation readings (Moyes 1998; Woodrow 1999; Clinton 2003).

- **Nail varnish.** Nail varnish, particularly those with blue, green or black tones, will absorb light at the same wavelength as haemoglobin and oxyhaemoglobin and will cause erroneously low readings (Moyes 1998). Iodine skin preparations are also likely to cause error (Hatfield and Tronson 2001).

- **Skin damage.** Probes may cause tissue damage if left in place for too long. It is recommended that probes are removed regularly and skin inspected for burns or pressure ulcers. The Medical Devices Agency recommends that the probe site be changed every four hours and the skin underneath carefully inspected (Medical Devices Agency 2001).

Finally, it is vital to remember that pulse oximeter readings on their own are of limited value and oximetry should be used in conjunction with other physiological parameters and patient assessments.

Invasive haemodynamic monitoring techniques

There are many invasive methods of monitoring which are employed with critically ill patients, but the value of each must be measured against the attendant complications and risks associated with each. Complications for patients occur during insertion, during continuous monitoring and as a result of long-term insertion. While it is the medical practitioners who decide upon the utility of using these techniques and are responsible for their insertion, it is frequently the anaesthetic practitioner who is responsible for maintaining the equipment, ensuring the patient's safety and comfort and finally obtaining and collating the data. In many cases the devices provide essential patient information and the patient's treatment will rely heavily upon the data acquired. It is essential therefore that practitioners are aware of common technical and physiological variables which might influence the data and are able to work comfortably with the equipment and, where necessary, able to troubleshoot commonly encountered problems.

Pressure transducers

Most invasive monitoring systems incorporate a pressure transducer system. Pressure transducers are electromechanical devices that detect pressure changes and convert (transduce) them to electrical signals which can be displayed onto a monitor. In haemodynamic monitoring they detect changes in intravascular pressure and transduce them into digital read-outs and electrical waveforms.

A cannula is inserted into the patient and pressure changes are transmitted via a fluid-filled pressure tube to a supple diaphragm located in a transducer dome. The fluid passes through the transducer dome and pressure waves are transmitted to the diaphragm, which is connected via an electrical cable to the monitor. The fluid-filled tubing is maintained under continuous pressure of 300 mmHg (greater than arterial pressure) using a 0.9% solution of saline. This maintains a continuous flush of approximately 3 ml of fluid per hour, which prevents backflow and ensures patency of the line. Previously, heparinised solutions were used, but saline is cheaper and effective and is not linked with any of the attendant risks associated with heparinised solutions (Thacker and Williams 1997). The transducer system is calibrated to atmospheric pressure (zeroed) and the zero stopcock should be positioned at the fourth intercostal space in order to measure accurately (Clinton 2003).

Manometry and central venous pressure

While invasive monitoring generally employs transducers to measure the intravascular pressure, manometry is still frequently used in many clinical situations and in particular for monitoring central venous pressure (CVP). The CVP is a manometer line inserted percutaneously under aseptic technique into a central neck vein, usually the subclavian or jugular vein. The line is advanced to lie in the superior vena cava where it can be used to measure the pressure in the right atrium.

The principle of manometry in this situation is to balance a column of water in the manometer tubing with the pressure in the right atrium using a continuous column of water. The manometer should be positioned with the baseline at the level of the patient's right atrium. The baseline may be at zero on the scale although it is often preferable to set it at a higher level (e.g. 10 cm) in order to facilitate measuring negative pressures (Jowett and Thompson 2003). The device is attached to a fluid-filled bag, which is used to keep the line patent, and also for hydration purposes. This fluid should *never* have drugs added to it as checking the CVP may result in large boluses of the fluid being delivered to the patient (Hatchett 2002). The equipment is calibrated in line with the right atrium and this is usually achieved with a spirit level using the mid-axillary line as the reference point. It is often helpful to mark the spot with a pen to ensure that the same mid-axilla point is used for each measurement.

For CVP measurement the three-way tap is turned in order to allow the fluid to fill the vertical manometer line. The three-way tap is then turned so that the fluid column drips slowly into the central vein. When the fluid reaches resistance (from the central venous pressure), the infusion will stop and the top of the vertical column of fluid is then read against the cm measure. This is regarded as the CVP. Once the fluid column has settled, slight oscillations will be seen which relate to venous pulsations and respiration – it is usual to measure the CVP at the end of respiration and in a manometer system it will be expressed in cm/H_2O. Following CVP recording, the three-way tap should be returned to the normal point and the flow rate of the infusion readjusted accordingly.

Central venous pressure

The CVP is often used to measure the pressure in the right atrium; more accurately it is a direct measure of *right ventricular end diastolic pressure*. Blood volume, cardiac function and vascular tone will influence this. The CVP is also an indirect measure of left ventricular end-diastolic pressure in healthy individuals, but this correlation is not predictive in a patient who has right heart dysfunction. Conditions such as right heart valve defects (tricuspid or pulmonary valve disease), right ventricular myocardial disease (cardiomyopathy or right ventricular infarction) or right heart failure due to pulmonary conditions (pulmonary embolism, COPD or pulmonary hypertension) will result in poor correlation. Hence reliance upon CVP as an indication of left heart function is not advised (Darovic 2002).

As the CVP is a direct measurement of the venous pressure it is one of the main parameters to alter when there are changes to the fluid status and it is an invaluable aid in surgical patients. When there is fluid loss, a compensatory tachycardia will often result to maintain the cardiac output. The blood pressure may be maintained for some time, however, as a result of compensatory peripheral vasoconstriction and the CVP can be very useful in identifying covert bleeding following surgery. Normally, about 3 litres of blood volume is stored in the venous system, 1 litre in the arteries and 1 litre in the heart and lungs. When haemorrhage occurs, most of this blood comes from the veins and the first sign of low blood volume is a gently falling CVP. After about 500 ml of blood loss, a tachycardia appears; after 800 ml of blood loss, the CVP starts to fall rapidly and this is followed later by a fall in the arterial blood pressure (Hatfield and Tronson 2001).

Indications for insertion of a CVP are given in Figure 4.10, although the CVP is most valuable in the operating theatre for estimating the patient's fluid status and for the administration of fluids if required.

The normal range of the CVP is wide and varies according to the patient's pre-existing haemodynamic status. If a manometer system is used a normal range is 3–11 cmH$_2$O and this corresponds to 0–8 mmHg if the pressure is transduced onto a monitor. As the normal range is wide, it is essential that one-off readings are not used to make haemodynamic judgements – regular observations of trends are important to reflect the true status of the circulating volume. As with any other assessment technique a number of factors can limit the value of CVP recordings and prevent them from being an accurate index of the patient's haemodynamic status (Darovic 2002). The CVP is influenced by cardiac performance, venous tone and blood volume. Alterations in any of these factors will affect CVP measurements and may produce deceptively high or low recordings:

- Administration of fluids and electrolytes
- Administration of irritant drugs (amiodarone)
- Administration of blood and blood products
- Monitoring CVP
- Venous access for insertion of temporary pacemaker
- Administration of parenteral nutrition
- Inaccessible peripheral access – burns, patients in shock, thrombosed or inflamed peripheral veins
- Multiple infusions

Figure 4.10 Indication for central venous cannulation
(Adapted from Clinton 2003 and Darovic 2002)

Limitations to CVP monitoring

- **Systemic venoconstriction.** Venoconstriction occurs as a compensatory mechanism. In blood loss, for example, venous constriction will occur to maintain central circulation and this will initially elevate the CVP. Clearly this raised CVP is not a true indication of the circulating volume. Venoconstriction by the same mechanism will also occur in hypothermic patients.
- **Right ventricular dysfunction.** Many conditions affect the distensibility of the right ventricle (RV) and result in a stiff, non-compliant RV. Inability of the RV to expand to receive the venous return results in a CVP value which is deceptively high despite changes to the intravascular volume. Many chronic and acute conditions can result in RV dysfunction such as chronic heart failure, COPD, acute RV myocardial infarction and hypertrophy.
- **Respiratory effects.** Intrathoracic pressure varies during the respiratory cycle and hence normal breathing causes the CVP to rise and fall in the manometer tubing – the '*respiratory swing*'. This respiratory effect may be more accentuated if a patient is dehydrated. Similarly if the patient is receiving positive-pressure ventilation the CVP will be artificially elevated because of the cyclic positive-pressure ventilator breaths. Conversely, the externally applied pressure impedes venous return and reduces cardiac output. These effects are further compounded by the application of positive end-expiratory pressure (PEEP) to the ventilator circuitry.

The CVP is therefore a useful measure of the patient's fluid status and in particular it is invaluable in identifying covert haemorrhage earlier than other measured parameters. Limitations to its use are laid out above and these limitations, alongside the risks inherent in cannulation of a major vessel (air embolus, infection and inadvertent vascular or pleural puncture) must be borne in mind when managing the patient.

Arterial blood pressure monitoring

Arterial blood pressure (BP) monitoring is occasionally employed when there is a need for continuous monitoring of the blood pressure. Arterial lines designed for this technique are usually inserted into the radial artery, although brachial, dorsalis pedis or femoral arteries may also be used. The arterial line is attached to a fluid-filled manometer line, a pressurised bag of saline and a transducer. The equipment must be zeroed to atmospheric pressure and the baseline aligned to the level of the right atrium as previously described (*pressure transducers*). Invasive arterial monitoring when calibrated in this manner is generally more accurate than readings derived from auscultation, although it is important to compare a non-invasive blood pressure with an arterial recording at the initiation of treatment.

The characteristic arterial trace should be observed on the monitor and in addition a digital pressure will be recorded. The arterial waveform should demonstrate systole, diastole and a slight notch on the downward stroke – the dicrotic notch. The dicrotic notch corresponds with aortic valve closure during diastole as indicated in Figure 4.11.

It is important that the above trace is maintained, and practitioners should be familiar with the appearance of a dampened trace which may be caused by an air bubble trapped in the transducer system, blood clotting around the catheter tip or displacement of the catheter tip into the vessel wall (Figure 4.12). Indications for arterial BP monitoring are given in Figure 4.13.

In addition practitioners should remain constantly vigilant to the potential hazards associated with cannulation of a major artery. The line must be labelled clearly using red tape, close to the line's entry port. This is to ensure primarily that no drugs are administered into the line. It also alerts all practitioners that the artery is cannulated and to be cognisant of the risk of arterial exsanguination, ischaemia or infection.

Mean arterial pressure

The mean arterial pressure (MAP) is an additional value, which can be recorded with arterial monitoring. MAP indicates the average pressure in the arterial system throughout the cardiac cycle. However, the arithmetic mean (mid-point between the systolic and diastolic pressure) is not an accurate measure of the mean blood pressure and a formula is used to estimate the MAP (Figure 4.14). On the monitor the MAP will appear as a whole number in brackets below the

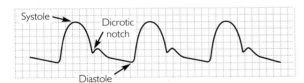

Figure 4.11 Normal arterial pressure trace

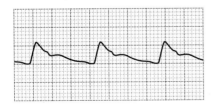

Figure 4.12 Dampened arterial pressure trace

- When there is a need for continual direct blood pressure measurement when the BP is either unusually low or high (hypovolaemia, phaeochromocytoma)
- When there is a need for regular arterial blood gas sampling (hypoxia, hypercarbia)
- To provide ongoing evaluation of treatments (inotropic drug therapy, vasoactive drug therapy or fluid resuscitation)
- In rapidly changing clinical circumstances (major surgery, major trauma, critical illness such as cardiogenic shock)

Figure 4.13 Indications for arterial monitoring

$$MAP = diastolic + \frac{(systolic - diastolic)}{3}$$

Example: Blood pressure = 110/50 mmHg

$$MAP = 50 + \frac{(110 - 50)}{3}$$

$$= 50 + \frac{60}{3}$$

$$= 50 + 20$$

$$MAP = 70 \text{ mmHg}$$

Figure 4.14 Mean arterial blood pressure calculation

systolic and diastolic pressure recordings. This digitally displayed value is derived from data averaged over several cardiac cycles (Darovic 2002; Hatchett 2002).

The normal MAP is usually in the range 60–80 mmHg. Increasingly MAP is viewed as a more accurate representation of the arterial pressure throughout the whole vascular system and therefore it is often used in preference to derived systolic and diastolic values.

Haemodynamic monitoring in the operating theatre is invaluable for recognising and assessing serious changes in the cardiovascular status of patients. In addition, haemodynamic monitoring provides a valuable means of evaluating the effects of prescribed therapies and directing further treatments. It is imperative that practitioners feel comfortable with the equipment used, that they are able to obtain and respond appropriately to the derived data and that they remain vigilant of the potential hazards and limitations inherent in each technique employed.

PHARMACOLOGY RELATED TO ANAESTHESIA

Experience has shown that practitioners' knowledge of pharmacology is poor. The reasons for this are multifactorial, but one may be that it is viewed as the domain of doctors. The argument against this is how can effective care be given to the patient if the practitioner does not have a working knowledge of the drugs they are to administer or be involved in administering? This knowledge will inform the practitioner of the effect on the patient. It will enable answers to be given to the patient's questions in a way that they will understand without having to defer to the medical practitioner. Pharmacology when approached in a logical manner is understandable and extremely fascinating.

When examining any pharmacological agent the same questions must be asked. For example how does the body react to the drug being given (pharmacokenetics)? What happens to the body when a drug is administered (pharmocodynamics)? In anaesthesia the drugs must be approached from a logical position. What does the anaes-

thetist want to do to the patient? What sequence do they want to do it in?

The first thing the anaesthetist will do is induce anaesthesia, in simple terms send the patient to sleep. This is usually done with intravenous induction agents, because these cause a rapid smooth induction. Inhalational agents can achieve induction but are less rapid. Intravenous anaesthesia is achieved by a bolus dose of the induction agent or by continuous intravenous infusion. The anaesthetist, based on clinical assessment of the patient, makes the choice of technique and agent.

Secondly the anaesthetist will wish to keep the patient asleep for the duration of surgery. This can be achieved by continuous infusion of the induction agent. However the use of volatile and gaseous agents remain popular for maintaining anaesthesia. Usually a mixture of 66% nitrous oxide in oxygen and low concentrations of a volatile agent are employed (Mushambi and Smith 2001).

Throughout the induction and maintenance of anaesthesia the patient will still be able to experience pain, noted by physiological signs such as increased pulse rate, blood pressure and sweating, so as part of the anaesthetic technique supplementary analgesia must be given. These analgesics will be given for intraoperative pain control, but the anaesthetist will also consider the overall surgical experience of the patient and as part of the anaesthetic technique will look at postoperative analgesia and may incorporate this in the intraoperative period.

Another decision the anaesthetist has to make is whether the patient should breathe spontaneously during surgery or be ventilated. This again is based on a number of factors such as clinical assessment of the patient and the type of surgery they are undergoing. Whether the patient is going to breathe spontaneously or be ventilated, the stages mentioned above will still be applicable. However to facilitate ventilation a neuromuscular blocking agent must be used. This will enable the anaesthetist to ventilate the patient in the absence of respiration (Table 4.3).

The anaesthetic practitioner in the UK does not administer any of the anaesthetic agents but will be

Table 4.3 Anaesthetic pharmacology in the spontaneous and ventilated patient

Patient breathing spontaneously	Patient ventilated
Induction	Induction
Maintenance	Maintenance
Analgesia including spinal and epidural	Analgesia including spinal and epidural
	Muscle relaxation

involved in the preparation of them. In order to be an effective advocate for the patient the anaesthetic practitioner must be knowledgeable about the agents available, indications for use and the pharmacodynamics and pharmacokenetics of them. This knowledge will aid in the appropriate preparation and administration. It will also enable the anaesthetic practitioner to answer any questions the patient may have regarding the possible side effects they may experience postoperatively and what measures will be taken to prevent them. At this point the anaesthetist and the anaesthetic practitioner should be working in collaboration to give the best possible care to the patient. The anaesthetic practitioner may be in the anaesthetic room with the patient, while the anaesthetist may be taking the previous patient to the post-anaesthetic care unit, and so at this point the anesthetic practitioner will be able to answer any questions the patient may have.

The following sections will look in depth at induction, maintenance, and at the analgesic and neuromuscular blocking agents that are used as part of current anaesthesia.

Induction agents

The induction agents examined in this section will include thiopental, propofol, etomidate and ketamine. It must be noted however that benzodiazepines and opioids can be used to induce anaesthesia, but large doses are required and this prolongs recovery from anaesthesia.

Thiopental sodium

Thiopental is the most commonly used intravenous agent in the world (Aitkenhead 2001). However in the UK its use has been superseded by the advent of propofol. Thiopental still is of clinical use and the anaesthetic practitioner must have an in-depth knowledge of this induction agent.

Thiopental was developed and came into use in the 1930s. It is a barbiturate anaesthetic induction agent, working in what is commonly phrased as 'one arm to brain' circulation time, this being slower in patients whose cardiac output is impaired. In quantitative terms eyelash reflex loss should occur within 30 seconds.

Thiopental comes in a 2.5% solution, which is usually dissolved in distilled water. This solution can then be kept for up to 24 hours (Aitkenhead 2001). In adults the dose is 4 mg kg^{-1}. In children the dose is 6 mg kg^{-1} and in the elderly the dose is considerably less at 2.5–3 mg kg^{-1}.

Effects on organ function

- **Central nervous system** – Consciousness after the initial dose of thiopental is usually achieved after 5–10 minutes, but because of its analgesic effect restlessness may be seen in the post-anaesthetic period. Bradycardia can be observed because sympathetic nervous system activity is depressed. However tachycardia is more likely to be observed because of hypotension and loss of vagal tone.
- **Cardiovascular system** – When larger doses are given combined with rapid administration peripheral vasodilation is observed due to myocardial contractility being depressed. If the patient has cardiac disease or is hypovolaemic, profound hypotension will occur, and although this does not make it an absolute contraindication in these patients, the drug must be administered slowly and special care must be taken. Consideration of alternative induction agents should be made.
- **Respiratory system** – A period of apnoea is usually observed after the administration of thiopental due to a reduction in the sensitivity of the respiratory centre to carbon dioxide. Obviously this is not a particular issue when inducing anaesthesia as all the equipment is available to ventilate the patient. Thiopental depresses the parasympathetic laryngeal reflex arc leading to laryngospasm in the presence of surgical stimulation.

Adverse effects

Besides those mentioned intra-arterial injection should be considered. This is obviously accidental and can happen in the presence of an arterial line. Also when performing venous cannulation the brachial artery can be inadvertently injected. The patient will complain of severe pain and the area will become blanched and blistering may occur. If untreated it will result in ischaemia and gangrene. The needle must be left in place and a vasodilator such as papaverine 20 mg administered. Heparin should be given intravenously and continued postoperatively.

Thiopental while not widely used in the UK is still part of the choice of drugs used to induce anaesthesia, particularly for rapid sequence induction (Cook and Morris 2002). Added to this it is a potent anticonvulsant and thus useful in epileptics undergoing surgery. It can also be used in the treatment of status epilepticus.

Propofol

Propofol was first released in the 1970s and Cremofor L was used as the solvent in the propofol solution. However there was an unacceptable amount of adverse reactions, and it was withdrawn. It was reintroduced in the 1980s in a 1% aqueous emulsion containing soya bean and egg phosphatide (Weksler *et al.* 2001). Due to the lipid nature of the drug it is painful on injection in the small veins of the hands, so 1% lidocaine is added prior to injection (Fryer 2001). However in a recent study it was found that adding ephedrine 30–70 micrograms reduced the incidence and intensity of propofol-induced pain. Added to this there was a lesser decrease in blood pressure (Cheong *et al.* 2002). Because of its lipid base propofol can support bacterial growth if contaminated (Seeberger *et al.* 1998), thus it should only be drawn up immediately prior to injection.

The dose for an adult is normally 1.5–2.5 mg kg^{-1} with a reduction in the elderly to 1.25 mg kg^{-1}. In children a dose of 3–3.5 mg kg^{-1} is required, but it is not recommended in children below one month of age. When using propofol as a continuous infusion the rates are different and this will be examined later.

Effect on organ function

- **Central nervous system** – Transfer of propofol to the sites of action in the brain is slower than thiopental. The loss of eyelash reflex is not seen as quickly as with thiopental, usually after about 20–40 seconds. However there are minimal 'hangover' effects seen postoperatively and patients regain consciousness rapidly. Convulsions have been reported with administration, and thus it should be avoided in epileptic patients (Ding and White 2002).
- **Cardiovascular system** – The hypotensive response seen after induction is greater than with thiopental, due in the main to vasodilation. The effect of this is reduced by slow administration. Bradycardia has been observed after administration, so an agent such as atropine or glycopyrrolate should be used in patients with pre-existing bradycardia. Care should also be taken in its use in the presence of drugs likely to cause bradycardia (Aitkenhead 2001).
- **Respiratory system** – Like thiopental, respiratory depression is observed on administration for the same reasons as previously mentioned. However it is likely to be more prolonged, but the same precautions should be taken. Laryngospasm is uncommon with a low incidence of coughing. For this reason it is the induction agent of choice when inserting a laryngeal mask airway.

Propofol is a uniquely flexible induction agent with rapid redistribution and metabolism, meaning it is the ideal agent to use in day surgery procedures. It is one of the anaesthetic innovations that has enabled day surgery to progress in the way that it has in the last 15 years. Added to this it can be used for sedation during regional anaesthesia procedures and for the sedation of patients in the intensive care environment; both can be achieved by a continuous infusion.

Total intravenous anaesthesia (TIVA)

Propofol is currently the only intravenous anaesthetic agent available suitable for use as TIVA. The advantage of using continuous infusion to maintain anaesthesia is that the doses required are small and cause minimal cardiovascular depression. Until recently the use of total intravenous anaesthesia in children would not have been the ideal. However with the use of TIVA the incidence of side effects from inhalational agents is reduced, and the use of EMLA cream and lidocaine reduce the pain on injection issue (Kretz 2002).

Advantages of TIVA
- Smaller doses are required to maintain anaesthesia and there is minimal cardiovascular depression.
- The patient recovers rapidly once the infusion has been discontinued.
- In patients who may easily become hypoxic, high concentrations of oxygen can be given.
- It can be used in procedures where inhaled agents may be difficult.
- It can be utilised where nitrous oxide is contraindicated, e.g. middle ear surgery.

The aim of TIVA is to reach a plasma concentration that will maintain anaesthesia. The problem with this is that each patient is an individual and it is only possible to estimate a dose. Thus a commonly used regime is a bolus dose of $1\,mg\,kg^{-1}$, infusion rate $10\,mg\,kg^{-1}$ for 10 minutes, $8\,mg\,kg^{-1}$ for 10 minutes, maintenance $6\,mg\,kg^{-1}$. However this would need to be adjusted dependent on patient need. This achieves a plasma concentration of 3 micrograms ml^{-1}. Added to this patients receive nitrous oxide and fentanyl. If these are not added higher infusion rates are needed.

Target controlled infusions (TCI)
More recently intravenous anaesthesia pumps have become more sophisticated. The pumps are now computerised and the target concentration, e.g. 3 micrograms ml^{-1} is input plus the patient's age and weight, and the computer will calculate and deliver the appropriate infusion rate. Throughout the anaesthetist has control of the pump and can adjust the target concentration according to clinical indication. These are known as target controlled infusions (TCI).

Advantages of TCI
- Simple intravenous technique
- Control of the depth of anaesthesia (can be done rapidly)
- Slowing induction means decreased hypotension and apnoea
- Ability to predict recovery accurately (Padford 2000)
- Implicated in a decrease in postoperative nausea and vomiting (Millar 2000).

Disadvantages of TCI
- Cannot be used in unconscious patients as the system assumes the patient is conscious on commencement of the infusion
- Induction time is longer, between one and two minutes
- It is necessary to use some form of monitoring to measure the depth of anaesthesia, as there is a risk of awareness.

Etomidate
Etomidate causes less cardiovascular depression than thiopental; it is therefore used in patients with a compromised cardiovascular system, but it has been superseded by propofol (Aitkenhead 2001). It acts rapidly and typically lasts for 2–3 minutes. It is metabolised in the liver and plasma, and 2% is excreted unchanged in the urine (Simpson and Popat 2002). Involuntary movement can be observed during induction of anaesthesia in up to 40% of patients, and in 10% coughing and hiccuping can occur. It is also painful on injection. It is presented in a one-off bolus dose of 20 mg in 10 ml. This is because the use of etomidate depresses the synthesis of cortisol and impairs the response to adrenocorticotrophic hormone (Simpson and Popat 2002). The effect of this can also be demonstrated on single dose and can last for several hours. It has been argued that the use of etomidate in patients requiring critical care must be questioned, and alternatives should be sought (Roberts and Redman 2002). Finally recovery from anaesthesia is not smooth. Patients are restless and there is a 30% incidence of postoperative nausea and vomiting. Aitkenhead (2001) concludes by saying, 'There are few positive indications for etomidate' (p. 177).

Ketamine

While ketamine does not have a widespread use in the UK, its use in North America and developing countries is more prevalent. In the UK it tends to be used in specialist areas and difficult locations, e.g. major incidents or when frequent change of dressings is required.

Effects on organ function

- **Central nervous system** – It can be given intravenously or intramuscularly. When given intravenously it induces anaesthesia within 30–60 seconds and lasts between 10–15 minutes. Intramuscularly it works between 3–4 minutes and has a longer duration of action of between 15–20 minutes. The major advantage is its analgesic effect. The main disadvantage is its hallucinogenic effects. This is termed as 'emergence delirium' and is particularly visible in the presence of noise. If a ketamine anaesthetic is administered all staff in the operating department must be made aware, and the patient should be recovered in a quiet area postoperatively.
- **Cardiovascular system** – Ketamine should not be used in patients with pre-existing hypertension, because on administration arterial pressure and heart rate increase. Added to this, cardiac output and myocardial oxygen consumption may also increase.
- **Respiratory system** – As mentioned previously ketamine can be used in difficult locations to carry out a procedure where pain control is required without the loss of pharyngeal and laryngeal reflexes; however this is not guaranteed and equipment must be available to maintain the airway.

Adverse effects

- Emergence delirium
- Hypertension
- Prolonged recovery
- Increased salivation
- Allergic reactions
- Increased intracranial pressure.

To summarise, intravenous induction agents produce unconsciousness in order to allow surgical anaesthesia. The agents reviewed here are the ones used in current clinical practice. The anaesthetic practitioner must be familiar with these and be aware of the current evidence available on which to base their practice.

As discussed previously, induction agents are not given in isolation; they are part of the overall anaesthetic technique. In the next section inhalational anaesthetic agents will be reviewed. Primarily these maintain anaesthesia, although they can be used for induction.

Inhalational anaesthetic agents

The agents explored in this section will be halothane, enflurane, isoflurane, sevoflurane and desflurane. Each of these is equally good at maintaining anaesthesia, but as a group they have related problems and risks (Kretz 2002). For example, the use of halothane has reduced because of the risk of halothane hepatoxicity, which although a rare complication can happen after repeated halothane anaesthetics. Sevoflurane is increasingly being seen as the ideal induction agent (Kretz 2002). The ideal inhalational agent has yet to be discovered. None of the ensuing agents are perfect, and each agent must be used in the appropriate situation, weighing up its advantages and its disadvantages.

Minimal alveolar concentration (MAC)

MAC indicates the potency of anaesthetic agents and can be measured. A definition of MAC is as follows, 'The minimum alveolar concentration (in volumes per cent) of an anaesthetic at 1 atmosphere absolute (ata) that prevents movement in 50% of the population to a standard stimulus' (Mushambi and Smith 2001, p. 152).

Boxes 4.1–4.5 summarise the properties, advantages and disadvantages of the five inhalational anaesthetic agents mentioned above.

Analgesics

This section will look at analgesics used for the duration of anaesthesia. There are many other analgesics, which are used as part of a balanced anaesthesia technique; however they are not within the scope of this chapter.

Box 4.1 Halothane

- MAC (in oxygen) = 0.75%
- Recovery is slow because of the high blood/gas solubility and the time of recovery is directly related to the length of anaesthesia
- 20% is metabolised in the liver
- It is non-irritant to the airway and useful to use for a gaseous induction
- It antagonises bronchospasm and resistance in patients with bronchoconstriction
- There is a decrease in myocardial contractility and hypotention is observed. Arrhythmias are very common during halothane anaesthesia
- Relaxes uterine muscle
- In caesarian section amounts of less than 0.5% are not associated with bleeding. The same does not apply in a termination of pregnancy
- Potentiates non-depolarising muscle relaxants
- Is associated with postoperative shivering leading to increased oxygen requirements
- Patients may get a derangement in liver function tests following halothane anaesthesia but these are transient
- What is more dangerous but extremely rare is a type 2 liver dysfunction following the administration of halothane and the likelihood of this is increased by repeated exposure
- It is recommended that halothane is not repeated within a 3-month period

Advantages
- Smooth induction
- Very little stimulation of salivary and bronchial secretions
- Bronchodilation thus is useful in asthmatic patients

Disadvantages
- Arrhythmias
- Slow recovery
- Liver toxicity which is increased with repeated administrations

Box 4.2 Enflurane

- MAC = 1.68%
- Recovery is faster than halothane but slower than isoflurane, sevoflurane and desflurane
- 2.5% is metabolised in the liver
- Inhalation induction is pleasant as it is non-irritant
- Does not increase salivary and bronchial secretions
- Dose dependent depression of the myocardium leading to a reduction in cardiac output and subsequent hypotension
- No vagal effects so hypotension can lead to reflex tachycardia
- Dose related uterine relaxation
- Should be avoided in epileptics because of the risk of seizures
- Potentiates non-depolarising muscle relaxants
- Trigger agent for malignant hyperthermia
- Can cause a derangement of liver enzymes

Advantages
- Low incidence of arrhythmias
- Low risk of hepatic dysfunction

Disadvantages
- Risk of seizures
- Contraindicated in patients with renal disease

Fentanyl

Fentanyl is a synthetic opioid derived from pethidine. Its use is mainly during anaesthesia, because it is short acting and it is a severe respiratory depressant, neither of which characteristics are desirable in the recovery phase of anaesthesia. With smaller doses of fentanyl, respiratory depression will last up to 30 minutes; with larger doses it may be prolonged for up to 2–3 hours. Fentanyl has relatively few side effects. The use of fentanyl in an epidural has gained widespread popularity. It appears that when given extradurally its action is potentiated and its analgesic action can last up to 4 hours (Pleuvry 2001).

Box 4.3 Isoflurane

- MAC = 1.15% in oxygen, 0.56% in 70% nitrous oxide
- Pungent on inhalation with coughing and breath holding
- 0.17% metabolised making the risk of hepatic and renal toxicity negligible
- Dose-dependent depression of respiration
- Reduction in systemic vascular resistance leading to systemic hypotension
- Coronary vasodilation
- Dose-related uterine contraction
- Potentiates non-depolarising muscle relaxants

Advantages
- Rapid recovery
- Less risk of renal and hepatic toxicity
- Less incidence of arrhythmias

Disadvantages
- Not the ideal agent to use as a gaseous induction
- It may be contraindicated in patients with coronary artery disease

Box 4.4 Sevoflurane

- MAC 1.7% in 2% oxygen 0.66% nitrous oxide
- Non-irritant to the upper respiratory tract
- Fast induction
- Recovery slower than with desflurane
- 5% of absorbed dose metabolised in the liver
- Dose-dependent respiratory depression
- Relaxes bronchial smooth muscle (not to the same extent as halothane)
- Mild myocardial depression, although cardiac output is well-maintained
- No excitory effects
- Renal blood flow well-preserved
- Potentiates non-depolarising muscle relaxants
- Trigger agent for malignant hyperthermia
- In the presence of low fresh gas flows and the use of carbon dioxide absorbers Sevoflurane should be avoided due to the theoretical risk of toxicity

Advantages
- Smooth fast induction – ideal for paediatrics
- Rapid recovery
- Conventional vapourisers can be used

Disadvantages
- Potential of producing toxic metabolites
- Instability with carbon dioxide absorbers
- Expensive

Alfentanil

The main use of alfentanil is in day surgery as it is very short-acting and is used as part of a total intravenous anaesthesia technique. It is a respiratory depressant, but unlike fentanyl, its respiratory depressant effects are less profound.

Remifentanil

This is a relatively new opioid analgesic designed for use as part of an intravenous anaesthesia technique. It is short acting and wears off within minutes of it being withdrawn. The side effects are similar to those of fentanyl.

Nitrous oxide

Nitrous oxide is a poor anaesthetic but a potent analgesic. It is commonly used in a 50:50 mix with oxygen to give Entonox (Serpell 2001). One of the side affects of nitrous oxide is diffusion hypoxia. At the end of anaesthesia, hypoxaemia may occur as the concentration of gases in the alveoli is diluted by nitrous oxide. This is transient lasting up to ten minutes, and it is essential to administer oxygen so that the patient does not desaturate.

Another problem with nitrous oxide is the effect it has on enclosed spaces. In enclosed spaces of the body the volume of nitrous oxide diffusing into the space exceeds the volume of nitrogen diffusing out. Thus the space will expand. However some spaces do not have room

Box 4.5 Desflurane

- MAC 6% in 3% oxygen, 60% in nitrous oxide
- Requires a special vaporiser which requires electric power to heat and pressurise it
- Pungent smell
- Rapid recovery rate
- Upper respiratory tract irritant, and when used as a gaseous induction agent causes coughing, breath-holding and laryngospasm
- Dose-related decreases in systemic vascular resistance, myocardial contractility and mean arterial pressure
- When inspired, concentration is increased rapidly. There is an increase in sympathetic activity leading to an increased heart rate and mean arterial pressure
- Dose-related increase in cerebrovascular resistance leading to an increase in intracranial pressure
- Trigger agent for malignant hyperthermia

Advantages
- Offers precise control of maintenance of anaesthesia
- Rapid recovery
- Non toxic to the liver and kidney
- Does not cause convulsions

Disadvantages
- Cannot be used for gaseous induction
- At high concentrations it causes tachycardia
- Expensive
- Requires a specialised vaporiser

for expansion, such as the middle ear, and this can cause surgical problems with pressure on the tympanic membrane. The volume can increase by up to three or four times the original volume. Nitrous oxide also diffuses into the endotracheal cuff in longer procedures, resulting in increased pressure on the tracheal mucosa. This can be avoided by inflating the cuff with saline or nitrous oxide (Mushambi and Smith 2001).

SPINAL AND EPIDURAL ANALGESIA/ ANAESTHESIA

Spinal and epidural analgesia can be used alone or in conjunction with general anaesthesia. The extent to which it is used as the sole method of anaesthesia is dependent primarily on the patient. There is a general expectation in the UK that patients will have a general anaesthetic (Simpson and Popat 2002). Because of this patients need to be well-prepared for the procedure. This section will look at spinal and epidural analgesia and will then briefly look at combined spinal/epidural and continuous epidural infusions.

Spinal analgesia/anaesthesia

The local anaesthetic for a spinal will be placed into the subarachnoid space. This is a fluid filled space containing cerebral spinal fluid (CSF). Because it is a fluid-filled space this has a direct impact on how this technique works. A spinal is usually performed at below the level of L1 to avoid mechanical damage to the spinal cord and the aim is for the local anaesthetic agent to act on the cauda equina and the spinal cord (Harrop-Griffiths 2001).

There are three types of nerves that can be blocked: (i) autonomic are not under conscious control and are involved with heart rate, the calibre of blood vessel and gut contraction; (ii) sensory nerves are involved with the sensations of touch and pain; (iii) finally motor nerves which control movement and when blocked the patient will not be able to move. Autonomic and sensory nerves are blocked first followed by the motor nerves. A spinal anaesthetic will block all of these nerves in approximately 5 minutes (Ankcorn and Casey 1993).

In order to understand the effect of a spinal it can be looked at in the following categories: factors that affect the spread of the solution in the subarachnoid space or factors affecting the height of the block; the complications of spinal analgesia; and contraindications.

Factors affecting the spread of the solution in the subarachnoid space (factors affecting the height of the block)

Specific gravity, i.e. the density of the solution, is an important factor in the spread of the solution. When the anaesthetic solution is injected into the subarachnoid space the majority of it should go towards the feet rather than up towards the chest for reasons that will be discussed later in this section. This is achieved by using a local anaesthetic solution that has a density greater than CSF, a hyperbaric solution. Hence 'heavy bupivacaine' is the drug of choice. The local anaesthetic solution is made 'heavy' by the addition of glucose. Bupivacaine solution without the addition of glucose is termed as isobaric, meaning it has the same density as CSF and the spread of it is governed by the volume of solution injected. Solutions which are lighter than CSF are termed as hypobaric and this can be achieved by the addition of sterile water (Harrop-Griffiths 2001).

Added to the baracity of the solution is the position of the patient. If a spinal is performed in the sitting position using a hyperbaric solution the sacral nerve roots will be blocked; this is sometimes termed as a 'saddle block'. Once the spinal has been performed the level of the block can be manipulated to a certain degree by the patient's position, i.e. head down if a higher block is required and head up for a lower level block, being mindful of the additional hypotension which may follow.

The volume of the solution injected is directly proportional to the spread, so large volumes of local anaesthetic solutions will spread further and produce a denser block; this could be detrimental to the patient if not well-controlled.

Obviously the rate at which the solution is injected will have an effect on the extent of the block. However the slower the injection the more predictable the block. A controlled turbulence in the CSF can be set up termed as 'barbotage' but the effect of the block is less predictable.

Complications of spinal analgesia

- **Cardiovascular system** – Hypotension will be demonstrated due to vasodilation and functional decrease in circulating volume. It is important that the patient is preloaded with crystalloid and colloid solutions, and a vasoconstriction agent such as ephedrine should be available. It has been suggested that the latter is more important and there is a move to use vasoconstriction agents routinely (Harrop-Griffiths 2001).

- **Respiratory system** – Breathing will cease if the spread of the solution reaches the mid-cervical level or the fourth ventricle of the brain, where the respiratory centre is. This is termed as a 'total spinal'. The treatment for this would be in the first instance to reassure the patient if they are conscious, as this is very frightening for them. They will need to be anaesthetised quickly, ventilated and blood pressure maintained with fluids and vasopressors.

- **Post-dural puncture headache (PDPH)** – This is caused by the hole that is made in the dura and leakage of CSF, and is related to the size of the hole (Sudlow and Warlow 2002). The incidence of this can be up to 90% (Williams *et al.* 1998). This can be reduced if a smaller bore needle is used, usually size 25G, 27G and 29G. The shape of the needle is also important: a conical needle is less likely to cause a PDPH than a cutting tip. The treatment for PDPH is in the first instance bedrest with good analgesia and hydration. If this is not effective, a blood patch should be considered. This involves the injection of about 10–20 ml of the patient's blood into the extradural space around the site where the original dural puncture was performed. Coagulation of the blood is thought to stop the leakage of CSF. An abolition of PDPH occurs in 90% of cases when using this technique (Sudlow and Warlow 2002). The use of prophylactic epidural blood patch as a method to prevent PDPH has also been explored (Serpell *et al.* 1998; Berger *et al.* 1998), but further evidence is required to support this practice (Sudlow and Warlow 2002). It is postulated that with bedrest, hydration and analgesics PDPH will resolve itself within three days; this being the case the necessity for a blood patch has been questioned (Williams *et al.* 1998).

- **Rare complications** – Meningitis is a very rare complication of spinal analgesia because of the potential risk of infection of the meninges. Short-term deafness and cranial nerve dysfunction have also been reported (Harrop-Griffiths 2001).

Contraindications

- Lack of patient consent
- Raised intracranial pressure
- Patients with coagulation disorders
- Local or systemic sepsis
- Neurological disorders
- Children as their co-operation is required
- Operations lasting over 2 hours
- Operations above the thorax
- Shock.

Epidural

The epidural space is between the dura mater and the vertebral canal. It is a potential space filled mainly with fatty areolar tissue and veins. Epidural analgesia has the advantage over spinal analgesia because it can be performed at any level, although it is usually carried out at L3/4 (Lee 2001).

Indications for epidural analgesia/anaesthesia

- Surgery
- Postoperative analgesia
- Trauma
- Labour
- Acute ischaemic pain
- Intractable back pain.

Factors affecting the spread of the solution in the epidural space (factors affecting the height of the block)

As mentioned previously the epidural space is filled with fat and veins and this has a direct bearing on the spread of the solution. Baracity of the

solution does not play a part and so isobaric bupivacaine is used. The rate of injection does not really play any part as the use of fine-bore catheters makes it virtually impossible to inject with any sort of speed (Simpson and Popat 2002).

Complications of epidural analgesia

- **Cardiovascular system** – Hypotension will be observed for the same reasons as a spinal. However the effects of these will be slower in onset (Lee 2001).
- **Respiratory system** – As previously mentioned an epidural can be performed thoracically. This is useful in the treatment of chest trauma. It means that the anaesthetist will be able to make the patient pain free without inhibiting respiration. This is achieved by only blocking the autonomic and sensory nerves; the motor nerves are not blocked meaning the patient will be able to breath, but be pain free. The benefits of this are immediately obvious. Thoracic epidurals are performed to control pain after surgery particularly post-thoracotomy, known to be one of the most painful surgical procedures, where it has been found to be more effective than intravenous patient controlled analgesia (Macias *et al.* 2002).
- **Total spinal** – this can happen if the Tuohy needle is advanced too far and there is inadvertent puncture of the dura and the needle enters the subarachnoid space. The anaesthetist will check for cerebral spinal fluid, a test dose will be given and the effect on the patient noted. If a total spinal occurs, treatment is as detailed in the spinal analgesia section.

Other considerations that can lead to complications following epidural analgesia are toxic doses of the local anaesthetic solution. This is an issue because larger volumes are being used and there is a danger of exceeding the maximum safe dose of the local anaesthetic solution. Where the epidural is being topped up on a regular basis, there is a danger of accumulation to toxic doses. The use of a continuous infusion will solve this as smaller doses are being given over a longer period (Russell 2001).

Another complication of epidural analgesia is the risk of infection, particularly when the catheter is left in place for a few days. The incidence of infection at the epidural entry site or deep catheter track infections is between 1% and 6% (Breivik 1999). The incidence of meningitis is only 3:3,000,000, and the incidence of epidural abscess in obstetric patients was found to be 1:505,000 (Scott and Hibbard 1990). Epidural abscess is a serious complication requiring surgical decompression, although the use of antibiotic therapy has been described in the absence of neurological symptoms (Kindler *et al.* 1998).

Contraindications

- Lack of patient consent
- Sepsis anywhere near the site of the injection
- Lack of patient co-operation; children may fit into this category although an epidural can be performed once they are anaesthetised (Mazoit and Baujard 2002)
- Shock
- Demyelinating conditions of the spinal cord such as multiple sclerosis. This is not an absolute contraindication, but subsequent episodes of the condition may be blamed on the block, although there is no evidence to support this (Simpson and Popat 2002)
- Bleeding tendency.

Combined spinal/epidural (CSEA)

This technique is gaining popularity and special packs where the combined spinal/epidural needle is provided have been developed. The technique consists of advancing the epidural needle into the epidural space and then advancing the spinal needle through this and pushing it into the subarachnoid space and performing the spinal. The spinal needle is then withdrawn and the epidural catheter is inserted, and the epidural needle withdrawn. The advantage of this technique is that the epidural can be used for postoperative pain management. However the failure rate for the technique is approximately 10% (Russell 2001).

The anaesthetic practitioner's role in caring for a patient undergoing spinal and epidural analgesia/anaesthesia

If possible the anaesthetic practitioner should see the patient prior to surgery. This is particularly relevant if the patient is going to be awake during their surgery. This means that the patient will not only be familiar with the anaesthetist, who would have assessed them, but they will also be familiar with the anaesthetic practitioner who is going to care for them.

The reason for seeing the patient prior to surgery is mainly for psychological purposes. The anaesthetist will have carried out a physical assessment, past anaesthetic history and explained the procedure in terms of the anaesthetic, but little emphasis will have been put on the psychological preparation of the patient. Added to this, the patient may mention to the anaesthetic practitioner something they omitted when speaking to the anaesthetist. This is where the anaesthetic practitioner and the anaesthetist should be working in collaboration for the benefit of the patient and share information.

As mentioned at the start of this section, patients in the UK expect to be asleep for their surgery and they need support if they are going to be awake during it. The anaesthetic practitioner can explain in simple terms what they may feel when having surgery under local anaesthesia. One of the simplest explanations is to equate it with having an injection at the dentist where a degree of pulling and pushing is felt but they do not feel pain.

The anaesthetic practitioner can explore what will happen to the patient in the anaesthetic room, gaining their confidence and co-operation. They can also tell the patient what they will see upon entering theatre and who will be there. Finally they can inform the patient of what will happen in the recovery area.

With time constraints the reality is that most anaesthetic practitioners will not be able to visit the patient prior to surgery; however all that has been detailed previously can be done on reception of the patient into the anaesthetic room. This is where the skill of the anaesthetic practitioner can be demonstrated.

PRACTICE EXEMPLAR 4.1: CAESARIAN SECTION

Sue is 36 and was admitted to theatre for a caesarean section under epidural analgesia/anaesthesia. The anaesthetist had seen her but the anaesthetic practitioner had not met her before. The epidural was inserted and the operation commenced. Sue kept saying she could feel it. The anaesthetic practitioner took time with her to ascertain whether she was in pain or could just feel the movement of the surgeon. Sue was so distressed that in the end she had to be anaesthetized as she was unable to articulate what she was feeling.

Would this have happened if the anaesthetic practitioner had seen Sue before her surgery and gone through what was going to happen to her step by step? Or would it have happened anyway?

Prior to the patient's arrival all equipment needed must be prepared. This will leave time when the patient arrives to communicate and develop a rapport with them. The anaesthetic practitioner can help the patient get into the right position either sitting or lying on their side with their back curved. The anaesthetist can be given all their equipment on a sterile trolley, and then the practitioner can go back to the patient, encouraging them to lie still and informing them of what is happening to them; again the anaesthetist and the anaesthetic practitioner should work as a team.

Once the procedure is completed the patient can be helped onto their back and should be encouraged to explain the sensations they are feeling. Once the block has been established the patient can move into theatre and be made comfortable on the table. At every stage an explanation should be given as to what is being done to them and why. It is the anaesthetic practitioner's role to stay with the patient throughout the procedure, and you should not be afraid to hold their hand, if this is what the patient wants you to do. A skilful practitioner will quickly establish the level of support each patient may need.

Obviously the patient will be fully monitored and the practitioner must watch that this is done in conjunction with observing the patient for any change in their condition. The reality is that the anaesthetist should also be present throughout, and teamwork should pervade the whole patient experience.

NEUROMUSCULAR PHYSIOLOGY AND MUSCLE RELAXANTS

Physiology of neuromuscular transmission

Nervous impulses arise in the cells in the anterior horns of the spinal cord, and the equivalent cells in the brain for the cranial nerves. Muscle tone in the body is maintained by continuous nervous impulses. Each impulse travels down the nerve axon by electrical conduction, jumping in myelinated nerves from one node of Ranvier to the next. The nodes of Ranvier are excitable and participate in the propagation of the action potential. The axon branches into nerve terminals each of which comes into contact with one muscle cell. The nerve structure closest to the muscle is the synapse, which is opposite the endplate. The junction between the end of the nerve and the motor endplate of the muscle fibre is called the neuromuscular junction (Figure 4.15). A chemical transmitter, acetylcholine, brings about conduction of the impulse across the neuromuscular junction. Acetylcholine is produced in the axon of the nerve and stored in the junction of the nerve, and small amounts are continually being produced. When a nerve impulse arrives at the junction, acetylcholine migrates across the synaptic cleft and binds selectively to nicotinic acetylcholine receptors at the endplate, producing an alteration in the membrane permeability. The action potential does not carry information to other cells, but triggers the contraction process. Sodium (Na^+) ions rush into

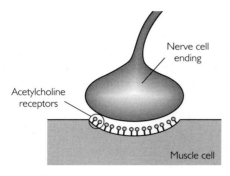

Figure 4.15 Neuromuscular junction

the cells and potassium (K$^+$) ions are released, bringing about a change in the voltage known as endplate potential (Kervin 2002). Depolarisation spreads through the muscle fibre, calcium ions are released from the endoplasmic reticulum and the muscle contracts. Acetylcholine is destroyed by the enzyme cholinesterase thus enabling the next impulse to be effective. Acetylcholine is broken down into choline and acetic acid (Donati 1995).

Depolarising muscle relaxants

Suxemethonium (Scoline)

Suxemethonium is similar to a double molecule of acetylcholine joined together. It mimics the action of acetylcholine and attaches itself to the acetylcholine receptors on the motor end plate causing increased membrane permeability. This results in the characteristic fasciculation and flaccid paralysis. The motor endplate will remain depolarised for a period of 3–5 minutes and no further transmission of impulses can occur. Suxemethonium is destroyed slowly by the enzyme pseudocholinesterase or plasma cholinesterase (Harper 1995a).

Advantages
- Optimal intubating conditions are obtained within 30 seconds.
- The effects only last for 3–5 minutes.

Disadvantages
- 'Scoline apnoea' may occur. 1 in 2800 people may experience prolonged apnoea for up to 3 hours following administration.

- Contraindicated in patients who are pregnant, on haemodialysis or who have hepatic failure, because they tend to have low levels of plasma cholinesterase.
- Bradycardia – atropine should be administered before giving large doses of suxemethonium.
- Muscle pains – up to 50% of patients experience pain after suxemethonium. In particular young ambulant women develop muscle pains on the day after receiving suxemethonium. This is thought to be due to the fasciculation, which produces tearing of the muscle fibre and small hemorrhages.
- Hyperkalaemia – the depolarisation produced by the suxemethonium leads to a reduction in intracellular potassium. Some patients may exhibit very large potassium fluxes and develop dangerous increases in serum potassium concentrations. Groups susceptible to this are: patients with severe burns, patients with extensive muscle damage, paraplegic patients and patients with peripheral neuropathies.
- Suxemethonium causes a transient increase in intra-occular and intracranial pressure. This is due to an increase in arterial and venous pressures and prolonged contracture of the exoccular muscles.
- Intragastric pressure is also increased as a result of the fasciculation so increasing the risk of regurgitation.
- There is no antidote!
- Dual block – with prolonged administration the characteristics of the depolarisation block changes to resemble those seen with non-depolarising agents.
- Suxemethonium is a trigger agent for malignant hyperpyrexia (Harper 1995a).

Non-depolarising muscle relaxants

This type of block works by blocking the nicotinic receptor sites on the motor endplate, and prevents the transmission of the impulse by acetylcholine. There is therefore no change in the membrane permeability and no depolarisation. Each produce the characteristic block described previously but they differ in potency, duration of action and side effects (Pollard 1995).

Advantages
- Long-term muscle relaxation
- Their action may be reversed.

Disadvantages
- Have to wait longer to obtain optimal intubating conditions
- Although the action may be reversed, this can only be done after a variable length of time.

Mivacurium

This is a relatively new short-acting non-depolarising muscle relaxant. It produces good to excellent intubating conditions within 2.5 minutes. The duration of neuromuscular blockade is obviously related to dosage, but the range is between 10 and 15 minutes. Additional dosages produce another 15 minutes of neuromuscular blockade without the accumulation of neuromuscular blocking effect. It can be reversed in the normal way, but because spontaneous reversal is rapid, reversal may not be routinely required (Pollard 1995).

Patients who are sensitive to suxemethonium are likely to be sensitive to mivacurium. It should be used with caution in asthmatics because of the release of histamine. Furthermore caution should also be taken when administering it to patients who are hypovolaemic. Other side effects associated with mivacurium are skin flushing, mild transient hypotension, transient tachycardia and bronchospasm, which are obviously dose-related.

Atracurium

This is a non-depolarising muscle relaxant similar in onset and duration to vecuronium. It is unique in that it is broken down at a plasma level by a process called 'Hoffman elimination' which occurs by plasma pH and body temperature. The termination of action of this drug is not dependent on metabolism or excretion by the liver or kidneys, so it is useful in cases of hepatic or renal failure. Anaesthetic agents (halothane), or surgical manoeuvres (peritoneal traction) which cause vagal stimulation are more likely to produce bradycardia when a cardiovascularly inactive drug like vecuronium is being used than agents which produce tachycardia like pancuronium (Pollard 1995).

Vecuronium IV

Non-depolarising muscle relaxant of medium duration of action: 20–30 minutes. It has very little effect on the cardiovascular system causing neither tachycardia nor hypotension. It does not promote histamine release. It is excreted mostly in the bile and to a small extent through the kidneys; therefore it is useful in cases of renal failure (Pollard 1995).

Pancuronium

One of the newer synthetic non-depolarising muscle relaxants. Rapid onset lasting 20–30 minutes. It causes slight tachycardia and a slight increase in blood pressure. It does not release histamine or cross the placental barrier in significant amounts. Excreted largely in the kidneys, metabolism in the liver and excretion in the bile are alternative excretory mechanisms (Pollard 1995).

Rocuronium

A steroid-based non-depolarising muscle relaxant, which has been relatively recently introduced into clinical practice. It is eliminated principally in the liver unchanged, thus in patients with hepatic dysfunction the duration of action is increased. Intubation is possible within 60 seconds and its duration of action is about 30–40 minutes. Reversal is with an anticholinesterase. As yet few side effects have been reported (Pollard 1995).

Reversal of non-depolarising muscle relaxants

Kervin (2002) notes that non-depolarising agents are not actually 'reversed'. Instead an anticholinesterase such as neostigmine is administered which allows the build up of acetylcholine levels at the neuromuscular junction, thus enabling the block to be overcome. This is achieved by a decrease in the metabolism of cholinesterase, which in turn increases the availability of acetylcholine. Neostigmine has certain muscarinic effects, stimulating the parasympathetic nervous system, which include: (i) an increased peristaltic action; (ii) bradycardia; and (iii) increased salivary activity. Therefore an anticholinergic agent such as glycopyrolate is always given in conjunction with neostigmine (Harper 1995b).

Neostigmine

An anticholinesterase, which inhibits the action of cholinesterase. The excess acetylcholine produced possesses muscarinic effects, which stimulate the parasympathetic nervous system causing increased salivation, increased gut activity and bradycardia. It also has nicotinic effects which are exerted on the skeletal neuromuscular junction, therefore they agonise the effects of the non-depolarising muscle relaxants (Kervin 2002).

Glycopyrolate

Glycopyrolate is used in preference to atropine because there is less cardiovascular stimulation since it does not cross the blood–brain barrier, and so excitatory side effects do not occur. It is given to counteract the muscurinic effects of neostigmine.

EMERGENCY ANAESTHESIA

The classification of an emergency is broad, but for the purpose of this section, patients with life-threatening conditions who are admitted to the operating department for immediate surgery will be classified as an emergency.

For the patient undergoing emergency anaesthesia the most important potential problem relates to the need to protect the airway from aspiration during anaesthesia, because they are usually not fasted for the required period of time. If aspiration of the stomach contents occurs the patient is at risk of aspiration pneumonitis (Dawson and Cockcroft 1996).

Mendelson's syndrome was first described by a New York obstetrician, and because of this when applied to the obstetric population it is referred to as Mendelson's syndrome. For all other emergencies it is commonly referred to as acid aspiration syndrome although the terms are interchangeable.

The patients at risk are usually obstetric patients; trauma patients; patients with a history of reflux or hiatus hernia; patients with gastrointestinal obstruction; obese patients and any patient where there is a history of delayed gastric emptying.

The aim of any emergency induction is to prevent the aspiration of stomach contents. This can be achieved in a number of ways such as emptying the stomach contents prior to induction; inducing anaesthesia in the head-up tilt position; inhalational induction in the left lateral head-up tilt position; consideration of a local anaesthetic technique if possible. However the most common form of anaesthetic technique for emergency anaesthesia is a combination of neutralising the stomach contents and rapid sequence induction.

Rapid sequence induction

The process of a rapid sequence is often referred to as a 'crash' induction; however this is not a practice that should be encouraged. The anaesthetic practitioner must remember that due to the nature of this induction the patient will be awake and listen to all that is being said; discussing a 'crash' induction will increase their anxiety further.

The whole procedure revolves around the use of cricoid pressure or Sellick's manoeuvre. The cricoid cartilage is compressed, which in turn is pressed against the 5th or 6th cervical vertebrae. Sellick described the application of cricoid pressure with three fingers: the thumb and the middle finger either side of the cricoid and the forefinger applying the pressure (Sellick 1961). The rationale for the use of the cricoid cartilage is because it is the only complete ring; all the others are C-shaped.

Discussion has ensued about the force with which the pressure is applied (Palmer and Ball 2000). It is now generally accepted that 30 Newtons of pressure is sufficient to prevent regurgitation; a force greater than this will cause airway obstruction (Vanner 2001; Hartsilver and Vanner 2000). Rapid sequence induction is a skilled procedure at a time when the patient is at greatest risk. The anaesthetic practitioner must demonstrate skill and an ability to be calm under pressure and empathetic to the needs of the patient. All anaesthetic practitioners will be aware of the procedure, but it is worth noting that if the patient vomits the anaesthetist will make the decision to remove the cricoid pressure. If removed the patient is at risk of aspirating. If it is maintained they are at risk of a ruptured oesophagus (Boerhaave syndrome) (Andrews 1992).

Emergencies in anaesthesia

This section will look briefly at two of the uncommon emergencies encountered in anaesthesia – prolonged neuromuscular blockade following suxemethonium and mivacurium, and malignant hyperthermia.

Prolonged neuromuscular blockade following suxemethonium and mivacurium

As alluded to previously, if plasma cholinesterase is structurally abnormal due to either inherited or acquired factors, prolonged neuromuscular blockade will be observed following administration. In the structure of plasma cholinesterase, abnormalities have been identified in the amino acid sequence. Firstly a patient who is heterozygote for the atypical gene will have prolonged neuromuscular blockade for up to 30 minutes. Secondly a patient who is a homozygote for the atypical gene may have prolonged neuromuscular blockade for up to two hours. A final rare abnormality has been identified where the neuromuscular blockade can last up to three hours. These patients have little or no capacity to metabolise suxemethonium and mivacurium, and they are broken down by non-specific esterases (Hunter 2001).

In clinical terms, it will be observed that the patient will not commence breathing after the required period of time. The real danger in this situation is awareness as the anaesthetic may have been withdrawn upon completion of surgery. The treatment will therefore be to keep the patient anaesthetised and ventilated, usually transferring them to the intensive care or high-dependency unit. The degree of blockade should be monitored until there is full recovery from the neuromuscular blockade. It has been suggested that a further treatment would be to administer fresh frozen plasma (a source of plasma cholinesterase) or to give neostigmine as the neuromuscular block will have developed into a dual block (Hunter 2001).

Following an episode of suxemethonium or mivacurium apnoea, the patient and their immediate family must be screened. This should not be carried out immediately after the prolonged neuromuscular blockade, as plasma cholinesterase levels will be reduced because of the presence of suxemethonium and mivacurium.

In order to detect the atypical gene, plasma is tested, and when dibucaine is added it will inhibit the action of the benzoycholine in the plasma. The dibucaine number is the percentage to which there is inhibition of benzoycholine (Table 4.4). In a recent study it was suggested that this method may misidentify genotypes, and the use of molecular biology was advocated to improve the accuracy of diagnosis (Cerf *et al.* 2002).

Malignant hyperthermia

Malignant hyperthermia is an inherited condition. The estimated incidence is 1:12,000 in children and 1:40,000 in adults (Stoelting and Dierdorf 2002). The trigger agents are suxemethonium and all the inhalational agents, although halothane is the most potent. A defect in the calcium release channels result in a susceptibility to malignant hyperthermia, and the mortality rate is about 5% (Hobbs 2001).

Essentially Malignant hyperthermia is characterised by increases in the patient's metabolic rate. The earliest signs will be an unexplained tachycardia and an increasing end-tidal carbon dioxide. In some patients the signs of malignant hyperthermia will manifest themselves within ten minutes of induction of anaesthesia, while in others several hours may elapse. A rise in temperature is not a feature seen in all patients, but if it does it will rise by more than 2°C/hour, exceeding 40°C. Alternatively a primary sign may be masseter spasm connected to the administration of suxemethonium, although less than 10%

Table 4.4 Dibucaine number for the different genotypes

Normal plasma cholinesterase	Heterozygote for atypical gene	Homozygote for atypical gene
77–83	45–68	Less than 30

Table 4.5   Clinical signs of malignant hyperthermia. Adapted from Hopkins 2000

Initial clinical signs	Secondary clinical signs	Third clinical signs
Masseter spasm	The patient will feel hyperthermic	Skeletal muscle rigidity
Tachypnoea	Cyanosis	Prolonged bleeding
Rapid exhaustion of soda lime	Cardiac arrhythmias	Dark urine
Tachycardia		Oliguria
Increase in end tidal carbon dioxide		Cardiac arrhythmias

of patients who exhibit this sign progress to full malignant hyperthermia syndrome (Hobbs 2001) (Table 4.5).

Management

- All trigger agents should be discontinued and 100% oxygen administered.
- Intravenous dantrolene should be given 1–2 mg/kg^{-1} every five minutes. Dantrolene is a skeletal muscle relaxant. Unlike anaesthetic muscle relaxants it works on the junction of the nerve endings with the muscle surface. The use of this has contributed to the decrease in mortality rate. Dantrolene comes in powder form and takes some minutes to reconstitute.
- Sodium bicarbonate should be administered to counteract acidosis.
- The patient should be actively cooled with ice packs and if necessary gastric and rectal lavage performed with iced saline.
- A vapour-free anaesthetic machine should replace the original machine and circuits.
- Once a patient has had an episode of malignant hyperthermia they must be tested. This is done with a halothane and caffeine induced contracture of a muscle specimen.

CONCLUSION

Anaesthetic practice is a vast subject. It is impossible in one chapter to cover every aspect, but here the principles have been examined. The work has been supported by the evidence available to enable the reader to develop their knowledge further by indicating the breadth and depth of information upon which they can base and develop their practice.

REFERENCES

Aitkenhead AR (2001) Intravenous anaesthetic induction agents. In: Aitkenhead AR, Rowbotham DJ and Smith G (eds) *Textbook of Anaesthesia*, 4th edn. London: Churchill Livingstone.

Andrews PLR (1992) Physiology of nausea and vomiting. *British Journal of Anaesthesia* 69 (Suppl 1): 2s–19s.

Ankcorn C and Casey WF (1993) *Spinal Analgesia – A Practical Guide*. Issue 3 http://www.nda.ox.ac.uk

Association of Anaesthetists of Great Britain and Ireland (1989) *Assistance for the Anaesthetist*. London: The Association of Anaesthetists of Great Britain and Ireland.

Association of Anaesthetists of Great Britain and Ireland (1997) *Checklist for Anaesthetic Apparatus*. London: The Association of Anaesthetists of Great Britain and Ireland.

Association of Anaesthetists of Great Britain and Ireland (2000) *Recommendations for Standards of Monitoring during Anaesthesia and Recovery*. London: Association of Anaesthetists for Great Britain and Ireland.

Bailey R (1995) What's in a name? *Nursing Standard* 10(8): 23–24.

Berger CW, Crosby ET and Grodecki W (1998) North American survey of the management of dural puncture occurring during labour analgesia. *Canadian Journal of Anaesthesia* 45(2): 110–114.

Breivik H (1999) Infectious complications of epidural anaesthesia and analgesia. *Current Opinion in Anaesthesiology* 12(5): 573–577.

Brimacombe J (1993) The laryngeal mask airway: tool for airway management. *Journal of Post-Anesthesia Nursing* 8(2): 88–95.

British Hypertension Society and the Practitioners Hypertension Association (1997) *Blood Pressure Measurement. Recommended Techniques*. London: St George's Hospital.

Brown GW, Patel N and Ellis FR (1991) Comparison of propofol and thiopentone for laryngeal mask insertion. *Anaesthesia* 46(9): 771–772.

Cerf C, Mesguish M, Gabriel I, Amselem S and Duvaldestin P (2002) Screening patients with prolonged neuromuscular blockade after succinylcholine and mivacurium. *Anesthesia Analgesia* 94(2): 461–466.

Cheong MA, Kim KS and Choi WJ (2002) Ephedrine reduces the pain from propofol injection. *Anesthesia Analgesia* 95(5): 1293–1296.

Clinton H (2003) Haemodynamic monitoring in theatre. *British Journal of Anaesthetic and Recovery Nursing* 4(1): 10–16.

Cook TM and Morris J (2002) Use of thiopental for rapid sequence induction – a reply. *Anesthesia* 57(4): 414–415.

Croft PR and Cruickshank JK (1990) Blood pressure measurement in adults: large cuffs for all? *Journal of Epidemiological and Community Health* 44(2): 170–173.

Darovic GO (2002) *Haemodynamic Monitoring: Invasive and Noninvasive Clinical Application*, 3rd edn. Philadelphia: WB Saunders.

Davies P and Warwick J (2001) Regurgitation, vomiting and aspiration. *Anaesthesia and Intensive Care Medicine* 2(9): 358–361.

Dawson PR and Cockroft S (1996) Anaesthesia and aspiration pneumonitis. *British Journal of Theatre Nursing* 6(6): 37–39.

Ding Z and White PF (2002) Anesthesia for electroconvulsive therapy. *Anesthesia Analgesia* 94(5): 1351–1364.

Donati F (1995) Physiology: nerve, junction and muscle. In: Harper NJN and Pollard BJ (eds) *Muscle Relaxants in Anaesthesia*. London: Edward Arnold.

Erickson KM, Keegan MT, Kamath GS and Harrison BA (2002) The use of the intubating laryngeal mask endotracheal tube with intubating devices. *Anesthesia and Analgesia* 95(1): 249–250.

Fox N (2002) Pulse oximetry. *Nursing Times* 98(40): 65.

Fryer JM (2001) Intravenous induction agents. *Anaesthesia and Intensive Care Medicine* 2(7): 277–281.

Hand H (1999) Cardiopulmonary resuscitation: the laryngeal mask airway. *Nursing Standard* 13(43): 48–54.

Harper NJN (1995a) Suxemethonium. In: Harper NJN and Pollard BJ (eds) *Muscle Relaxants in Anaesthesia*. London: Edward Arnold.

Harper NJN (1995b) Reversal of neuromuscular blockade. In: Harper NJN and Pollard BJ (eds) *Muscle Relaxants in Anaesthesia*. London: Edward Arnold.

Harrop-Griffiths W (2001) Spinal anaesthesia. *Anaesthesia and Intensive Care Medicine* 2(3): 103–106.

Hartsilver EL and Vanner RG (2000) Airway obstruction with cricoid pressure. *Anaesthesia* 55(3): 208–211.

Hatchett R (2002) Clinical observation and monitoring devices. In: Hatchett R and Thompson D (eds) *Cardiac Nursing. A Comprehensive Guide.* Edinburgh: Churchill Livingstone.

Hatfield A and Tronson M (2001) *The Complete Recovery Room Book*, 3rd edn. Oxford: Oxford University Press.

Hill DW and Summers R (1994) *Medical Technology – A Nursing Perspective*. London: Chapman and Hall.

Hobbs G (2001) Complications during anaesthesia. In: Aitkenhead AR, Rowbotham DJ and Smith G (eds) *Textbook of Anaesthesia*, 4th edn. London: Churchill Livingstone.

Hopkins PM (2000) Malignant hyperthermia: advances in clinical management and diagnosis. *British Journal of Anaesthesia* 85(1): 118–128.

Hunter JM (2001) Muscle function and neuromuscular blockade. In: Aitkenhead AR, Rowbotham DJ and Smith G (eds) *Textbook of Anaesthesia*, 4th edn. London: Churchill Livingstone.

Huszar RJ (2002) *Basic Dysrhythmias: Interpretation and Management*, 3rd edn. London: Mosby.

Jacobson C (1998) Protocols for practice: applying research at the bedside. Bedside cardiac monitoring. *Critical Care Practitioner* 18(3): 82–85.

Jevon P and Ewens B (2002) *Monitoring the Critically Ill Patient*. Oxford: Blackwell Science.

Jowett NI and Thompson DR (2003) *Comprehensive Coronary Care*, 3rd edn. Edinburgh: Balliere Tindall.

Kallar SK and Everett LL (1993) Potential risks and preventative measures for pulmonary aspiration: new concepts in perioperative fasting guidelines. *Anesthesia Analgesia* 77(1): 171–182.

Kervin MW (2002) Residual neuromuscular blockade in the immediate postoperative period. *Journal of Perianesthesia Nursing* 17(3): 152–158.

Kindler CH, Seeberger MD and Staender SE (1998) Epidural abscess complicating epidural anaesthesia and analgesia. *Acta Anaesthesiology Scandanavia* 42(6): 614–620.

Kretz FJ (2002) The future of paediatric anaesthesia is total intravenous anaesthesia. *Current Opinion in Anesthesiology* 15(3): 305–307.

Lee A (2001) Local anaesthetic techniques. In: Aitkenhead AR, Rowbotham DJ and Smith G (eds) *Textbook of Anaesthesia*, 4th edn. London: Churchill Livingstone.

Macias A, Monedero P, Adame M, Torre W, Fidalgo I and Hidalgo F (2002) A randomized double-blind comparison of thoracic epidural ropivacaine, ropivacaine/fentanyl or bupivacaine/fentanyl for post-thoracotomy analgesia. *Anesthesia Analgesia* 95(5): 1344–1350.

MacRae W (1996) The team approach to anaesthesia. *British Journal of Theatre Nursing* 6(4): 9–10.

Maskrey N (1999) Has the rule of halves in hypertension been replaced by the rules of (almost) two-thirds and (almost) three-quarters? *Cardiology* 2(4): 12–13.

Mazoit JX and Baujard C (2002) Paediatric caudal and epidural analgesia. *Current Opinion in Anesthesiology* 15(5): 533–536.

McConnell E (2001) Applying cardiac monitor electrodes. *Nursing* 31(8): 17.

Medical Devices Agency (2001) *Tissue necrosis caused by oximeter probes*. SN 2001 (08). London: Medical Devices Agency.

Millar JM (2000) Postoperative nausea and vomiting. In: Padford NL. *Total Intravenous Anaesthesia*. Oxford: Butterworth Heinemann.

Millar JM, Rudkin GE and Hitchcock M (1997) *Practical Anaesthesia and Analgesia for Day Surgery*. Oxford: Bios.

Moriarty A (1999) ECG interpretation: misplacement of limb leads. *British Journal of Cardiology* 6(1): 50–52.

Moyes J (1998) *Pulse Oximetry: Principles and Practice*. London: BMJ Publishing.

Mushambi MC and Smith C (2001) Inhalational anaesthetic agents. In: Aitkenhead AR, Rowbotham DJ and Smith G (eds) *Textbook of Anaesthesia*, 4th edn. London: Churchill Livingstone.

NHS Management Executive (1996) *Professional Roles in Anaesthetics: A Scoping Study*. London: HMSO.

NHS Modernisation Agency (2002) *Changing workforce programme. New ways of working in health care*. London: NHS Modernisation Agency.

O'Brien E, Beevers D and Marshall H (1995) *ABC of Hypertension*. London: BMJ Publishing.

Oakley M (1999) The anaesthetic practitioners' perception of their role. *British Journal of Anaesthetic and Recovery Nursing* 5(1): 6–8.

Owens TM, Robertson P, Twomey C, Doyle M, McDonald N and McShane A (1995) The incidence of gastroesophageal reflux with the laryngeal mask: a comparison with the face mask using esophageal lumen pH electrodes. *Anesthesia and Analgesia* 80(5): 980–984.

Padford NL (2000) *Total Intravenous Anaesthesia*. Oxford: Butterworth Heinemann.

Palmer JH and Ball DR (2000) The effect of cricoid pressure on the cricoid cartilage and vocal cords: an endoscopic study in anaesthetised patients. *Anaesthesia* 55(3): 260–287.

Pleuvry BJ (2001) Opioid mechanisms and opioid drugs. *Anaesthesia and Intensive Care Medicine* 2(11): 450–455.

Poets CF, Seidenberg J and Von Der Hardt H (1993) Failure of pulse oximeter to detect sensor detachment. *Lancet* 341(8839): 244.

Pollard BJ (1995) Non depolarising muscle relaxants. In: Harper NJN and Pollard BJ (eds) *Muscle Relaxants in Anaesthesia*. London: Edward Arnold.

Roberts RG and Redman JW (2002) Etomidate, adrenal dysfunction and critical care. *Anaesthesia* 57(4): 413.

Russell R (2001) Pain relief in labour: regional, epidural and patient controlled analgesia. *Anaesthesia and Intensive Care Medicine* 2(5): 185–189.

Scott DB and Hibbard BM (1990) Serious non-fatal complications associated with extradural block in obstetric practice. *British Journal of Anaesthesia* 64(5): 537–541.

Seeberger MD, Staender S, Oertli D, Kindler CH and Marti W (1998) Efficacy of specific aseptic precautions for preventing propofol-related infections: analysis by a quality-assurance programme using the explicit outcome method. *Journal of Hospital Infection* 39(1): 67–70.

Sellick BA (1961) Cricoid pressure to control regurgitation of stomach contents during induction of anaesthesia. *Lancet* 2: 404–406.

Serpell M (2001) Inhalational analgesia anaesthesia. *Anaesthesia and Intensive Care Medicine* 2(11): 446–447.

Serpell MG, Haldene GH, Jamieson DRS and Carson D (1998) Prevention of headache after lumbar puncture: questionnaire survey of neurologists and neurosurgeons in the UK. *British Medical Journal* 316(7146): 1709–1710.

Shields L and Werder H (2002) *Perioperative Nursing*. London: Greenwich Medical Media.

Simpson PJ and Popat MT (2002) *Understanding Anaesthesia*, 4th edn. Oxford: Butterworth Heinemann.

Soliz J, Sinha A and Thakar D (2002) Airway management: a review and update. *The Internet Journal of Anesthesiology* 6(1): 1–16.

Spiers CM (2002) Arrhythmia interpretation in the perioperative arena. *British Journal of Anaesthetic and Recovery Nursing* 3(3): 12–18.

Spiers CM and Stinchcombe E (2002) An introduction to cardiac monitoring and rhythm interpretation. *British Journal of Anaesthetic and Recovery Nursing* 3(1): 8–14.

Stoelting RK and Dierdorf SF (2002) *Anesthesia and Co-Existing Disease*, 4th edn. London: Churchill Livingstone.

Stone B, Leach A, Alexander C *et al.* (1994) Results of a multicentre trial. The use of the laryngeal mask airway by practitioners during cardiopulmonary resuscitation. *Anaesthesia* 49: 3–7.

Sudlow C and Warlow C (2002) Epidural blood patching for preventing and treating post dural puncture headache. *Cochrane Review*. In: The Cochrane Library, Issue 3, Oxford. Update software found at http://www.update-software.com/CLIB

Sykes JB (ed) (1982) *The Concise Oxford Dictionary*, 7th edn. Oxford: Oxford University Press.

Thacker D and Williams TW (1997) Effect of heparinised saline versus normal saline on maintaining patency of a peripherally inserted central catheter. *National Association of Vascular Access Networks* 2(2): 16–18.

Vanner R (2001) Techniques of cricoid pressure. *Anaesthesia and Intensive Care Medicine* 2(9): 362–363.

Weksler N, Rozentsveig V, Tarnoploski A and Gurman GM (2001) Commercial propofol solutions: is the more expensive also the most effective? *Journal of Clinical Anaesthesia* 13(5): 321–324.

Williams E, Beaulieu Jenkins G and Fawcett W (1998) Efficiency of epidural blood patches in obstetrics. *Canadian Journal of Anaesthesia* 45(10): 103.

Woodrow P (1999) Pulse oximetry. *Nursing Standard* 13(42): 42–46.

Useful websites

Association of Anaesthetists of Great Britain and Ireland
www.aagbi.org

British Anaesthetic and Recovery Nurses Association
www.barna.co.uk

National Association of Theatre Nurses
www.natn.org

Royal College of Anaesthetists
www.rcoa.ac.uk

5 PRINCIPLES OF SURGICAL PRACTICE

Amanda Parker

CHAPTER AIMS

- To examine surgical aspects of infection control
- To introduce appropriate surgical equipment
- To explore issues surrounding patient care
- To discuss the need for suitable and up-to-date documentation.

INTRODUCTION

Surgery has always been practised; what has changed over the years is the extent of surgery and its complexity, from Homer's reference to battlefield surgery in 800 BC, to bladder and plastic surgery operations in India in 650 AD, with the first manual of surgery produced by Paracelsus, 'Die Kleine Chirurgia' in 1528. Today's surgery has developed from the days of the barber to advanced techniques including the use of lasers, endoscopes and microscopes. Surgical techniques now allow 'free tissue transfer' due to advances in microsurgical techniques and cardiac surgery to the 'beating heart' rather than utilising bypass techniques. These techniques and others allow surgery to benefit individuals who may previously not have been offered this option.

The advances in perioperative care and the use of evidence-based practice ensure that care throughout the perioperative period is optimal. Also appreciation of the morbid events that affect the outcome of surgery, specifically inadvertent hypothermia and pressure injuries, improve the quality of care.

Throughout surgery there has been the presence of an assistant to the surgeon. This is currently a surgical practitioner, either a nurse or operating department practitioner. Their role is multifunctional, to provide quality care for individual patients, manage resources related to surgical episodes, act as the patient's advocate, all the time ensuring that teamworking is practised.

This chapter intends to explore further some of the principles that aid in enabling the success of surgery and without which would result in an increase in the morbidity or mortality of surgical patients.

INFECTION CONTROL

Infection control within the theatre environment covers a vast area. This section intends to review basic infection control issues within the environment, explore infection transmission and examine how the obtaining and maintaining of a sterile field reduces the risk of transmission. Finally sterilisation and disinfection methods in current use will be discussed.

Management of infection control is the responsibility of all staff under health and safety guidelines (Health and Safety Executive 1999); therefore it essential that everyone has a good understanding of the rationale behind practice and takes individual responsibility for implementing policies. Policies and guidelines should be in place to guide individuals, minimising the risk of infection transmission to both staff and patients.

Design of the operating theatre has an impact on the ability of the environment to prevent the transmission of infection. Ventilation, humidity and baseline temperature all affect the presence and spread of micro-organisms within the operating environment. Assuming that these factors are externally controlled, what actions could surgical practitioners take to affect the incidence of surgical infections?

In the 1500s Fracastorius stated that disease was spread via three methods: direct contact;

handling articles that infected patients had handled; and distance transmission. Today the focus remains the same; it is recognised that there is a chain of events that needs to be broken to prevent transmission (Figure 5.1). Transmission of infection requires: the presence of a pathogenic organism; a reservoir; method of exit-transmission; portal of entry; plus susceptibility of the host. Only by breaking this chain can infection be prevented.

While environmental design is out of the practitioner's control, the management of reservoirs is certainly within their domain. Surgical practitioners can ensure that zoning for unrestricted, semi-restricted and restricted access is fully maintained. They must ensure that within all these areas adequate cleaning of the environment occurs; this is essential to break the reservoir link of the chain. This requires the removal of obvious surface dirt and the thorough disinfection of floors. Additionally, in restricted areas the scrubbing of floors daily and

disinfection of all equipment and surfaces is required (Woodhead *et al.* 2002).

There should be liaison with the hospital infection control team and an evidence-based department policy devised. Where new staff are introduced, the provision of education and the use of competencies ensures their understanding of the environmental cleaning requirements, plus the impact of their non-compliance with policies. In addition to routine cleaning there should be local policies on the management of spillages that prevent these from acting as a reservoir of infection.

Equipment is a reservoir that potentially places patients at risk and practitioners have the responsibility for ensuring that all equipment used during surgery is sterile. Methods of sterilisation will be examined later. Besides ensuring equipment is sterile prior to use, practitioners need to maintain its sterility when handing to a sterile area, additionally ensuring that they retain appropriate information to ensure traceability of the equipment at a later date. For much equipment this requires the retention of the adhesive label supplied by their sterile service provider. Where departmental equipment is used for sterilisation, this may entail noting date and time of activation, length of immersion and staff members involved. However equipment has been sterilised prior to use, this information should be made available within each individual patient's notes. This demonstrates good practice, ensures standards are maintained and provides a resource for identifying equipment used on individuals should recall of equipment or patients be required.

Following use equipment still remains a reservoir, having the potential to place other patients and staff at risk. All equipment once finished with should be removed from the surgical site, handled with gloves and returned to the sterile service supplier as soon as possible to allow decontamination to occur. Supplementary sharps such as blades, needles etc. should be handled with care, placed in a neutral zone on the practitioner's trolley, and a solid disposal case used.

Practitioners, patients and other staff within the perioperative environment are potential reservoirs of infection. It is each practitioner's

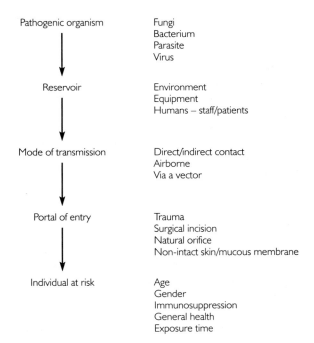

Chain of infection

Pathogenic organism	Fungi
	Bacterium
	Parasite
	Virus
Reservoir	Environment
	Equipment
	Humans – staff/patients
Mode of transmission	Direct/indirect contact
	Airborne
	Via a vector
Portal of entry	Trauma
	Surgical incision
	Natural orifice
	Non-intact skin/mucous membrane
Individual at risk	Age
	Gender
	Immunosuppression
	General health
	Exposure time

Figure 5.1 Chain of infection

responsibility to recognise and report any infection or open lesion that may place susceptible individuals at risk. They should also recognise that infection or open lesions place themselves in the position of being the susceptible recipient of pathogenic organisms.

Transmission

Contact, be it direct or indirect, is essential to manage when attempting to break the infection chain. The wearing of gloves is good practice but only if worn appropriately, i.e. when at risk of being in contact with blood or body fluids. Once gloves have been in contact they should be discarded and hands washed before commencing other activities. Good quality hand hygiene is regarded as the single most important factor and essential in combating spread of infection (Meeker and Rothrock 1999). It is recognised that it is the quality of washing and sufficient drying rather than the cleaning product used that reduces the potential of spreading infection (Davey and Ince 2000). All staff should remember that good hand hygiene not only protects patients but also individuals and their work colleagues.

Other methods of transmission that specifically affect staff are splashes and aerosolisation during surgery; this could be from irrigation, drills or the transfer of specimens. To protect themselves all staff should be routinely wearing facemasks and goggles and local policies should be in place.

Airborne

The dispersion of microbes is increased with movement, the majority of these microbes from staff (Woodhead *et al.* 2002). Practical aspects to reduce dissemination require the reduction of movement. During surgery doors should remain closed preventing the ingress of corridor air plus utilising only the required number of staff for surgery and restricting the number and movement of visitors.

While it is recognised that practitioners cannot affect the ventilation system in place, they should ensure it is working on the day of surgery. Those practising in areas with laminar flow have additional responsibilities to ensure they utilise it effectively and contain all trolleys and equipment within the laminar flow area.

Vector

A vector may be any mechanical agent that picks up an infectious agent and then carries it to a susceptible host. Glove powder is considered a vector, though powdered gloves are now not used. In surgery practitioners need to be aware of the principles of vector contamination (McCulloch 2001).

Portal of entry

Patients undergoing a surgical incision all have a potential entry site for infection. Those who arrive for surgery following a traumatic accident will have increased their opportunity for infection

---

PRACTICE EXEMPLAR 5.1: CONTAMINATED GLOVES

Mr X, a patient with a chest infection requiring emergency surgery, was admitted to theatre. The theatre practitioner donned a pair of gloves and assisted with cannulation and intubation of Mr X. Once in theatre while wearing the same gloves the theatre practitioner removed the temporary dressing applied to Mr X's wound. While removing the dressing the oxygen saturation probe fell to the ground so the practitioner immediately replaced it to ensure monitoring continued.

Mr X's wound was placed at risk from direct contact; the practitioner may have contaminated their gloves during cannulation or intubation. The direct contact may have placed Mr X or other staff or patients at risk once contaminated gloves were used to handle the saturation probe.

Within your own work area – stop and look, observe practitioners' practice with their hands. Do they remove gloves? Do they contaminate equipment? Do they wash their hands?

development due to contamination of the wound. Additionally patients with multiple injuries develop the risk of contamination from one site to another. With multiple operation sites the scrub practitioner can influence and reduce the risk of cross-site contamination by preparing wound sites in a logical sequence, starting with the least contaminated or from a non-open surgical site.

Natural orifices are also an entry site for infection; therefore staff should ensure they remain vigilant during procedures that involve any natural body opening. Opportunities remain frequent with endotracheal tubes inserted nasally/orally, urinary catheters and cystoscopes used urethrally, and gastroscopes used via the oesophagus, to name a few opportunities for the introduction of infection. Alongside the protection of patients, staff must remain vigilant for their own wellbeing, protecting open wounds that may act as an entry gate.

Individuals at risk

Those who may be at risk from infection are wide and varied, an individual's general health and nutritional state playing a large part. Those whose risk is increased are young children due to their immature immune system, the elderly who have a diminished immune response so cannot respond appropriately to infection, and those whose immune system has been damaged or compromised. Additionally others whose immune system may be affected and thus susceptible to infection are those who have undergone a large emotional or physical stress. This would include those involved in a major trauma, major burns or those undergoing extensive surgery. Patients considered not to be at risk initially may become at risk due to local factors affecting blood supply to a wound, such as oedema or ischaemia (McCulloch 1999). The longer the length of surgery the more there is an increased risk of infection due to the opportunities from exposure to the environment, the invasive use of equipment and handling of body tissue.

Combined with the principles of infection control is the need to obtain and maintain a sterile field for surgical procedures. Actions to this effect will enable a break in the transmission of infection.

OBTAINING AND MAINTAINING A STERILE FIELD

The obtaining and maintaining of a sterile field is designed to reduce the risk of infection transmission to individual patients and at the same time to protect staff from infection. This is achieved by combining a number of practices: staff dress and preparation; patient preparation; utilisation of sterile equipment; and etiquette during surgery.

Staff dress

All staff working within the theatre complex commence their day by changing into a cotton-based theatre suit, with trousers preferable to skirts to reduce the shedding of skin cells to the environment. Shoes must be impervious to allow for cleaning, protect toes and enable safe working practice. Therefore backless shoes/clogs are not suitable as there is the risk of stepping out. Theatre caps are provided for all staff to wear to prevent the shedding of hair, though the evidence would suggest that this is only a requirement for scrubbed staff or those working within laminar flow theatres during implant surgery (Woodhead *et al.* 2002). Scrub staff clothing during surgery consists additionally of masks, eye protection, and following scrubbing the donning of gowns and gloves.

Masks

Masks are donned prior to scrubbing and while their benefit in preventing infection is questionable they do prevent bacterial shedding onto the wound site (Woodhead *et al.* 2002) though an alternative view is that the wearing of masks causes rubbing and the release of potentially harmful skin flakes (Xavier 1999). Currently there is insufficient research to prove or disprove either theory. Recommendations indicate that all staff involved in prosthetic implant surgery under laminar flow should wear masks to protect the patient (Woodhead *et al.* 2002). Where masks are worn they should be changed at the end of each case.

Masks provide the wearer with protection from body fluid and blood splashes, also providing protection from inhaling smoke and laser plume. The wearing of masks by scrub staff following risk assessment of invasive procedures is that masks should be worn at all times by all scrub staff (Health and Safety Commission 1999).

Eye protection

Eye protection is donned prior to scrubbing and may be in the form of a visor, spectacle or goggle. Though not worn to protect the patient they protect the scrubbed individual from penetration injury, conjunctival contact with blood or body fluid splashes, or aerosolisation (Collins *et al.* 2000). The increasing usage of power tools and lavage would suggest following risk assessment that for the majority of surgical cases scrubbed staff should wear eye protection.

Scrubbing

Preoperative hand scrubbing is used to reduce the bacteria count on the hands of scrub staff and is the first defence for preventing transmission of pathogens. Prior to scrubbing all jewellery with the exception of a single plain band should be removed as they may be a source of micro-organisms (AORN 1999). The wearing of false nails should be prohibited due to the evidence supporting the presence of pathogens (Hedderwick *et al.* 2000). For the same reason the wearing of nail polish should also be prohibited (Schroeter 1998). The recommended length of scrub time remains debatable and is influenced by the antimicrobial agent used, two minutes viewed as the minimum time acceptable. The first scrub of the day must include cleaning beneath the nails (AORN 1999).

Methodology of scrubbing should ensure that hands and arms are scrubbed effectively from fingertips to elbows and that hands are held higher than elbows. Subsequent hand cleaning can utilise an alcoholic hand rub (Jones *et al.* 2000; Woodhead *et al.* 2000; AORN 1999).

Gowns

Gowns are worn during sterile procedures to prevent bacteria from the scrubbed practitioner passing through the fabric to the environment or

Box 5.1

Consider the scrub practices within your workplace:

- Do you have policies in place for all staff to follow?
- Is there compliance with these policies – if not why not?
- What can you as an individual do to improve your practice and the practice of others?

the operation site. When wet the fabric needs to prevent the transfer of bacteria through the fabric.

Gowns currently supplied are made from polyester cotton, microfilament or a disposable impermeable material. Best practice would suggest that only gowns that are waterproof and disposable should be used (Woodhead *et al.* 2002). Where material gowns are used they should be checked for faults and aprons worn underneath to protect the wearer from contamination. Microfilament gowns should be checked for faults, observed for strike-through and monitored to ensure appropriate disposal following the maximum number of uses. Gowns may be back-fastening or wrap around. Back-fastening gowns should never be exposed to the operation site as the area is unprotected. Wrap around gowns should only be considered sterile at the commencement of a procedure; after this they are at risk of contamination and are not visible to the wearer (Meeker and Rothrock 1999). All gowns are supplied sterile and donned following the scrubbing of hands. They should be handled with dry hands, by the inside only, then assistance given to secure by a circulator. Hands do not protrude from the cuffs until gloves have been donned.

While the main rationale for gown wearing is to protect the patient, they have the additional benefit of providing protection to the wearer from contamination from blood or body fluids. Theatre gowns are considered as medical devices and in the future will have to comply with legal minimum standards. These standards will include wet and dry microbial penetration and a requirement to meet performance standards in relation to wet and dry tensile strength and resistance to penetration and linting (Line 2003). The same regulations will apply to drapes as these are also considered to be medical devices.

Gloves

Gloves are worn to create a barrier that prevents the transmission of pathogens to the patient and also to protect the wearer from contamination from blood or body fluids. Gloves should be donned using the closed glove technique; this allows the glove to be handled only through the gown, preventing contamination. Once applied, the gloves should fully cover the cuffs of the gown.

Surgical gloves are generally manufactured from latex because of its effective barrier properties. Due to the increase in latex allergies suffered by both staff and patients alike there are now latex-free alternatives available for use by latex-allergic staff or for use during surgery on a latex-allergic individual. (Latex allergy is covered later in this chapter.)

Evidence demonstrates that the wearing of double gloves, though reducing manual dexterity and sensation, increases protection to the wearer from needlestick injuries (Patterson *et al.* 1998) and reduces hand contamination (Fisher *et al.* 1999). The patient is also increasingly protected from glove leaks.

Once fully dressed, only the areas below the shoulders, above the waist and from the elbow to the hands are considered sterile. Therefore posture and positioning by the practitioner should support this. Hands should remain below the shoulders and above the waist without folding them under the arms; elbows should be held close to the body and unless surgery is to be performed in a seated position, practitioners should avoid sitting or leaning on unsterile surfaces (Meeker and Rothrock 1999).

On completion of surgery all equipment worn must be removed without contaminating the wearer or other individuals, disposed of correctly or decontaminated if appropriate. Handwashing or the use of an alcoholic hand rub should then decontaminate hands.

Patient preparation

Patient preparation incorporates skin preparing and draping. Shaving of skin prior to surgery has been shown to cause injury and increase infection risk. Studies demonstrate that where possible patients who require hair removal to provide access to the incision site should (where possible) use a depilatory cream on the day prior to surgery, otherwise clippers should be used to remove hair (Woodhead *et al.* 2002).

Skin preparation at the time of surgery is performed to prevent bacteria entering the incision site. Solutions used vary widely but they should all be rapidly effective, broad spectrum and effective against both Gram-negative and Gram-positive bacteria plus fungi and viruses. They need to remain active when in contact with blood or body fluids/secretions/excretions. No known toxic or allergic solutions should be used on an individual. Solutions should ideally be available in single-use containers. Ideally only one solution should be applied to prevent inactivation. Current recommendation is that alcoholic solutions are the most effective, though care must be taken to prevent pooling and time allowed to ensure the solution is dry prior to application of the drapes or the use of electrocautery – due to the risk of combustion (Woodhead *et al.* 2002). Additionally pooling under pneumatic tourniquets, around ECG electrodes and diathermy plates can result in chemical burn injury to the patient (Choudhary *et al.* 1998).

Preparation should not commence until all non-scrubbed staff have completed all care requirements for the individual. Prior to commencing the scrub, the practitioner needs to have ensured the patient has no allergy to the solution to be applied.

Cleansing commences with the cleanest area moving to less clean areas, working from the incision site outwards, unless this is a contaminated area (NATN 1998a). Where open wounds, or areas such as anus or vagina, are to be prepared, these areas are prepared last, the sponges used once and immediately discarded. Following skin preparation all sponges and holders are discarded and never returned to the instrument

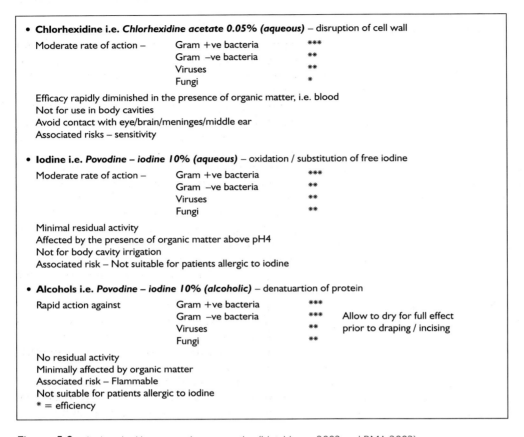

- **Chlorhexidine i.e. *Chlorhexidine acetate 0.05% (aqueous)*** – disruption of cell wall

Moderate rate of action –	Gram +ve bacteria	***
	Gram –ve bacteria	**
	Viruses	**
	Fungi	*

  Efficacy rapidly diminished in the presence of organic matter, i.e. blood
  Not for use in body cavities
  Avoid contact with eye/brain/meninges/middle ear
  Associated risks – sensitivity

- **Iodine i.e. *Povodine – iodine 10% (aqueous)*** – oxidation / substitution of free iodine

Moderate rate of action –	Gram +ve bacteria	***
	Gram –ve bacteria	**
	Viruses	**
	Fungi	**

  Minimal residual activity
  Affected by the presence of organic matter above pH4
  Not for body cavity irrigation
  Associated risk – Not suitable for patients allergic to iodine

- **Alcohols i.e. *Povodine – iodine 10% (alcoholic)*** – denatuartion of protein

Rapid action against	Gram +ve bacteria	***	
	Gram –ve bacteria	***	Allow to dry for full effect
	Viruses	**	prior to draping / incising
	Fungi	**	

  No residual activity
  Minimally affected by organic matter
  Associated risk – Flammable
  Not suitable for patients allergic to iodine
  * = efficiency

Figure 5.2 Antiseptic skin preparation properties (Hutchinson 2002 and BMA 2003)

trolley (Meeker and Rothrock 1999). Care must be taken to ensure spongeholder tips are protected, solutions are not allowed to pool and any wet linen/protection is removed prior to draping.

The use of adhesive sheets with or without antiseptic impregnation and wound guards to prevent postoperative wound infection and intra-operative contamination have been shown to provide no clear benefits to patients in either the prevention of postoperative infection or in reduction of contamination; therefore their use can be questioned (Woodhead *et al.* 2002).

Draping

As with gowns, theatre drapes should prevent bacteria from the scrubbed practitioner or from non-sterile areas of the patient passing through the fabric to the environment or the operation site. Should the fabric become wet it needs to prevent the transfer of bacteria through the fabric. Drapes are supplied currently made from cotton fabric, microfilament or a disposable impermeable material. Best practice would suggest that only drapes that are waterproof and disposable should be used (Woodhead *et al.* 2002). Where material drapes are used they should be checked for faults and protection applied underneath to protect the patient from self-contamination and to protect the skin from excess moisture. With microfilament gowns these should be checked for faults, observed for strike-through and monitored to ensure that following the maximum number of uses they are disposed of.

Before applying drapes, skin preparation solutions should have been allowed to dry. Care must be taken with adhesive drapes to ensure patients have no allergies. Where drapes have no adhesive they should be secured using towel clips that do not perforate the fabric. Additional care should be taken to ensure that the patient's skin is not injured by the use of towel clips.

When applying drapes practitioners should ensure they have sufficient drapes folded and prepared. These need to be held at waist height until placed on the patient with controlled movements that minimally disturb the air, ideally by two people to reduce the risk of contaminating the drapes or practitioners involved. Practitioners need to protect their hands by folding the drape over them to prevent contamination. Draping commences from the incision site working out towards the peripheries. Once in place drapes should not be moved; any drape below the edge of the operating table is considered unsterile (Meeker and Rothrock 1999).

Drapes should not be removed until the completion of surgery and until after the application of the wound dressings. Drapes should then be removed and disposed appropriately by the scrub practitioner; this prevents contamination of others and ensures that all equipment has been removed prior to drape removal.

Utilisation of sterile equipment

Prior to the commencement of surgery all required and anticipated equipment for surgery is collected and checked for sterility. The scrub practitioner prepares the equipment once scrubbed in a sterile manner ensuring at all times the sterile integrity of equipment. If any set is found to contain moisture on opening it is discarded, as its sterility cannot be guaranteed. Any equipment found to be contaminated is discarded; if this is a part of a tray the whole tray is discarded. The circulating practitioner ensures that they maintain a wide berth around the sterile trolley and provide all supplementary equipment to the scrub practitioner in a manner that maintains sterility. Preparation of equipment should only occur immediately prior to commencement of surgery; this reduces the risk of contamination of equipment to be used. All equipment should be laid out in a manner that facilitates ease of recognition and availability for immediate use.

Once at the operating table all trolleys and tables should be positioned adjacent to the operating table ensuring access to the surgeon. Positioning also needs to ensure there is sufficient space around the trolleys to reduce the risk of contamination of equipment or practitioners. When positioning care must be taken to ensure no pressure is placed on any part of the patient. During use all equipment should be replaced on trolleys or tables to reduce the risk of equipment falling to the floor or becoming contaminated in error.

Equipment used to removed tumours or used on 'dirty' areas, for example open bowel, should be used for these areas only and contained on separate trolleys or separate demarcated areas of a trolley. They must only be used on these areas and not moved to potentially contaminate other surgical areas.

Following completion of surgery, once all equipment is accounted for it is immediately sent for decontamination following hospital policy.

Theatre etiquette

Once in theatre and operating has commenced there are etiquettes that should be maintained. Some of these assist in maintaining the sterile field, others in reducing the introduction of infection while some simply aim to maintain order and control.

In relation to maintaining a sterile field, once scrubbed, practitioners should where possible position their trolley close to the surgical site and opposite the operating surgeon. This allows easy access for the passing of instrumentation and close observation of the operation site, increasing the scrub practioner's ability to anticipate surgical requirements. Once scrubbed, practitioners should ensure they pass back-to-back to keep the gown fronts sterile. Other health-care workers within the theatre environment should desist from passing between the patient and scrubbed staff; this avoids accidental desterilisation of scrubbed practitioners and also of the sterile field.

To reduce air movement within theatre and reduce the risk of turbulence of room air and the risk of contaminating sterile areas, staff should reduce general movement as much as possible. Theatre doors should remain closed during any procedure and opening and closing of theatre doors should be kept to a minimum.

Lines of communication need to remain open. Etiquette would suggest that at times general conversation or radios might disturb the operating surgeon; conversely music may enhance the operating atmosphere for both the surgeon and patient. Practitioners therefore need to be sensitive to the needs of operating surgeons and of the appropriateness of music and conversation. When messages need to be passed to the operating surgeon, best practice is to approach the scrubbed practitioner to impart the message or to request whether it is an appropriate time to interrupt surgery.

STERILISATION AND DISINFECTION

Patients admitted for surgery expect to find a clean, safe environment and to be protected from preventable infections. All practitioners have a professional responsibility to ensure that where possible practices in relation to sterilisation and disinfection are carried out and monitored.

Decontamination

Cleaning, disinfection and sterilisation are all forms of decontamination. Decontamination is

Box 5.2

- Within your work area, observe the amount of movement by practitioners and the frequency of door opening during one surgical procedure.
- Consider why the movement/door opening took place and whether action could have been taken prior to surgery commencing to avoid this.

Box 5.3

- Write a short description of decontamination, cleaning, disinfection and sterilisation.
- Identify methodologies within each process and when it is appropriate to utilise a specific process.

Many individuals, while using these terms, are unaware of their meaning and when each process should be utilised.

---

the process that removes organic matter and removes or destroys micro-organisms, allowing equipment to then be safe for handling or for use on patients. Methods used for decontamination on equipment are dependent upon the equipment's susceptibility to heat, chemicals, moisture and corrosion. Equipment design is also relevant, if it is fine-bored or porous. Other factors that may affect the process instigated are time, cost and safety.

Cleaning

Cleaning is a process that physically removes contamination, namely, dirt, grease, tissue etc. and does not necessarily destroy micro-organisms. It is essential to perform before disinfection or sterilisation of equipment as physical contamination reduces the ability of disinfectants or sterilants to achieve contact with the equipment. Failure to perform cleaning prior to disinfection and sterilisation places patients at risk of infection and thus potentially an increased hospital stay, an increased risk of mortality plus increased costs to the hospital. Additionally, practitioners and sterile service staff handling equipment are placed at increased risk of acquiring infections. Further consequences to equipment will result if cleaning is not performed, resulting in blockage of fine-bore equipment or malfunction. Cleaning may be performed manually; here appropriate protection should be worn: gloves, aprons and goggles. Cleaning may also be carried out with automated washers utilising water, detergent and heat, or ultrasonic cleaners where cavitation agitates the liquid and results in cleaning (Parkhouse and Warwick 2001). Cleaning as a final process is appropriate for use where there is low risk, items do not come into contact with patients, or with healthy skin. Therefore the process is suitable for items such as furniture, walls and floors. In some instances disinfection may be preferable.

Disinfection

Disinfection results in the reduction of viable micro-organisms to the extent they are not harmful to health. Disinfection does not achieve the same microbial reduction as sterilisation and does not inactivate some 'slow' viruses or bacterial spores. The main methods of disinfection are: boiling; washer disinfectors; chemical disinfection; and low-temperature steam.

Disinfection is suitable where there is an intermediate risk, i.e. contact with mucous membranes during endoscopy or for respiratory equipment, though in some instances sterilisation may be preferable.

- **Boiling** should occur in soft water at 100°C for 5 minutes; items should then be allowed to dry and cool. This lack of rigour, the time allowing for recontamination, and risk of injury from boiling water renders this method inappropriate within the surgical setting.
- **Washer disinfectors** achieve physical cleaning with heat disinfection of equipment. All micro-organisms bar some heat-resistant viruses and bacterial spores are inactivated.
- **Chemical disinfection** may be achieved via a washer disinfector that utilises chemicals:
  - Chlorine dioxide (Tristel®) – rapidly bacteriocidal, virucidal and – mycobactericidal; high level disinfection is achieved in 5 minutes and sporicidal in 10 minutes.
  - Electrolysed water (Sterilox™) – freshly generated solutions are sporicidal and mycobactericidal. The solution is produced by electrolysing a salt solution.
  - Glutaraldehyde 2% (Cidex®) – most bacteria and viruses are inactivated in 10 minutes. Mycobacteria require 20 minutes

and spores 3 hours. Potential harm to practitioners is well-recognised and use is being curtailed within most surgical areas and alternatives used.
  - Peracetic acid (Nu Cidex®) – bacteriocidal, virucidal and mycobactericidal within 5 minutes and sporicidal within 10 minutes.

For all chemical disinfectants practitioners should be aware of COSHH (Control of Substances Hazardous to Health) implications for staff. They should also be aware whether the chemical disinfectant of choice is corrosive to the equipment to be immersed and that all equipment should be rinsed to remove toxic residues prior to use. The advantage of chemical disinfectants is that they can be used at the point of use, although practitioners should be able to apply traceability principles in case an infection develops requiring patient or equipment recall. When using chemically disinfected equipment on patients, equality of care should be practised. If some patients have sterilised equipment while others receive similar equipment that has been disinfected, this demonstrates that patients are receiving differing standards of care.

Further chemical disinfectants available are hypochlorites. Different concentrations achieve differing outcomes, for example when used for blood spillages and environmental disinfection. Alcohol is bacteriocidal and mycobactericidal, but is not active against spores and has the advantage of leaving surfaces dry. Solutions of 60% and 70% (isopropanolol and ethanol) are more effective than absolute alcohol. Care is required due to flammability (Steer 2002).

Sterilisation

Sterilisation achieves inactivation of micro-organisms including viruses and bacterial spores. Sterilisation is required where there is a high risk to individuals, i.e. where equipment is introduced into a normally closed body cavity or is in contact with broken skin/membranes. Therefore surgical equipment and sundries require sterilising. It can be achieved via a number of methods including:

- **Dry heat sterilisation** – Here temperatures need to reach 160°C for 2 hours, 170°C for 1 hour or 180°C for 30 minutes. This method is used for the sterilisation of solids, non-aqueous liquids and items damaged by steam. The main disadvantage of the method is the length of cycle time and the temperature that may affect items containing some rubbers and plastics.
- **Ethylene oxide** – This is active against bacteria, viruses and spores though it is toxic, irritant, explosive and expensive. Microbiological monitoring is required to ensure efficacy of the process, therefore use is generally limited to industrial use with single-use plastic items frequently sterilised by this method.
- **Irradiation** – used industrially to sterilise single-use items. Gamma rays or electron beams are used to achieve sterilisation.
- **Low temperature steam and formaldehyde** – dry saturated steam and formaldehyde are used together at sub-atmospheric pressures to kill bacteria, spores and most viruses. Hollow items may be damaged due to the pressure, and formaldehyde is corrosive to some materials. A process that is toxic and irritant, and expensive.
- **Steam** – This is effective, non-toxic and non-corrosive. This form of sterilisation is achieved within an autoclave where steam is placed under pressure and air removed. Air may be removed by displacement or vacuum. Direct contact needs to occur between the steam and the items for sterilisation. Autoclaves reach 134°C for three minutes or 121°C for 15 minutes to achieve sterilisation. Equipment that is wrapped is managed within porous load autoclaves where air is removed by vacuum, so allowing steam to penetrate wrapping and also hollow items. Performance testing monitors the effectiveness of autoclaving with visual evidence available to end-users via indicators/tape that changes colour on completion of effective processing.
- **Sporicidal chemicals** (discussed previously), though considered disinfectants can act as sterilising agents if used for an extended period of time. Sporicidal chemicals that may be used

include: chlorine dioxide – sporicidal in 10 minutes; glutaraldehyde 2% – sporicidal in 3–10 hours; and peracetic acid – sporicidal in 10 minutes (Wilson and Jacobson 1999).

When any form of sterilisation has been used on surgical equipment and sundries all practitioners need to be aware of observing indicators and expiry dates of equipment and ensure these are monitored prior to use of equipment to reduce the potential risk to patients. Where tracing is applicable, local policies should be followed to ensure patients or equipment can be recalled in the future. Practitioners additionally have a responsibility to ensure that all single-use items are used for their original purpose and disposed of, not returned to sterile service departments for resterilisation (MDA 2000).

EQUIPMENT

Equipment required during surgery is wide and varied; this section intends to examine suture and instrument design that caters for a wide variety of surgical requirements. Individuals need to be aware of the physical properties of the variety of suture materials available for use and alternatives that may be available, plus the body's response to the various materials used. With regard to instruments, practitioners need to be aware of what an instrument is designed for to avoid inappropriate use and thus injury to patients or damage to the instrument resulting in costly repair or replacement bills. The use of electrosurgery and laser equipment will also be explored, highlighting the need for practitioner knowledge in order to prevent injury to patients when using these pieces of equipment.

Sutures

The use of sutures enables wound closure and allows for the removal of dead space, realignment of tissue planes and the securing of tissue edges until healing by first intention has occurred (Castille 1998). This section will examine suture use in more detail, though practitioners should also be aware of other closure methods available i.e. tissue adhesive, staples and adhesive strips. Whatever the choice of closure material, practitioners should be knowledgeable as to the properties of the option of choice and of the alternatives should the first choice be unavailable. Thought should be given to any tissue reaction, the final cosmetic result and removal. The age of the patient may be a significant factor; paediatric patients require a smaller suture size than adults, and dependent upon age the method of removal should be considered. Older patients require consideration, as their skin may be less elastic, more friable and prone to bruising or damage; these changes are dependent upon age, concurrent disease or pharmacological agents.

Suture categories

Sutures are divided into two categories: absorbable and non-absorbable.

Absorbable sutures are designed to hold the wound together and withhold normal stresses until healing has occurred. Presentation is as a synthetic material, which is hydrolysed by body fluids; it may be a braided or monofilament suture. Length of time taken to be hydrolysed will vary; dependent upon the suture of choice the minimal time varies from 40 to 90 days, with complete absorption varying from 60 to 210 days.

Non-absorbable sutures are not affected by body fluids and once within a body cavity become encapsulated (Newlands 1998/9). Presentation may be as a natural or synthetic material and either twisted, braided or monofilament.

Gauge of suture ranges from 1 mm to as fine as 15 microns (7–11/0); best practice indicates that the finest gauge that will hold tissues securely should be used (Newlands 1998/9). Castille (1998) recommends 5/0 for faces, scalp and upper limbs; 4/0 and 3/0 for trunk and lower limbs.

Needles

In addition to decisions about suture type there is the choice of needle; these again are varied (Figure 5.3).

The shape of needle used is restricted by the surgeon's degree of access to the site to be sutured. Besides shape there is also the bore description to be considered. This may be round-bodied to separate tissues rather than cut them, cutting to address dense tissue, or spatulated as in the case of needles for ophthalmic use.

Having identified the appropriate suture material and size plus needle shape, errors can still occur that will reduce the effectiveness of the suturing or cause damage to wounds. The most common errors include: (i) pulling sutures too tight, so causing swelling and reducing vascularity to the wound edges; (ii) allowing sutures to be too loose resulting in the wound gaping and not healing by first intention; (iii) placing sutures too near the wound edge, so that they may pull out; (iv) overlapping of the wound edges, which can result in wound dehiscence (Castille 1998). These

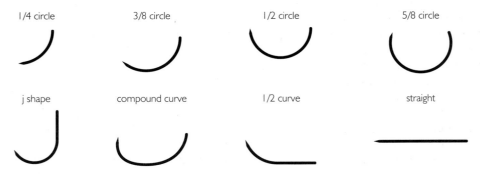

Figure 5.3 Needle shape

aspects can be identified easily on final skin closure, but may cause irreparable damage or complications if involving internal sutures. The type of suturing technique used is the choice of the surgeon and may include interrupted, continuous, subcuticular and endoscopic sutures. Additionally, they may include a secondary suture line, retention sutures and traction sutures.

All practitioners involved with suturing have a responsibility to have a working knowledge of sutures in use within their practice area plus knowledge of alternative materials available. They also must ensure that all sutures within the surgical field are accounted for and added to the visible swab count. On closure of each layer, a further count should be undertaken to ensure all sutures and their packaging are accounted for. On completion of surgery this count should be documented within the patient's care plan/surgical record.

Instruments

Instrumentation within all surgical specialities is wide and varied, but the role practitioners take with their management is the same. All practitioners need to be competent to use the equipment, be able to recognise their instruments, be aware of their uses and understand the principles of how to care for them. Misuse of instrumentation can place the patient and practitioners at risk of injury and may become costly if instruments become damaged or broken when used incorrectly or inappropriately. Practitioners involved in the buying of equipment need to ensure that any equipment bought/supplied to their department conforms to current Medical Devices Agency (MDA) guidelines and is Conformity European (CE) marked (MDA 2000).

Presentation of instruments may come in a variety of forms from preset instrument and drape packs, Edinburgh pre-set trays or via a container system. Whatever the format of presentation all practitioners should be aware of how they identify that their equipment is sterile and within its usable date. They should also know how they identify the traceability of the set should there be a need to track and identify

equipment used on a specific patient at a later date (NATN 1999). Prior to use the practitioner must ensure that they have checked which instruments are present against the set checklist and also that all components of instruments are accounted for. Any supplementary instruments should be recorded and checked prior to use. Items identified as faulty should be removed and replaced where possible. Faulty items should then be tagged to identify them to sterile service staff as requiring repair or replacement. Prior to commencing surgery, practitioners should ensure they have all the instrumentation they need, along with any additional instrumentation that may be required in the event of unanticipated extension of planned surgery or emergency.

Instruments can be broadly discussed under five categories: cutting instruments; artery forceps; clamps; tissue forceps; and retractors. Instrumentation additional to these can be considered as accessory equipment.

Cutting instruments

Cutting instrumentation includes both scalpel handles (BP handles/Barron handles) and scissors. Scalpel handles come in a variety of sizes and require blades to be attached. To reduce the risk of sharps injury, blades should be attached and removed using appropriate tools/aids and not by hand. Prior to use the blade should be checked for security to ensure no injuries occur due to blade slippage.

Scissors vary from extremely fine to large and heavy, being angled, straight or curved. All scissors are designed for a specific use and should only be used for that purpose. Misuse could result in damage to the patient and to instrumentation. Prior to use these should be checked for smooth action and sharpness; blunt scissors must be identified for repair/resharpening.

Artery forceps

Artery forceps (haemostats/haemostatic forceps) are utilised for clamping blood vessels, blunt dissection, handing or holding supplementary items, i.e. ties/pledgets. These come in a variety of sizes and may be curved or straight, giving the user the ability to vary the pressure applied via the ratchet lock. Prior to use the tips should be inspected to ensure they meet.

Clamps

A variety of clamps are available and those used are dependent upon the surgery to be undertaken. Vascular clamps are designed to be atraumatic and, as with artery forceps, may have a ratchet lock to allow variable degrees of pressure to be applied. Bowel clamps are designed to be crushing for application to distal and proximal ends, or non-crushing for application at the site of anastamosis. In use crushing and non-crushing must be clearly identified by practitioners to ensure accurate identification and usage.

Tissue forceps

Tissue forceps may be for tissue dissection or holding. Dissecting forceps are supplied in a variety of lengths and weights and may be toothed or non-toothed. The former are presented as interlocking grooves or teeth. Heavy teeth allow for the holding of heavier tissues such as muscle, while finer teeth are utilised on finer tissues. Plain, non-toothed forceps are for holding very delicate tissues such as vessels. Prior to use all dissection forceps should be checked for approximation of the tips.

Holding forceps are of various sizes and weights from the finer Allis to the heavy Lanes, again for use on various weights of tissue. Again inspection of alignment is required. Within this category are included needleholders and spongeholders. Needleholders are provided in different weights and lengths to balance the depth of suturing and the weight of the needle in use. Care should be taken to use an appropriate weight of needleholder for each needle used; too heavy a needle within a fine needleholder will result in strain on the joint and tips leading to costly damage of the needleholder. Passing of loaded needleholders should ideally occur via a 'safe transfer zone' to reduce the risk of accidental injury to scrubbed practitioners or the patient.

Retractors

Retractors may be hand-held or self-retaining, allowing access to the site of surgery. Where self-retaining retractors are used any screws should be confirmed as present prior to and on commencement of surgery. Retractors are provided in a variety of lengths and widths to allow for accurate retraction and with those that contain teeth, additional care should be taken to ensure no accidental injury is caused to the patient or to scrubbed personnel.

This has provided an insight into types of instrumentation in use; a wide variety are available and their use will be dependent upon the surgical speciality undertaken. During use instruments should be maintained in an organised manner to allow for immediate identification and allow for prompt retrieval. Any question as to the sterility of an item should result in its being removed from use and returned for sterilisation at the end of surgery with the remainder of the set. Throughout surgery the practitioner should ensure that all instruments are handled carefully and passed to users in a safe manner, sharp instruments ideally via a 'safe transfer zone' such as a receiver. Instruments other than blades and needles should be considered as sharps as many scissors and retractors have aspects that can inflict injury to receiving personnel. Items found to be blunt should be identified and notified to the sterile service department; the items should then be sent for sharpening.

Following completion of surgery, instruments should be counted against the initial set list along with supplementary items to confirm all instruments are present and accounted for following surgical closure. Instruments should then be returned to the sterile service departments following local policy guidelines and utilising the systems and processes in place to identify the location of equipment sets. The patient's individual care plan/documentation should be completed to indicate who has accounted the instrumentation used.

Practitioners need to be aware of their professional accountability with regard to surgical counts. While no legal requirement exists to perform a surgical count, practitioners have a duty of care to their patient to ensure that they come to no harm (NMC 2002). For this reason the National Association of Theatre Nurses has provided a number of documents that indicate what can be considered best practice when performing a surgical count (NATN 1998a,b). Within these they indicate the necessity to ensure the following:

- All swabs, instruments and sharps are accounted for prior to the commencement of surgery and as they are added to the surgical field.
- Counts should be performed by two staff members who can identify and recognise all items to be counted; one of these must be a qualified staff member.
- Counts to be audible.
- Counts should be recorded clearly within the theatre.
- No items to be removed from theatre until the final count has been completed and confirmed as correct.
- Counts to be performed at the commencement of any cavity closure
- On completion a verbal acknowledgement that the count was correct is made.
- At the end of surgery the count is documented and signed for by the scrub and circulating staff performing the count (NATN 1998a).

During use equipment that is sharp has the potential to injure patients and staff; therefore appropriate handling is essential. Practitioners need to ensure that sharp prongs, scissor tips etc. are maintained within a 'safe transfer' area away from the patient and staff when not required, but convenient to access safely. Should injury occur to the patient or staff member this should be documented and appropriate action taken under hospital policy.

Education on the use and handling of equipment is essential. Practitioners new to theatre practice can benefit from handling and passing clean instrumentation away from the surgical field. This is an opportune time to consider equipment against set lists with discussion from experienced practitioners.

ELECTROSURGERY

Electrosurgical units to provide haemostasis during surgery have been used since the 1930s (Meeker and Rothrock 1999). It is the process by which an electrical current is passed to tissues to achieve cutting, coagulation and haemostasis during surgery. Methods of electrosurgery include monopolar diathermy and bipolar diathermy. Additionally, ultrasonic devices are also available to provide options for coagulation and cutting.

Risks from the use of electrosurgery include: (i) electrocution due to insulation failure or faulty equipment; (ii) accidental burns as a result of negligence, alternative pathways taken by electrical current, direct coupling and capacitive coupling; (iii) fire following ignition of alcohol based fluids or drapes; (iv) inhalation of surgical plume; and (v) interference with other electromedical devices (NATN 1998a).

Monopolar electrosurgery

During monopolar electrosurgery electrical current is passed from a generator through the patient via a live electrode in the form of forcep or pencil to a return electrode, usually in the form of a patient plate, and then back to the electrosurgical generator to complete the circuit (Figure 5.4). The return electrode must be of sufficient size, and contact maintained to prevent concentration of the energy and the associated heat generated, which can result in a burn injury to the patient. Application of the return electrode should be on a well-vascularised area close to the site of surgery and avoiding bony prominences. The current use of isolated units as opposed to older technology grounded units reduces, but does not eliminate the risk of burn injury to alternative sites other than the return electrode site, as the electrical energy is caused to return to the generator by the use of a transformer within the generator unit (NATN 1998a).

The ability to vary the waveform, power setting, exposure time and electrode size allows for different effects on tissue to be achieved. The use of a high frequency and low voltage delivered slightly above the tissue to increase the heat generated will result in a cutting mode that continually bombards tissue producing heat and cell rupture, and the tissue is cut (Meeker and Rothrock 1999). Due to the speed, heat is produced which dissipates as steam and plume. A lower frequency and higher voltage intermittently supplied produces heat more slowly, and allows coagulation via desiccation or fulguration to occur. The size of active electrode also dictates the effect on tissue; small electrodes will have the maximum tissue effect due to the concentration of electrical energy, while larger electrodes require more power to produce a lesser effect.

Bipolar electrosurgery

In bipolar electrosurgery, the active and return electrode are combined within the delivery instrument, though separated by insulation (Figure 5.5). One tine of the forcep will contain the active electrode with the other tine containing the return electrode; as tissue is grasped, current is able to pass from the active electrode through the tissue to the return electrode, heat is generated and coagulation occurs. Because the current passes from one tine to another, no current passes through the patient's body, thus eliminating the need for a patient return plate.

Hazards of electrosurgery

Due to the risk associated with electrical equipment, staff should check electrosurgical equipment prior to use, observing for the integrity of insulated power and delivery cables.

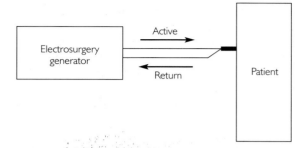

Figure 5.5 Bipolar electrosurgery

With monopolar equipment the patient plate (return electrode) must be observed for security and accurate siting; it should not be allowed to dislodge or become wet. Pooling of flammable solutions should be avoided due to the risk of fire. The active electrode should be held within a non-conductive holder when not in use to prevent burn injury caused by accidental triggering of the equipment. When possible a smoke evacuator should be used to remove electrosurgical plume.

The use of electrosurgery in minimal invasive surgery has the risks of insulation failure and coupling. Insulation failure can occur due to damage by other instruments, or due to frequent use. Coupling can be direct as electrical energy passes to a non-insulated instrument or capacitive where the electrosurgical energy is transferred through insulation to other conductive equipment nearby. All of these aspects can result in accidental damage to internal organs; therefore practitioners need to be aware of the risks (NATN 1998a).

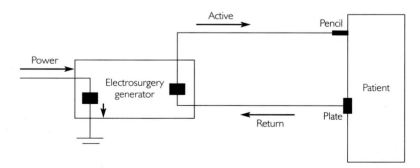

Figure 5.4 Monopolar electrosurgery – isolated circuit

On completion of surgery all patients should be observed for injury from both the active and return electrode sites, and information regarding the electrosurgical equipment used, power settings and site of any return electrode should be documented in the patient's care plan/file.

For perioperative practitioners the issue of electrosurgical plume is becoming a major concern. Currently no legislation exists to ensure mandatory action is taken to protect practitioners from the effects of plume, though plume is recognised as a hazard. It is known that following thermal destruction smoke is a byproduct. This smoke is known to contain toxic gases and vapours such as benzene and hydrogen cyanide, plus dead and live cellular matter and viruses (AORN 2002). In high concentration this plume can cause irritation to the upper respiratory tract and eyes while presenting surgeons with poor visibility at the sight of surgery. Current methods available for practitioners enabling them to avoid the potential hazards of electrosurgical plume are the use of high filtration masks and smoke evacuators, of which a number are currently available. These methods are preferable over the current practice of using wall suction units with in-line filters.

LASER

The use of laser technology within the operating theatre is wide and varied, and it is essential that practitioners have an understanding of their responsibilities in relation to the use, action and complications associated with laser use.

Laser is an acronym for Light Amplification by Stimulated Emissions of Radiation. Laser technology has the advantages of producing minimal tissue damage, reduced scarring and less postoperative pain, and allows for the use of local anaesthesia so reducing the complications associated with general anaesthesia and recovery.

Lasers utilise light in the form of electromagnetic energy from the shorter ultraviolet to the longer infrared wavelengths within the electromagnetic spectrum. Stimulation of a particle of laser medium within a resonating chamber produces a photon (a portion of electromagnetic energy). The original particle of laser medium may come from a number of different sources: carbon dioxide and argon are gaseous examples with the neodymium:YAG (Nd:YAG) a solid medium example. Stimulation occurs by passing a current through the gas or in the Nd:YAG by the use of high power lamps (Shields and Werder 2002).

The one photon produced can then trigger the particle to emit further identical photons (stimulated emission) that will travel in the same direction with the same wavelength. Amplification then occurs, as mirrors within the resonating chamber reflect the photons; these are then directed by mirrors to produce a laser beam. This laser beam has the ability to cut, coagulate, vaporise and weld. The radiation from laser technology is described as non-ionising, and as such does not present a radiation risk to health-workers or individuals, though their use does not come without hazards and practitioners need to be aware of the associated risks of eye injury, plume inhalation and fire (Davey and Ince 2000). Because of these associated risks only authorised staff should use the laser and appropriate training should be provided with a laser protection supervisor appointed to supervise day-to-day safety aspects.

Once the laser beam is delivered to the target area, four interactions occur: (i) it may be reflected in order to reach difficult to access areas; (ii) it may scatter as the beam is spread over a larger area as it disperses; (iii) transmission occurs when the beam passes through fluid or tissue without thermally altering them to reach the target area; (iv) absorption results when tissue is altered as a result of the laser beam. Absorption is dependent upon the laser wavelength, power setting, spot size and length of application time (Meeker and Rothrock 1999).

Laser mediums

Different laser mediums produce different wavelength beams and are suitable for different types of surgery. Carbon dioxide produces a powerful infrared, coaxial output highly absorbed by water that is suitable for cutting, coagulation and vaporising and is frequently used in plastic surgery, general surgery and gynaecological surgery (Shields and Werder 2002).

Argon gives a blue light of a lesser wavelength than carbon dioxide, that can be delivered via flexible fibrescopes. This beam is readily absorbed by haemoglobin and can pass through the eye without causing damage. It is therefore very suitable for coagulation, so is frequently used in gastroenterology, gynaecology and ophthalmic surgery (Davey and Ince 2000).

The Nd:YAG produces an infrared beam that can be utilised within fibreoptic cables and provides deep penetration, though not as well-focused as carbon dioxide. The beam is able to transmit through clear fluids with tissue coagulating without the vaporisation; as a result the Nd:YAG is generally used for endoscopic surgery and ophthalmic surgery (Meeker and Rothrock 1999). Following firing of the laser, its use should be recorded and documented within the patient's medical records.

Laser safety

Laser safety involves being aware of hazards to the surgical staff, other health professionals within the theatre, and to the patient. The hazards associated with laser use involve the risk of injury following exposure to the beam, fire and plume containment.

To protect staff, warning signs should be placed outside the area of laser use. Dependent upon the laser type in use, windows or openings should be appropriately covered. The laser should be maintained in the standby mode and when not in use the key should be stored in a locked area away from the laser machine. At all times the surgeon should ensure they are aware of the location of the laser foot-pedal and avoid accidental firing.

Eyes require specific protection from laser radiation; all staff involved should be supplied with appropriate goggles dependent upon the type of laser being used. Where endoscopes are being used they should have the eyepiece protected with a special cover. The wearing of goggles or the use of specifically designed eye-shields should be used to protect patients' eyes.

The skin surrounding the site of surgery on the patient should be protected and staff should be aware of the risk of skin burn injury to the patient and themselves following accidental firing of the laser (Meeker and Rothrock 1999).

The risk of fire is associated with both direct and reflected laser beams. Water or saline should be available to douse any small fire and a fire extinguisher available within the theatre. Non-reflective equipment should be used, with any reflective items removed from the local vicinity and covered. Alcoholic prep' lotions should not be used and other combustibles avoided. Where this is unavoidable as in the case of some drapes, these should be kept moist throughout the procedure and frequently monitored (Shields and Werder 2002). Endotracheal tubes designed for laser use should be used.

Health professionals also need to be protected from the risks associated with laser plume. Smoke evacuation systems should be used with their filters changed as recommended by the manufacturer. High filtration (0.3–0.1 μm) masks are also available.

PATIENT CARE

Within this section the aim is to discuss aspects of care that if not addressed by practitioners could cause harm to patients, extend their hospital stay, or result in morbidity or death of their patient. These areas are: pressure area management; thermoregulation; wound management; and the management of a patient with a latex allergy.

Pressure area care

Pressure ulcer development has been identified as costing the health service millions of pounds per year. Collier (1999) calculated that the treatment cost for one individual with a grade 4 pressure sore was approximately £40,000 in addition to their original treatment. These costs have resulted in the National Institute for Clinical Excellence (NICE) producing risk assessment and prevention guidelines (NICE 2001). This evidence has been used to inform the Department of Health in their production of the Essence of Care benchmarks of which one category specifically benchmarks pressure area care management (DoH 2001). Incidence within surgical patients is estimated at between 12 and 66% (Schultz et al. 1999).

Associated factors

There are a number of factors that affect the causes of pressure sores. Extrinsic factors include pressure, friction and shear. Intrinsic factors may include increasing age, low blood pressure, reduced mobility, poor oxygen perfusion and a poor nutritional status. Additional to these, external factors can further exacerbate and add to the risk of pressure sore development. These external factors include length of surgery, positioning, restraints/positioning devices and lifting and handling techniques to name a few. An individual undergoing surgery already increases their risk of developing a pressure injury with the hard operating surfaces increasing compression. Friction and shear are also a risk as individuals are transferred onto and off the operating table. This aspect also includes the manual handling technique used; these are identified as the commonest cause of friction (Dealey 1997). Intrinsic factors may be exacerbated as patients are often maintained with a low blood pressure during surgery and mobility is removed by anaesthesia or reduced by the need to operate under local or regional anaesthesia. Additional to this nothing can prevent individuals who are elderly or in a poor nutritional state from requiring surgery; they in all probability account for a large amount of surgery undertaken.

Practitioners need to be aware that patients who are inappropriately positioned or supported, not repositioned or have no actions taken to reduce pressure are at risk of pressure injury. This injury may take many forms, for example, alopecia as a result of pressure to the occiput; neuropathies ranging from minor sensory motor loss to paralysis; reactive hyperemia; or pressure sore development ranging from stage 1 to stage 4 (McEwen 1996). It is essential that individuals are assessed and individualised integumentary precautions instigated. Thus actions need to be taken to consider how pressure area care can be considered a priority within the operating environment.

Individuals over 65 and under five years of age are particularly at risk. The older adult has changes in the elasticity and resilience of their skin; in addition cardiovascular disease reduces microcirculation and increases the risk of pressure ulcer development. Those under five are at risk as their skin is still maturing and their head to body weight is disproportionate, the areas particularly at risk being the head, ears and heels. The use of oxygen saturation probes and repeated heel pricks can also cause damage.

Assessment

To prevent pressure sore development it is essential to assess who may be at risk so that appropriate preventative measures can be taken. Areas for consideration are skin condition, the general status of the individual and their physical and mental status. To assist individuals there are a number of risk assessment tools available, including the Norton Score, Knoll Score, Waterlow Score and the Braden Score (RCN 2001) plus many others. These are aimed at different groups of patients and utilise different variables to score an individual's risk in a numerical format.

The Waterlow Score can be considered appropriate for surgical patients as it is aimed at acute care patients and incorporates weight and build, skin type, continence, mobility, sex, age, appetite, skin damage, surgery and medication within its variables. Here the higher the patient's score the more at risk of pressure sore development they are considered to be.

- 10–14: at risk
- 15–19: high risk
- 20+: very high risk.

Essentially it does not matter which scoring system is used provided audit is undertaken to establish the effectiveness of the scoring system in use.

Once a patient has been identified as at risk of developing a pressure sore, action needs to be taken to reduce this risk.

Preventative actions

With pressure considered to be the main cause of pressure sore development, the initial action considered has to be how to reduce pressure. The main method of relieving pressure is traditionally regular repositioning of the patient. During surgery this is deemed to be impractical and disruptive. Options such as tilting again are also considered impractical, though both should be utilised on patients identified at risk if there is an opportunity to incorporate them. One suggestion is that small body shifts can achieve some degree of pressure relief (Antle and Leafgreen 2001) and these should be considered where possible as a part of the care given to patients undergoing surgery that is anticipated to extend over a long period of time.

Additional to repositioning or movement (where possible) is the use of pressure-relieving mattresses. Standard operating table mattresses have been identified within a number of studies as a major risk factor in pressure sore development, as has the use of warming mattresses under the patient (Ratliff and Rodeheaver 1998). The use of pressure-reducing mattresses has been found to reduce the pressure on tissues and reduce pressure sore development. While risk assessment can be used to identify who would benefit from their use, the most effective method should be their introduction as standard care for all individuals undergoing surgery. To limit their use to cases estimated to last over a specified period of time or those scoring appropriately on an assessment will eliminate some individuals who may benefit and allows equality of care to all individuals.

It is already recognised that moist skin is at increased risk from maceration, friction and shearing forces and therefore at increased risk of breakdown and pressure sore development. To prevent this, a number of actions can be taken. Patients known to be incontinent can be catheterised prior to surgery along with patients known to be undergoing extensive surgery or those who will be immobile following surgery. Scrub practitioners can ensure that they avoid the use of excess skin preparation lotions that may pool under the patient. Where it is likely that lotion pooling will occur, action should be taken to protect the patient's skin prior to preparation and protection provided and then removed prior to draping so leaving the patient's skin dry. Any protection provided and left in position should not interfere with any distribution devices in use (RCN 2001).

Positioning

In order to reduce friction and shear it is essential that sufficient practitioners are present during positioning, and that any devices used to aid in transfer and positioning are sufficient. Practitioners need to be aware of current manual handling techniques and how positioning equipment functions. There should be sufficient support equipment to allow all patients the maximum degree of protection that the individual requires; supplementary equipment should be maintained and cleaned after use. When buying equipment or protection devices consideration should be given to size, durability, hypoallergenic properties, ease of use, ease of cleaning, methods of handling, storage requirement and its ability to maintain normal capillary interface pressure (AORN 2001).

When protecting patients' prominences it should be noted that foam pads, towels and rolled bedding are not effective at reducing pressure and may cause friction, as opposed to gel pads that redistribute pressure over a wider area (AORN 2001). Static air mattresses with multiple compartments are considered to provide pressure relief to individuals, though practitioners need to ensure these are re-inflated and maintain adequate air volumes. Dynamic air mattresses are available, though these are currently considered to require further research to determine their value in relieving pressure and maintaining the patient's position during surgery (Armstrong 2001). Recommendations from the 2001 clinical practice guidelines *Pressure Ulcer Development Risk Assessment and Prevention* (RCN 2001) clearly state:

Pressure redistribution mattresses/overlays should be used on the operating table of individuals assessed to be at risk of pressure ulcer development.

(p. 16)

Practitioners need to additionally ensure that extraneous devices/equipment attached to the patient are positioned in such a manner that it does not result in pressure injury. This may include: intravenous lines, catheters, tourniquets and diathermy cables plus many other pieces of equipment.

Thermoregulation

The maintenance of a normal body temperature during surgery is essential in reducing the risks associated with inadvertent hypothermia. Inadvertent hypothermia occurs in patients whose normal protective reflexes have been suppressed. Within the perioperative environment hypothermia is generally defined as a core temperature below 36°C (Ensminger 1999). The incidence of hypothermia is identified as being as high as 70% of surgical patients (Sessler 2000; Arndt 1999). Paediatric and older adults are identified as being at greater risk. Others more at risk would include those with insufficient energy stores due to their debilitated state or those with an impaired metabolic rate.

Older adults are more at risk due to reduced subcutaneous adipose tissue that acts as insula-

tion, and a reduced basal metabolic rate that affects the ability to generate heat. Ageing affects the circulatory system, and heat distribution around the body will become compromised with neurological control of vasoconstriction and vasodilatation also affected.

Paediatric patients, particularly the newborn and very young children, have an increased risk due to their underdeveloped thermoregulatory system. They have a large surface area compared to their body mass and only small stores of subcutaneous fat. Additionally as opposed to shivering in response to hypothermia, young paediatric patients increase their metabolism of brown fat to produce heat; this results in an increased oxygen requirement.

Consequences of hypothermia

The consequences of hypothermia are wide-ranging and include: reduced tissue perfusion that can result in postoperative wound infection and pressure sore development; venous stasis that may lead to development of deep vein thrombosis; reduced coagulability of platelets that may allow bleeding to occur either intraoperatively or postoperatively.

A patient's basal metabolic rate is reduced by 5–7% for every degree centigrade lost. Poor perfusion and low metabolism may affect the kidneys, brain and liver and thus affect drug excretion (Arndt 1999). Patients recovering

---

PRACTICE EXEMPLAR 5.2: NERVES AT RISK FROM PRESSURE INJURY

Mrs Smith has attended theatre for abdominal surgery. She will be in a supine position for approximately three hours and has a Waterlow score of 16. From the time Mrs Smith enters the anaesthetic room identify which of Mrs Smith's nerves may be at risk from pressure injury.

During anaesthesia, the nerves to the eye, the supraorbital and facial nerves are at risk from compression by facemasks, catheter mounts and anaesthetist's hands.

During surgery, the ulnar nerve is at risk due to compression of the humerus and the edge of the operating table, the radial nerve from compression between the edge of the table or armboard. The humerus and the sciatic nerves are at risk from direct compression onto the operating table (Warwick 2000).

from anaesthetic who shiver increase their oxygen consumption by 300–400% at a time when their basal metabolism is reduced and cardiac output is increased by 400–500% (Bernthal 1999). The provision of additional warming to perioperative patients in order to prevent hypothermia developing is proven to reduce the risk of morbid cardiac events by 55% (Kurz *et al.* 1996). Research by Scott *et al.* (2001) demonstrated that the warming of patients intraoperatively produced a relative risk reduction in the development of pressure ulcer development of 46%.

Methods of heat loss

Before practitioners consider what warming techniques to apply to their individual patient they need to consider how patients lose heat. The majority of heat loss occurs via radiation, the transfer of heat from one surface to another via infrared waves. Heat loss due to conduction occurs due to direct contact with another object within the perioperative environment; this will be from the patient's skin to the operating table and instruments.

Convection heat loss is dependent upon air currents and is considered the second most important source of intraoperative heat loss. Practitioners should be aware of the air changes within their environment and consider the hypothermic implications to the patient when using laminar flow systems. Evaporation from surgical wounds and from alcoholic skin preparation lotions also contributes to an individual's heat loss. The inhalation of unheated unhumidified gases will also lead to heat loss due to evaporation (Bernthal 1999).

An additional significant factor that can contribute to a marked afterdrop in body temperature is following the isolation of a limb by tourniquet; during use of the tourniquet the limb is isolated and distal tissue becomes cold. Following the release of the tourniquet there is a drop in body temperature as heat from the core is redistributed (Sessler 2000).

The induction of a general anaesthetic encourages vasodilation as it reduces the patient's ability to vasoconstrict while additionally causing direct peripheral vasodilation allowing core body heat to reach the peripheries. Spinal and epidural anaesthetics also affect thermoregulation by affecting the control centrally as peripheral, sympathetic and motor pathways are blocked, so preventing vasoconstriction and shivering from occurring (Sessler 2000).

During both general and regional anaesthesia, it is the redistribution of body heat decreasing the core temperature that is the primary cause of hypothermia during the first hour of either method of anaesthesia, though the core is decreased twice as much during general anaesthesia as opposed to during regional anaesthesia. During longer procedures patients undergoing regional anaesthesia will develop a greater degree of hypothermia as the temperature of patients undergoing general anaesthesia will plateau, while those under regional anaesthesia continue to lose body heat (Sessler 2000). Patients undergoing combination anaesthesia involving both general and regional techniques are at the greatest risk of hypothermia as the combination of factors affect thermoregulation and prevent the patient from actively being able to vasoconstrict or shiver in response to the reduced body temperature (Buggy and Crossley 2000).

Active hypothermia is often instigated during cardiac and neurosurgery to reduce metabolic activity and protect the patient from cardiac and cerebral ischaemia with the patient's temperature being cooled to the region of 28°C (Bernthal 1999). Cardiac patients often suffer from 'afterdrop' whereby there is a large differential in the core and peripheral temperatures resulting in a significant temperature drop following redistribution. This can be overcome by increasing the length of rewarming time, though this time has to be balanced against the associated risks in relation to cardiopulmonary bypass (Sessler 2000).

Methods of warming

Methods of intraoperative warming have to first reduce the causative factors as much as possible. Therefore exposure of the patient should be reduced prior to and during surgery. The patient should be kept covered until surgery commences; during surgery more than one layer of drapes may be used and the theatre temperature should be maintained above 24°C; this will assist in maintaining the patient's body temperature (Bernthal 1999). Ensminger (1999) promotes the use of reflective jackets and hats, which have resulted in patients becoming less hypothermic, while absorbent reflective blankets are now also available for use.

Active warming of the environment can be considered alongside forced air warmers, radiant lamps, and warmed bedding postoperatively. The warming of intravenous fluids reduces the direct action of adding cooled fluids direct to the heat transport system, plus the use of humidified moisture exchangers for volatile gases. Intraoperatively, staff can consider the use of warming skin preparation solutions, excluding those that are alcohol-based, irrigation fluids and cleaning lotions.

Carli and Macdonald (1996) discuss the benefits that can be achieved by the prewarming of patients' skin prior to anaesthesia, though currently this does not appear to have become routine practice.

Taking into account that the majority of patients are known to become hypothermic during a surgical procedure, best practice would suggest that all surgical patients should have their temperature monitored pre-, intra- and post-surgery to ascertain their warming requirements. Practitioners should additionally be aware that the recovery to normothermia can be slow and take in the region of two to five hours (Sessler 2000). Regular audit of patients' temperature will indicate the incidence of inadvertent hypothermia and allow for a review of current practice.

Wound management

Surgical wound infections are recognised as a major cause of morbidity, extended surgical stay and increased hospital costs (Nortcliffe and Buggy 2003); thus wound healing is essential to a patient's overall recovery. While the majority of infections are recognised as exogenous, coming from patients, perioperative practitioners can

Box 5.4

> Consider the perioperative practices and protocols you currently have in place and review these against the incidence of patients with inadvertent hypothermia.
>
> **What actions did you need to take?**
> - An audit to determine the incidence of hypothemia
> - Introduce monitoring of patient's temperature
> - Review the department thermoregulation protocol
> - Review the equipment available to promote patient warming
> - Review the education provided to perioperative practitioners.

benefit care from an increased awareness of identifying those at risk. Surgical site infections are those that occur within 30 days of surgery assuming no implant is involved and can be categorised as superficial incisional, deep incisional or organ/space. The current incidence of all postoperative infection has been identified as 4.3%, 25% of these deep or organ/space infections (Dixon 2002). The majority of surgical wounds heal by first intention following direct closure, though a number may be left to heal purposefully by second intention. Where an implant is involved in surgery the implant material should be inert in body fluids (Rubin and Yaremchuk 1997). Implant materials used are generally metals, i.e. stainless steel, titanium, polymers such as polythene, dimethylsiloxane (silicone), or ceramics such as hydroxyapatite (Eppley 1999). During healing involving an implant there is formation of fibroconnective scar tissue that envelopes the implant or fibrous encapsulation of the implant (Eppley 1999).

Influencing factors

A number of factors increase an individual's risk of acquiring a surgical site infection; these relate to the patient, their operation, length of surgery and their wound classification.

Patient factors include age, where evidence would suggest that infection is associated with a higher degree of mortality with a deterioration in immunity in those over 70. The very young have a poorly developed immune system. Additional factors include nutritional status with protein calorie malnutrition associated with surgical site infection (Dixon 2002) and smoking which affects the immune system and reduces oxygen delivery. The following factors also influence a patient's risk of surgical infection: diabetes; obesity; co-existent disease/infection; anaemia; malignancy; and immunosuppression (Dixon 2002).

The type and length of surgery are factors plus the effects of surgery and anaesthesia. The stress response to surgery is indicated to result in immunosuppression that lasts for several days following surgery. Anaesthesia may influence oxygen delivery due to hypovolaemia, hypotension, or introduction of infection other than surgical site following the insertion of vascular access or when introducing epidural/spinal anaesthesia.

The type of surgery has an influence; where the surgical site is the head/neck, or the thorax normal body flora includes *Staphylococci aureus*. This bacterium has been identified as a leading pathogen in surgical site infection (Mangram *et al.* 1999). The length of surgery increases the risk of surgical infection due to hypothermia, a reduction in the quality of the surgical environment with an increased risk of wound contamination from colonised personnel, respiratory droplets, dust, skin squames or other airborne matter (Dixon 2002).

Wound classification taking into account wound contamination is indicative of the likelihood of surgical site infection development. Four categories include:

1 **Clean** – an uninfected operative wound not involving respiratory, gut or urinary tracts.
2 **Clean-contaminated** – where the respiratory, gut and urinary tracts are incised but no unusual contamination occurs.

3 **Contaminated** – open or accidental wounds or where sterility is broken or gut contents spilt.
4 **Dirty/infected** – old traumatic wounds including devitalised tissue (Dixon 2002).

Considering the three factors, patient, surgical aspects and wound classification, it is transparent that while practitioners can reduce the risk to patients they cannot eliminate them totally, but all steps taken to reduce the associated risks will impact on a patient's development of a surgical site infection and therefore their postoperative recovery.

Where implants have been used, soft tissue coverage should be as thick as possible to reduce the risk of exposure or thinning of the dermis (Eppley 1999). Additional precautions to reduce the risk of infection can be taken by perioperative staff. These include: avoiding exposure of the implant – do not remove from packaging until required; avoiding extensive handling of the implant – use clean instruments and minimal contact with gloves; change gloves if handling is necessary; plus avoid contact with surrounding skin or the oral cavity where the risk of bacterial transmission will be increased (Eppley 1999).

Dressings

Wound dressings need to promote healing by providing a moist environment while protecting the wound from injury or harm (Casey 2002). Morison (1992) described the criteria a good wound dressing should fulfil. These include:

- Non-adherent
- Impermeable to bacteria
- Ability to maintain a high humidity at the wound site
- Able to remove excess exudates
- Thermally insulating
- Non-toxic and hypoallergenic
- Comfortable and conformable
- Able to protect the wound
- Require infrequent changing.

Dressings materials are wide and varied and as a wound changes it should be remembered that dressing materials might need to be changed:

- **Alginates,** e.g. Kaltostat®, are considered to be interactive and are suitable for exuding wounds but should not be applied to non- or minimally exuding wounds. Once applied they may require an additional dressing.
- **Foams,** e.g. Lyofoam®, are for use on exuding wounds requiring a change once saturated.
- **Hydrocolloids,** e.g. Duoderm®, are effective on medium to low-exuding wounds; they are absorbent and self-adhesive, not requiring a secondary dressing, able to remain in place for up to 5 days.
- **Hydrogels,** e.g. Intrasite®, have the ability to either hydrate a wound or to absorb exudates, so are useful on necrotic wounds facilitating debridement, or on exuding wounds. A secondary dressing is required.
- **Low adherent dressings,** e.g. Melonin®, are suitable for sutured wounds or wounds with minimal exudates, often used with hydrogels to provide a moist environment or additional padding to absorb exudate.
- **Medicated dressings,** e.g. Inadine®, are low adherent and impregnated with povidone-iodine; suitable for wounds with superficial wound infection.
- **Semi-permeable films,** e.g. Tegaderm™, are designed to stay in place for several days, provide a moist environment with no absorbency and are suitable for covering superficial wounds such as skin graft donor sites and superficial wounds.
- **Vapour permeable membranes,** e.g. Tegapore™, require a secondary dressing as they allow exudates to pass through them to the secondary dressing, allowing for the primary dressing to remain intact until healing is complete. Suitable for wounds anticipated to require a number of weeks to heal.

Besides standard dressing materials, alternative options are available: maggot and larval therapies are currently undergoing a new resurgence. Larvae are identified for use on necrotic wounds as they reduce the number of bacteria found within a wound by feeding on the necrotic tissue and exudate. Claxton *et al.* (2003) would also suggest that the saliva and digestive secretions from maggots contain antibacterial properties. While there appear to be benefits from the use of larval therapy, patients are not always accepting of the method (Chalmers and Muir 2003).

Vacuum-assisted closure is increasing in popularity for deep cavity wounds, pressure ulcers, traumatic wounds and following skin grafting. Here negative pressure is applied to a wound to promote blood flow and increase the rate of granulation. The disadvantages of vacuum-assisted closure are the difficulties in practice of achieving a seal, and the reduced mobility of the patient during the period of use (Milne and Houle 2002).

Tissue culture is an alternative option in the management of burn patients where a full-thickness skin graft from the patient or a donor is harvested and cultured to grow larger sheets of cells; these are then grafted to a granulating wound bed (Boyce *et al.* 2002). Cadaveric skin may be used as a temporary dressing until cells are grown, or until already accessed split skin sites are available for re-cropping (Robb *et al.* 2001).

Identification of an appropriate dressing is essential and should take into account the patient's age and skin condition. The elderly may have thin friable skin which adhesive dressings may damage, while children require a dressing that allows them to continue their normal behaviour as much as possible. A dressing therefore needs to be adaptable and secure, with consideration given to how it is removed.

Latex allergy

The incidence of latex allergy has been recognised since 1979, gaining more attention since the 1990s following the introduction of Universal Precautions (Carroll 1999). The introduction of Universal Precautions resulted in an increased exposure to latex and is recognised by many as a trigger for the increased number of people with latex allergy (Bowyer 1999; Carroll 1999; Johnson 1999). Within the health-care setting, latex allergy has implications for both staff and patients.

The term latex has become recognised as referring to natural rubber latex (NRL). Products containing NRL are widely available within the domestic environment. Within the health-care setting the most common items recognised as containing NRL are gloves. NRL is used within the manufacture of gloves because of the protection it provides to the wearer, for its flexibility and durability (NATN 2000). Within the perioperative environment the use of products containing latex has been widespread; where possible many products have been replaced with NRL-free products for the benefit of both patients and staff. All products that do contain latex vary in their allergenic potential due to the extractable proteins and accelerators contained within the product and the quality of the product following the manufacturing process.

Reactions

Reactions to NRL are not all immunological; irritant contact dermatitis is a non-immune response largely associated with glove use, which results in a localised reaction. Symptoms from a localised reaction occur shortly after exposure and may produce itchiness, red skin and cracks, limited to the area exposed. This localised response may not be a response to latex, but as a result of perspiration within gloves, incomplete rinsing of soap products or insufficient drying of hands.

Chemical sensitivity dermatitis (type IV reaction) is a delayed hypersensitivity to chemicals used within the manufacturing process. The reaction occurs 6–48 hours after the latex exposure producing a localised blistering reaction that may extend away from the exposed area. Individuals who develop a type IV sensitivity are at risk of going on to develop a type I hypersensitivity if they continue to be exposed to the allergen, i.e. latex gloves (NATN 2000).

Latex allergy (type I reaction) is an immediate immunological reaction due to the extractable natural proteins found in NRL. The reaction occurs immediately following exposure to the allergen; an individual's response will vary depending upon their level of sensitivity and degree of exposure and may be mild or extend to an anaphylactic response. An allergic response is common in people who already have allergies to

avocados, bananas, chestnuts and kiwi fruit.

Exposure can occur via a number of routes and perioperative practitioners need to be aware of how their patients may come into contact with NRL. Exposure may be via contact with the skin, mucous membranes and internal tissues or via inhalation, intravascular or intrathecal exposure (NATN 2000).

Perioperative care

All organisations need to identify a protocol for recognising those patients at risk of latex allergy. This should ideally occur via a screening tool at the outpatient stage of admission; this approach identifies patients prior to procedures that may expose them to NRL products and enables early identification of patients who are due for surgery within the operating department.

Early identification of surgical patients with a latex allergy allows preventative action to be taken by the perioperative team. These actions include:

- Removal of NRL products from theatre prior to patient entry
- Place patient first on theatre list to reduce risk from aerosolisation of NRL
- Staff wear NRL-free gloves
- Only NRL-free products used on the patient following admission to the theatre suite
- Products known to contain NRL products that cannot be avoided, e.g. tourniquet/mattress covers should be covered with a NRL-free barrier material.

Due to the design and management of theatres it is essential to ensure that all members of the perioperative team, namely, anaesthesia staff, theatre staff and recovery staff, are aware of patients with a latex allergy. This will allow appropriate actions to be taken in all the areas where the patient will be.

For patients admitted as an emergency knowing they have a latex allergy, surgery should be delayed where possible until all actions to provide a latex-free environment can be achieved. Where this is not feasible, all possible preventative actions should be taken to achieve the optimum environment for the individual.

Communication and education is essential in ensuring that patients are protected from the risks associated with latex allergy. All organisations should ensure they have readily available policies available for staff to consult, which inform on how to provide and maintain a latex-free environment.

Recommendations include: the provision of a data-base of latex-free products; a centralised stock of latex-free products; a list of available alternatives; instructions for obtaining and maintaining a latex-free environment, including common sources of departmental latex and emergency drugs. It is suggested that all these recommendations are sited within an identified trolley or box readily available for staff to use (NATN 2000).

DOCUMENTATION

Documentation provides the indicator for the quality of care a patient receives. Reports produced by NCEPOD (1999) repeatedly indicate the need for an improvement in the documentation of patient care. This position is supported by the Essence of Care benchmarks (DoH 2001); these include documentation within the first eight standards. NATN (1999) and AORN (2000) have both produced recommended practices for perioperative documentation reflecting the importance of documentation within professional communication. The need for clear concise documentation is compounded by the increased litigation occurring within the NHS. Documentation is often required many years after an event; it aids the judging of the validity of complaints and supports professional accounts of events. Further influences affecting the need for accurate documentation are: clinical effectiveness, audit, risk management and quality assurance.

Clear documentation provides the basis for interprofessional communication, evidences care provided to patients and provides a permanent record of care and activity. Poor documentation is evidenced in a number of ways. Examples include:

- Incomplete records
- Inadequate/no record of observations
- Omission of date/time/names/signatures
- Failing to record care provided or recording care when none was provided
- No assessment/evaluation of a patient's condition.

Criticisms of poor standards of record-keeping suggest that it is given a low priority. Practitioners have a lack of awareness of the importance of good record-keeping, with poor information sharing occurring between staff.

Documentation related to patients within the operating department should remain secure and confidential and may be manual or computerised, and include X-rays, photographs and videos, all of which may identify patients. The Data Protection Act (1998) regulates the use of personal information and introduces standards of privacy. Organisations are required to ensure compliance with the Data Protection Act, and the role of the Caldicott Guardian was recommended in 1997 (Caldicott 1997). The Caldicott Guardian has to be either responsible for clinical governance promotion, a senior health professional or a member of the hospital management board. Their role is to ensure that the use of patient information is justified, patient data is not saved unnecessarily, and that a minimum patient data set is used and is only made available on a 'need to know' basis. They are also responsible for ensuring that those involved with patient information know their responsibilities and comply with the law (McHale and Tingle 2001).

Guidelines have been produced that indicate the content and style that enables effective record-keeping. Records should be:

- Factual, consistent, accurate
- Clearly written and not erasable
- Written as soon as possible after the event and providing current information on the care and condition of the patient
- No abbreviations, jargon or speculation
- Accurately dated and signed
- Identify problems that arise (UKCC 1998).

All practitioners should consider that where care is not documented there could be the assumption that care was therefore not provided. Care provided may include both physiological and psychological care. Within the perioperative field abbreviations are frequently used; this may be deemed acceptable where an organisation provides a list of acceptable abbreviations for use. These should be made available to patients to ensure they understand the use of abbreviations.

Patient care records during the perioperative period require practitioners to utilise documentation provided by other areas such as the ward staff, and to then document fully the care provided. Records may include preoperative checklists, consent forms, ward patient assessments for mobility and pressure scores.

Practitioners need to record interventions and actions taken during surgery; the format for this is varied among organisations and may be manual or computerised. The format adopted should provide the opportunity for practitioners to assess required care, be able to document care provided, and to then evaluate that care. It must ensure that it provides an overall picture of care, indicating who provided that care. Within the perioperative environment this is essential as much care provided is to prevent potential injury/complications to patients (NATN 1999) and includes positioning and protection used, electrosurgery use, and deep vein thrombosis prophylaxis. In addition to this is the recording of surgical counts, traceability of equipment and recording of implants; all these aspects have been previously discussed.

At any time should staff have any concerns regarding the availability of information supplied to them, the information data set they are recording or methods of transmitting confidential information, they should contact their Caldicott Guardian for clarification.

In addition to the completion of patient record documentation, practitioners may additionally be required to complete accident/incident documentation related to patients. This should be completed as soon as possible after an event via the organisations reporting mechanisms and written in a chronological order, including

Box 5.5

> - Do you know who your Caldicott Guardian is?
> - Does your patient care record document physiological and psychological care provided to patients? Does this include support provided to patients undergoing local/regional anaesthesia?
> - Are department papers containing patient details disposed of via confidential waste?

the facts with no assumption or supposition included (NATN 1999).

Within the workplace there should be policies, guidelines and competencies available to guide staff in relation to all aspects of surgical care. While these do not promote 'best' practice they aid in the identification and elimination of poor practice and promote safe practice. The active encouragement of audit will also indicate the effectiveness of current practice and should become a part of each individual practitioner's work practice.

CONCLUSION

It can be seen that the management of the surgical patient within the perioperative environment is multifaceted and complex. It requires practitioners to have a working knowledge of an array of relevant areas. Without the comprehension of infection control management, patients would be at risk of transmitted infections, while the ability to utilise and manage essential equipment effectively ensures patient safety during surgery. A practitioner's knowledge, risk assessment and actions related to patient care aspects such as pressure management and thermoregulation are the key to providing quality care for surgical patients, reducing a patient's risk of associated complications. Finally the completed documentation of the care provided by a practitioner summarises the care delivered and allows others to recognise the degree of risk assessment undertaken and the quality of the care provided.

REFERENCES

Antle D and Leafgreen P (2001) Reducing the incidence of pressure ulcer development in the ICU: nurses at one facility take the initiative. *American Journal of Nursing* 101(5): 24EE–24JJ.

AORN (1999) Recommended practices for surgical hand scrubs. *AORN Journal* 69(4): 842–850.

AORN (2000) Recommended practices for documentation of perioperative nursing care. *AORN Journal* 71(1): 247–250.

AORN (2001) Recommended practices for positioning the patient in the perioperative practice setting. *AORN Journal* 73(1): 231–238.

AORN (2002) Hazards of polyvinyl chloride; hands-free passing; smoke evacuators; henna tattoos; mercury hazards. *AORN Journal* 76(4): 686–691.

Armstrong D (2001) An integrative review of pressure relief in surgical patients. *AORN Journal* 73(3): 645–648.

Arndt K (1999) Inadvertent hypothermia in the OR. *AORN Journal* 70(2): 203–222.

Bernthal EMM (1999) Inadvertent hypothermia prevention: the anaesthetic nurse's role. *British Journal of Nursing* 8(1): 17–25.

Bowyer R (1999) The implications of latex allergy in healthcare settings. *Journal of Clinical Nursing* 8(2): 139–143.

Boyce S, Kaga R, Yakuboff K, Meyer N, Reiman M, Greenhalgh D and Warden G (2002) Cultured skin substitutes reduce donor skin harvesting for closure of excised full thickness burns. *Annals of Surgery* 235(2): 269–279.

British Medical Association and Royal Pharmaceutical Society of Great Britain (2003) *British National Formulary* 45. London: BMA.

Buggy DJ and Crossley AWA (2000) Thermoregulation, mild perioperative hypothermia and post-anaesthetic shivering. *British Journal of Anaesthesia* 84(5): 615–628.

Carli F and Macdonald IA (1996) Perioperative inadvertent hypothermia: what do we need to prevent? *British Journal of Anaesthesia* 76: 601–603.

Carroll P (1999) Latex allergy: what you need to know. RN 62(9): 40–46.

Casey G (2002) Wound repair: advanced dressing materials. *Nursing Standard* 17(4): 49–52.

Castille K (1998) Suturing. *Nursing Standard* 12(41): 41–48.

Chalmers J and Muir R (2003) Patient privacy and confidentiality: the debate goes on; the issues are complex, but a consensus is emerging. *British Medical Journal* 326(7392): 725–726.

Choudhary S, Koshy C, Ahmed J and Evans J (1998) Friction burns to thigh caused by tourniquet. *British Journal of Plastic Surgery* 51: 142–143.

Claxton M, Armstrong D, Short B, Vazquez L and Boulton A (2003) 5 Questions – and answers – about maggot debridement therapy. *Skin and Wound Care* 16(2): 99–102.

Collier M (1999) Pressure ulcer development and principles for prevention. In: Miller M and Glover D (eds) *Wound Management Theory and Practice*. London: Emap.

Collins D, Rice J, Nicholson P and Barry K (2000) Quantification of facial contamination with blood during orthopaedic procedures. *Journal of Hospital Infection* 45: 73–75.

Davey A and Ince C (eds) (2000) *Fundamentals of Operating Department Practice*. London: Greenwich Medical Media.

Dealey C (1997) *Managing Pressure Sores*. Wiltshire: Quay Books.

Department of Health (2001) *Essence of Care: Patient Focussed Benchmarking for Health Care Practitioners*. London: The Stationery Office.

Dixon G (2002) Sources of surgical infection. *Surgery* 20(8): 179–185.

Ensminger J (1999) Preventing inadvertent hypothermia – a success story. *AORN Journal* 70(2): 298–301.

Eppley B (1999) Alloplastic implantation. *Plastic and Reconstructive Surgery* 104(6): 1761–1785.

Fisher MB, Reddy VR, Williams FM, Link Y, Thacker JG and Edlich RF (1999). Biomedical performance of latex and non-latex double glove systems. *Journal of Biomedical Meter Research* 48: 797–806.

Health and Safety Commission (1999) *Control of Substances Hazardous to Health Regulations. Biological Agents Approved Code of Practice*. Sudbury: HSE Books.

Health and Safety Executive (1999) *The Management of Health and Safety at Work Regulations 1999*. London: HMSO.

Hedderwick SA, McNeill SA, Lyons MJ and Kauffman CA (2000) Pathogenic organisms associated with artificial fingernails worn by healthcare workers. *Infection Control Hospital Epidemiology* 21: 505–509.

Hutchinson N (2002) Asepsis, antisepsis and skin preparation. *Surgery* 20(8): 190–192.

Johnson G (1999) Avoiding latex allergy. *Nursing Standard* 13(21): 49–56.

Jones RD, Jampani H, Mulberry G and Rizer RL (2000) Moisturizing alcohol hand gels for surgical hand preparation. *AORN Journal* 71(3): 584–599.

Kurz A, Sessler DI and Lenhardt R (1996) Perioperative normothermia to reduce the incidence of surgical wound infection and shorten hospitalization. *New England Journal of Medicine* 334: 1209–1215.

Line S (2003) Decontamination and control of infection in theatre. *British Journal of Perioperative Nursing* 13(2): 70–75.

Mangram AJ, Horan TC, Pearson ML, Silver LC and Jarvis WR (1999) Guideline for Prevention of Surgical Site Infection, 1999. Hospital Infection Control Practices Advisory Committee. *Infection Control Hospital Epidemiology* 20: 250–278.

McCulloch J (1999) Risk management in infection control. *Nursing Standard* 13(34): 44–46.

McCulloch J (ed) (2001) *Infection Control – Science, Management and Practice*. London: Whurr.

McEwen D (1996) Intraoperative positioning of surgical patients. *AORN Journal* 63(6): 1059–1079.

McHale J and Tingle J (2001) *Law and Nursing*, 2nd edn. Oxford: Butterworth Heinemann.

Medical Devices Agency (2000) *Equipped to Care – The Safe use of Medical Devices in the 21st Century*. London: Medical Devices Agency.

Meeker M and Rothrock (1999) *Care of the Patient in Surgery*, 11th edn. London: Mosby.

Milne C and Houle T (2002) Current trends in wound care management. *Orthopaedic Nursing* 21(6): 11–18.

Morison M (1992) Priorities in wound management: which dressing? In: *A Colour Guide to the Nursing Management of Wounds*. London: Wolfe.

National Association of Theatre Nurses (1998a) *Principles of safe practice in the perioperative environment*. Harrogate : NATN.

National Association of Theatre Nurses (1998b) *Safeguards for invasive procedures: the management of risks*. Harrogate: NATN.

National Association of Theatre Nurses (1999) *Operating department records*. Harrogate: NATN.

National Association of Theatre Nurses (2000) *Understanding latex in the perioperative setting*. Harrogate: NATN.

National Confidential Enquiry into Perioperative Deaths (1999) *Extremes of age*. London: NCEPOD.

National Institute for Clinical Excellence (2001) *Pressure ulcer risk assessment and prevention. Inherited clinical guideline B*. London: NICE.

Newlands P (1998/9) Theatre, surgery, clinical and patient care: surgical sutures. *Hospital Healthcare Europe* 1998/9: 21–22.

Nortcliffe S and Buggy D (2003) Implications of anaesthesia for infection and wound healing. *International Anesthesiology Clinics* 41(1): 31–64.

Nursing Midwifery Council (2002) *Code of Professional Conduct*. London: NMC.

Parkhouse D and Warwick J (2001) Cleaning, disinfection and sterilization of equipment. *Anaesthesia and Intensive Care* 2(9): 364–368.

Patterson JM, Novak CB, Mackinnon SE and Patterson CA (1998) Surgeons concern and practices of protection against blood borne pathogens. *American Surgery* 228: 266–272.

Ratliff CR and Rodeheaver GT (1998) Prospective study of the incidence of OR-induced pressure ulcers in elderly patients undergoing lengthy surgical procedures. *Advanced Wound Care* 11(Suppl): 10.

Robb E, Bechmann N, Plessinger R, Boyce S, Warden G and Kagan R (2001) Storage media and temperature maintain normal anatomy of cadaveric human skin for transplantation to full thickness skin wounds. *Journal of Burn Care and Rehabilitation* 22(6): 393–396.

Royal College of Nursing (2001) *Pressure ulcer risk assessment and prevention – recommendations*. London: RCN.

Rubin JP and Yaremchuk MJ (1997) Complications and toxicities of implantable biomaterials used in facial reconstructive and aesthetic surgery: a comprehensive review of the literature. *Plastic and Reconstructive Surgery* 100(5): 1336–1353.

Schroeter K (1998) Impact of a 5-minute scrub on the microbial flora found on artificial, polished, or natural fingernails of operating room personnel. *AORN Journal* 68(5): 880–884.

Schultz A, Bien M, Dumond K, Brown K and Myers A (1999) Etiology and incidence of pressure ulcers in surgical patients. *AORN Journal* 70(3): 434–449.

Scott EM, Leaper DJ, Clark M and Kelly PJ (2001) Effects of pressure warming on pressure ulcers – a randomized trial. *AORN Journal* 73(5): 921–938.

Sessler D (2000) Perioperative heat balance. *Anesthesiology* 92(2): 578–593.

Shields L and Werder H (2002) *Perioperative Nursing*. London: Greenwich Medical Media.

Steer J (2002) Decontamination. *Surgery* 20(8): 197–200.

UK Parliament (1998) Data Protection Act London: HMSO.

UKCC (1998) *Guidelines for records and record keeping*. London: UKCC.

Warwick J (2000): Positioning the surgical patient. *Anaesthesia and Intensive Care Medicine* 1(1): 37–40.

Wilson MP and Jacobson SK (1999) Sterilization and disinfection. *Surgery* 17:134–137.

Woodhead K, Taylor EW, Bannister G, Chesworth T, Hoffman P and Humphreys H (2002) Behaviours and rituals in the operating theatre. *Journal of Hospital Infection* 51:241–255.

Xavier G (1999) Asepsis. *Nursing Standard* 13(36): 49–53.

Useful websites

www.aorn.org
www.bads.co.uk
www.barna.co.uk
www.medic8.com
www.natn.org.uk
www.ncepod.org.uk
www.nelh.nhs.uk

6 Principles of recovery practice

Melanie Oakley and Christine Spiers

CHAPTER AIMS

- To explore the recovery practitioner's role in managing the patient's airway, fluid balance and cardiovascular status
- To expand the practitioner's knowledge of cardiac arrhythmias and necessary interventions
- To consider the problems of pain and postoperative nausea and vomiting and to review evidence-based practice for the management of these complications
- To briefly review the management of cardiac arrest in the recovery room.

INTRODUCTION

For many years the recovery unit has been viewed as the 'Cinderella' of the operating department. Indeed 25 years ago many hospitals did not have recovery units and post-surgical patients were recovered on the surgical wards directly from theatres. As a result nurses were confident in caring for the patient immediately post-anaesthesia and surgery and were confident in airway management, observation of cardiovascular status, fluid replacement and immediate wound and drain care. Thus when recovery units started evolving, nurses were well-placed to work in recovery with little or no further training. The thought that just because you were a nurse you could work in recovery has continued until recently, but as every recovery practitioner will know, recovery has now become a 'high tech' area that requires a skilled practitioner with the appropriate training.

The recovery practitioner now has to act autonomously, as many units do not have a dedicated anaesthetist placed in the unit. The practitioner will have to take decisions prior to the anaesthetist being called. They will have to be familiar with emergency procedures and the technology and keep updated with the current evidence that underpins recovery practice. They will need to have a sound knowledge of all the surgical procedures carried out in order to care for the post-surgery patient. Knowledge of the anaesthetic technique performed and how this will influence patient recovery is essential. An understanding of the unique needs and differences of the two ends of the life continuum (children and the older person) is essential in order to give a high level of individualised care.

From this description it can be seen that the recovery practitioner is a highly skilled individual working in a critical care area who should have had education and training to support their practice. This chapter will examine the main areas of knowledge needed for the practitioner working in recovery.

MANAGEMENT OF THE PATIENT'S AIRWAY IN RECOVERY

Obviously the most important part of caring for the post-anaesthetic patient is ensuring they have a patent airway. This is one of the reasons why the ratio of staff to patients in recovery should be one practitioner to one unconscious patient (Association of Anaesthetists of Great Britain and Ireland 2002). The airway can be obstructed for many reasons, and a patent airway can be maintained by many different methods.

Airway obstruction

Upon entering the recovery unit the patient will have had an anaesthetic and as a result of that they will have loss of muscle tone to a greater or lesser degree. This will mean that the tongue has a greater propensity to fall posteriorly and obstruct the airway. All humans have a tongue and so it follows that after anaesthesia this is the most common form of obstruction. If airway adjuncts are not in place the airway must be maintained manually. This is easy to do when the patient is on their back, but safer for the patient if they are on their side (Prowse 1999).

Added to this the patient may have excess blood and secretions, which will also obstruct the airway, and these must be removed by gentle suction. In the immediate post-anaesthetic stage the patient is at high risk of vomiting. The skilled recovery practitioner will be able to recognise the signs of this. The patient will become pale and clammy, the blood pressure will drop and there may be increased swallowing culminating in vomiting. Obviously if the patient is on their back they must be immediately turned on their side, the trolley tilted to the head down position and suction applied to decrease the risk of aspiration. If aspiration is suspected a chest X-ray must be performed (Hatfield and Tronson 2001).

Other more unusual forms of airway obstruction are caused by throat packs being left in place, teeth, particularly in children and the elderly, compression of the trachea by for example a haematoma, and oedema of the larynx caused by surgery or a traumatic intubation. Laryngospasm is a major form of obstruction, although not as common nowadays with the wider use of the laryngeal mask airway.

Laryngospasm

Mevorach (1996) cites Olsson and Hallen (1984) who found a mean incidence of laryngospasm of 8.6/1000 in adults and 27.6/1000 in children. From these figures it can be assumed that most recovery practitioners at some time in their career will encounter it. Prompt action is required, and knowledge of the physiological processes involved and an appreciation of the treatment options available is essential.

Anatomy

A series of cartilaginous rings held together by ligaments intertwined by many small muscles make up the larynx. The epiglottis prevents foreign objects such as food, blood and teeth entering the trachea (Murray-Calderon and Connolly 1997). When the larynx is viewed under direct vision the vocal cords appear as white lines with a triangular shape between them. This triangular space is known as the glottis.

The larynx is controlled by two sets of muscles – intrinsic and extrinsic. The intrinsic muscles are responsible for the framework of the larynx, which includes the opening of the cords on inspiration, alteration of cord tension during speech and finally as a protective mechanism during swallowing by closure of the cords. The extrinsic muscles are involved in the movement of the larynx as a whole, which includes swallowing (Odom 1993). Murray-Calderon and Connolly (1997) expand on the description of these muscles by discussing something called 'glottis shutter closure' which is occlusion of the intrinsic muscles. Closure of the area controlled by the extrinsic muscles is called a 'ball valve closure'. The clinical significance of these is that when there is intrinsic glottic closure this will result in partial obstruction, whereas complete obstruction is caused by extrinsic ball valve closure.

The external branch of the laryngeal nerve supplies the cricothyroid muscle, which innervates the vocal cords. The remaining muscular structure is innervated by the recurrent laryngeal nerve (Murray-Calderon and Connolly 1997). Stimulation of these produces reflex laryngeal closure which will protect the lungs from aspiration and foreign bodies (Nawful and Baraka 2002).

The reason for laryngospasm is not clear (Murray-Calderon and Connolly 1997), although distinction must be made between laryngospasm and laryngeal stridor. Laryngospasm occurs in the partially anaesthetised patient by irritation from blood and mucous, while stridor will occur only when the patient is making active ventilatory effort and is often conscious (Sukhani et al. 1993).

Laryngospasm post-anaesthesia

Most authors agree that patients are more prone to laryngospasm post-extubation (McConkey

2000; Murray-Calderon and Connolly 1997; Odom 1993), with a higher incidence in children (Nawful and Baraka 2002). Excessive secretions, blood and irritation of the oral airway may also precipitate laryngospasm. Sukhani *et al.* (1993) indicate there may be a psychological component to laryngospasm; they describe a patient who developed stridor postoperatively, in the absence of any respiratory effort or decrease in oxygen saturation. When an investigation was carried out under direct vision it revealed no underlying pathology. This patient's stridor resolved itself with reassurance alone. Golden (1997) has also identified this phenomenon and suggested the treatment could be the administration of midazolam on emergence from anaesthesia and reassurance. Patients at risk are often anxious adolescents and young adults. Numerous terms for this phenomenon are to be found in the literature including hysterical stridor; psychogenic stridor; functional stridor; Munchausen stridor and spasmodic croup (Sukhani *et al.* 1993).

Treatment of laryngospasm

Classically the treatment for laryngospasm is 100% oxygen with positive pressure ventilation. Establishing the cause of the spasm is also an important aspect of treatment. If mucous or blood are the cause, gentle suctioning may be required which will resolve the situation. However suctioning must always be used with caution as it may well exacerbate the situation (Murray-Calderon and Connolly 1997).

Delaying the treatment of laryngospasm can lead to hypoxaemia and hypercarbia and the use of suxemethonium under these conditions can lead to serious arrhythmias. The suggestion has been made that the answer to this is to give relatively low doses of suxemethonium, e.g. 0.1 mg kg^{-1} (normal intubating dose 1.5 mg kg^{-1}). With this dose it has been found that there is very little effect on spontaneous respiration and bradycardia is not manifested by repeated doses. The conclusion was that the laryngeal muscles must be very sensitive to the effects of suxemethonium (Chung and Rowbottom 1993). A further treatment described is the use of sub-anaesthetic

doses of propofol 25 mg/kg^{-1} (Nawful and Baraka 2002).

A treatment for laryngospasm that does not involve the use of drugs is digital pressure (Addei 2003). The technique involves placing the middle finger of each hand in the notch behind the lobule of the pinna of each ear. Pressure is then put very firmly with the fingers while at the same time using the 'jaw thrust' manoeuvre. Larson (1998) concludes that if carried out correctly it will convert laryngospasm within one or two breaths to stridor and then to normal respiration. No scientific reason is presented as to why this method works, but Larson (1998) suggests one of the reasons may be that it causes severe pain to the patient which will relax the vocal cords by way of either the sympathetic or parasympathetic nervous system. Rajan (1999) while using this technique and finding it effective, disagrees with Larson's (1998) explanation of how it works. He suggests it works because the painful stimulus increases the tone of the muscle groups which support the airway. Finally Johnstone (1999) describes the same technique but this time in a unilateral way by holding the mask with one hand and applying pressure with the other. This technique sounds effective in the treatment of laryngospasm and is worth consideration and would be a skill the recovery practitioner could learn.

Post-laryngospasm induced pulmonary oedema

Post-laryngospasm induced pulmonary oedema occurs more commonly than generally thought – the figures are between 0.05 to 0.1% of all anaesthetics. Post-laryngospasm induced pulmonary oedema is often unrecognised or misdiagnosed (McConkey 2000).

The exact cause is not clear; however several suggestions have been put forward. The age of the patient is thought to be a factor in its development. Very few cases have been reported in the elderly (Baltimore 1999). Cases in the main appear to be in young athletic individuals; this is thought to be due to thoracic musculature. These patients often have a well-developed musculature and have the ability to create very high negative intrathoracic pressures. As the patient attempts to breathe against an obstructed airway, the high pressure causes oozing of fluid from the capillaries which leads to capillary epithelial damage. This in turn will lead to movement of fluid out of the vascular space and into the surrounding tissues (Baltimore 1999). The high negative intrathoracic pressures are not sufficient to cause the condition and other factors may play a role such as the anaesthetic itself. There may be myocardial depression by residual anaesthetic agents in the early postoperative period which would make the patient susceptible to post-laryngospasm induced pulmonary oedema. Airway bleeding may be the dominant event rather than pulmonary oedema and this may lead to disruption of the high pressure bronchial (McConkey 2000).

Whatever the cause, when treating post-laryngospasm induced pulmonary oedema there appear to be standard treatments. However the use of suxemethonium early on in laryngospasm appears to negate the severity of the symptoms (McConkey 2000). Other treatment is oxygenation and reintubation to ensure airway patency (Murray-Calderon and Connolly 1997). The use of diuretics is controversial because the pulmonary overload is due to leaky capillaries rather than fluid overload (Baltimore 1999). Midazolam may be given to reduce anxiety, as patients will be concerned about this unplanned event. Patients have very little recall of the immediate postoperative period (Mevorach 1996).

What appears clear from the literature is that a patient suffering from post-laryngospasm induced pulmonary oedema rapidly stabilises once treated and their stay in hospital appears to be limited to 24 hours (Murray-Calderon and Connolly 1997).

Implications for the recovery practitioner

The practitioner working in the recovery has a key role to play in the treatment of laryngospasm. They must act promptly, making sure the patient is well-oxygenated and reassured – whether conscious or unconscious – while calling the anaesthetist immediately to come and assess the situation. The practitioner must work calmly and efficiently to make sure all equipment and drugs are available should they be required. Finally the practitioner must remember the patient and continue to communicate with them at all times. Assessing which patients may be at risk from laryngospasm is key to the role of the recovery practitioner. This should be underpinned with knowledge of the pathophysiology involved and the current treatments based on the evidence available. The practitioner should work in collaboration with the anaesthetist to bring about the best possible treatment for the patient.

Respiratory depression

Obviously breathing is important; however when a patient has an anaesthetic there are a number of pharmacological agents, which have a respiratory depressant effect. The main group is opioids and if a patient is receiving opioids the respiratory rate should be constantly monitored. Respiratory depression associated with opioids is termed 'Ondine's' curse. Ondine was a mythical water nymph who found out that her lover had been unfaithful to her. She cursed him so that he had to remember to breathe; however he fell asleep and died (Prowse 1999).

Residual neuromuscular blockade

The recovery practitioner must be able to recognise whether the patient has got full muscular function and therefore it is important to assess whether there are any residual effects from the muscle relaxant. The patient must be asked to lift their head and sustain it for more than 5 seconds and stick out their tongue for the same duration. The recovery practitioner must ensure that the patient can grip their hand for the same period of time. The other question the recovery practitioner should ask themselves is why there is prolonged neuromuscular blockade in the first instance. Numerous drugs and physiological conditions can potentiate the action of muscle relaxants (Kervin 2002) (Figure 6.1).

Antibiotics such as tetracyclines
Local anaesthetics and cardiac antiarrhythmics
Magnesium
Volatile anaesthetic agents
Hypothermia
Hypokalaemia
Respiratory acidosis
Myasthenia gravis

Figure 6.1   Pharmacological agents and physiological conditions which may potentiate the action of muscle relaxants

Should the post-anaesthetic patient be recovered in the supine position?

There is no doubt that an unconscious patient is at higher risk of aspiration if they are in the supine position rather than on their side. So why do the majority of patients arrive in the recovery unit on their back? The practice appears to have evolved with the advent of the laryngeal mask airway. These facilitate a patent airway and safe delivery of oxygen in the post-anaesthetic period. However one of the accepted limitations of the laryngeal mask airway is that it does not protect the patient from aspiration. In practical terms what this means is that if the patient vomits in the recovery unit while still unconscious they have to be turned on their side quickly. There are a finite number of staff in the recovery unit so it makes this manoeuvre difficult and even dangerous. Would it be more sensible to turn the patient in theatre prior to arrival in the recovery unit where there are often more staff and lifting equipment to do this? The arguments against this practice would be varied and one view might be that it is unnecessary as patients regain consciousness very quickly following the administration of propofol. This argument would be indefensible if a patient died following aspiration, and precautions to prevent this were not in place. Recovery practitioners must be aware of the risks to the patient of being in the supine position, and perhaps current practice should be reviewed in a critical manner.

Summary

To summarise, airway management is the most important part of caring for the post-anaesthetic patient. This takes priority over all other aspects of the patient's care. There are many reasons why the airway will become obstructed and the patient ceases to breathe. The recovery practitioner must be familiar with these and the actions to be taken. Airway adjuncts have not been discussed as they are covered in Chapter 4.

POSTOPERATIVE NAUSEA AND VOMITING (PONV)

Without doubt the most common and distressing problems following anaesthesia and surgery are pain and emetic problems. In the past decades pain has been well-researched and the practice of pain management has advanced significantly; official reports have been instrumental in this (Royal College of Surgeons and the College of Anaesthetists 1990).

Clearly pain is very distressing for the patient having undergone major surgery. However in some instances PONV can be more distressing. Diemunsch *et al.* (1999) found that patients were willing to accept pain in exchange for freedom from PONV.

Nausea and vomiting has been associated with general anaesthesia for many years. John Snow in 1848 observed that vomiting was more likely to occur when the patient had eaten and happened more frequently when the patient was moved following surgery. His treatment was wine and Battley's solution of opium (Andrews 1992).

With the advent of less emetic anaesthetics and refined surgical procedures, the incidence of PONV has decreased. However the level is still unacceptable. When applying the incidence to day surgery patients Hitchcock (1997) found that it ranged from 30 to 60%. In the general surgical population it can range between 8 and 92% (Arnold 2002). Consideration should also be given to patients who suffer PONV for the first 24 hours following surgery; the incidence of this appears to be up to 30% (Lerman 1992).

The mechanisms of nausea and vomiting are poorly understood and there are a number of reasons for this. Firstly in order to carry out well-controlled trials large amounts of patients would need to be involved and the number of variables would be considerable such as age, gender, type of anaesthetic, surgical and anaesthetic technique; thus well-controlled trials are problematic. Secondly many studies do not differentiate between nausea and vomiting, and retching and vomiting. Thirdly prior to the introduction of 5-hydroxytryptamine-3 ($5\text{-}HT_3$) receptor agonists the physiological emetic mechanisms were under-researched. Finally there is a lack of animal models on which to study the physiological and pharmacological emetic mechanisms. Rats and rabbits do not vomit irrespective of stimulus.

What is nausea and vomiting?

Nausea is an unpleasant sensation associated with the desire to vomit. It may occur prior to vomiting but it can be prolonged. Once a patient has vomited this may alleviate the sensation of nausea.

Vomiting is an active expulsion of the upper gastrointestinal contents and can be proceeded by retching, although not always. Vomiting should not be confused with reflux, which is passive (Arnold 2002). In the natural world nausea and vomiting is an important defense mechanism for the expulsion of ingested toxins (Tate and Cook 1996).

The detrimental effects of nausea and vomiting can be classified into three groups. The first of these are the physical effects. Vomiting as mentioned previously is an active process putting stress on the oesophagus leading to oesophageal tears. In extreme cases the oesophagus can rupture. This illustrates the strain put on the body when vomiting and is of particular importance when delicate surgery has been performed, e.g. ophthalmic surgery.

Obviously in the recovery area vomiting is a problem if the patient is unconscious because there is a high risk of aspiration and all the attendant issues with that (see Chapter 4).

If vomiting is prolonged it will lead to metabolic effects such as dehydration, alkalaemia and

anorexia. The final effect of nausea and vomiting is psychological. If a patient has vomited following previous surgery they are three times more likely to vomit on subsequent surgery (Andrews 1992). This in turn will lead to aversion to surgery as vomiting itself is an aversive stimulus.

Physiology of vomiting

The emetic centre is situated in the brainstem and receives input from the chemoreceptor trigger zone (CTZ). Four neurotransmitters are involved in mediating the emetic response: dopaminergic; histamine; cholinergic–mucurinic; and 5-hydroxytryptaminic ($5\text{-}HT_3$) (Arnold 2002; Tate and Cook 1996). These will be triggered by stimuli such as trauma, noxious chemicals and gut distension and these messages will be sent via the vagus nerve to the CTZ. This information is in turn relayed to the emetic centre in the medulla resulting in the patient vomiting. According to Tate and Cook (1996) toxic substances can directly stimulate the CTZ and emetic centre as can the higher cortical centres resulting in the feeling of nausea and even vomiting, although this mechanism is poorly understood (Figure 6.2).

Factors predisposing to PONV

- **Gender** – The incidence of PONV appears to be higher in women than men and there seems to be a direct correlation with the stage of the menstrual cycle. PONV appears to be more prevalent in the first eight days of the menstrual cycle and lowest on days 18, 19 and 20 (Beattie *et al*. 1991). The natural progression from this is that gynaecological patients have a higher incidence of PONV.
- **Age** – Related to gender it follows that from the age of the menarche to the menopause there is an increased incidence of PONV (Beattie *et al*. 1991). In the general population the peak age appears to be between 6 and 16 (Tate and Cook 1996).
- **Obesity** – There is a definite correlation between body weight and the incidence of PONV. This is thought to be due to an accumulation of anaesthetic agents in the body

because of the increase in adipose tissue (Thompson 1999).

- **Past medical history** – If a patient has a history of PONV or motion sickness this is likely to increase the incidence of PONV (Jolley 2001).
- **Preoperative fasting** – Food induces vagal afferent activity abdominally, which can produce emesis. A patient with a full stomach is highly likely to vomit on induction and post operatively (Andrews 1992). If minimal fasting times are used, i.e. 6 hours for food and 2–4 hours for clear fluids, there does not appear to be an increased incidence of PONV. However if these times are exceeded patients may feel nauseous because of hunger (Kenny and Rowbotham 1992).

- **Anxiety** – There appears to be a correlation between anxiety and PONV. This is thought to be due to the increase in circulating cate-cholamines which stimulate the doperminergic receptors and increase swallowing of air causing gastric distention and stimulation of the cholinergic receptors (Hawthorne 1995).
- **Pharmacology of anaesthesia** – Premedication, anaesthesia and postoperative analgesia are well-recognised for stimulating the emetic response. However there is less emetic response when the induction of anaesthesia is carried out using propofol as a bolus or as part of a total intravenous anaesthetic technique (Millar *et al.* 1997). Generally at all stages of the patient's experience, the use of opioids increases the

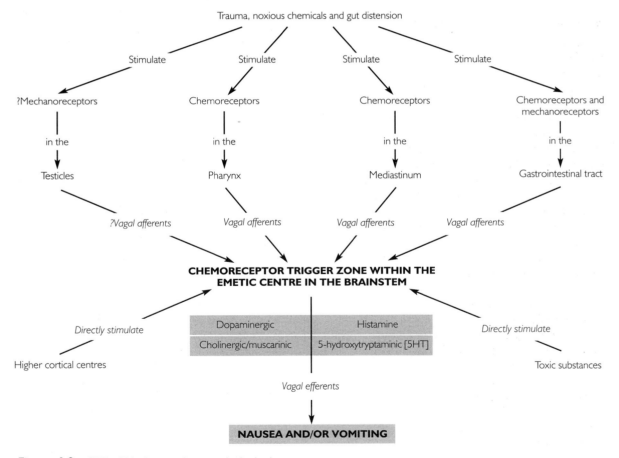

Figure 6.2 CTZ within the emetic centre in the brainstem

likelihood of PONV by stimulating the CTZ and the emetic centre (Thompson 1999).

- **Surgical factors** – Generally the relationship between surgical factors such as the site of operation remains unclear. There is no doubt however that as mentioned previously there is a higher rate of PONV in gynaecological patients particularly following laparoscopies. Again the reason is unclear because of the many variables. PONV rates are influenced by the duration of surgery: the longer the surgery the greater the incidence of emesis (Broomhead 1995).
- **Postoperative factors** – These include pain, hypertension, opioid analgesia and movement. There is a definite relationship between pain relief and the cessation of nausea (Thompson 1999). Antiemetics should always be given with opioid analgesia.

The management of PONV in recovery

To effectively manage PONV in recovery the practitioner must be familiar with all the possible risk factors. For example the patient should be pain free. Patients who suffer pain postoperatively are more likely to suffer from PONV (Sinclair *et al.* 1999). They should be well-hydrated, sudden movement should be avoided, the blood pressure should be maintained and the patient should be well-oxygenated.

PONV is usually treated by the use of an antiemetic. It is important however to select the most effective one. Two questions should be asked: (i) What prophylactic antiemetic was given as part of the anaesthetic, if any? (ii) What is the mechanism of action of that agent? From this a treatment plan can be derived. If an antiemetic has not been given, a dopamine receptor blocker such as metoclopramide is a good choice or a 5-HT$_3$ such as ondansetron. If this has not taken effect after 15–20 minutes, another antiemetic with a different mechanism of action should be administered. If an antiemetic has been given as part of the anaesthetic and is not effective in the postoperative period the same applies, choose an antiemetic with a different mechanism of action (Figure 6.3).

While antiemetic therapy is usually the first line of treatment for PONV, consideration must be given to non-pharmacological forms of treatment. Studies have examined the efficacy of peppermint oil (Tate 1997); ginger (Ernst and Pittler 2000); supplemental oxygen (Greif *et al.* 1999); isopropyl alcohol inhalation (Merritt *et al.* 2002); and acupressure (Ming *et al.* 2002). Some of these are simple to use and should be considered alongside conventional treatments.

It can be seen that a multimodal approach should be used to treat the patient suffering from PONV. Golembiewski and O'Brien (2002) proposed using a systematic approach to PONV.

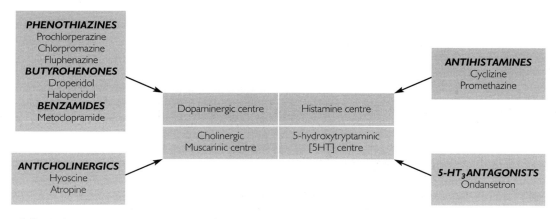

Figure 6.3 Antiemetics and their mechanisms of action

Firstly consideration should be given to the pre-operative risk factors the patient may have and this will give an indication of the potential risk of PONV, for example 1–2 risk factors = mild to moderate risk and more than 4 risk factors = very high risk. Consideration should also be given to the intraoperative period, employing techniques that will minimise the likelihood of PONV. The same is applied to the postoperative period. The algorithm is concluded with an examination of the treatment modalities, which could be given. In all cases non-pharmacological methods should also be considered (Figure 6.4).

In this section it can be seen that PONV is a problem for the patient and the recovery practitioner. Recognising patients at risk is essential in the effective treatment of PONV. There is no doubt that there is a definite link between pain and PONV (Chia et al. 2002). The management of pain is covered in the following section.

PAIN MANAGEMENT IN POST-ANAESTHETIC RECOVERY

Pain is defined in many different ways. Moline (2001) cited Merskey (1997) who defined pain as 'an unpleasant sensory and emotional experience associated with actual or potential tissue damage, or described in terms of such damage' (p. 389). The most clinically relevant definition of pain was proposed by McCaffery (1968) cited by Moline (2001): 'pain is whatever the experiencing person says it is, existing whenever he says it does' (p. 389). This definition is used widely and

---

Preoperative: assess risk factors (RF):
- 1–2 RF = mild – moderate risk: use single antiemetic prophylactically
- 3–4 RF = moderate to high risk: use a combination of antiemetics with differing modes of action
- More than 4 RF = very high: as with moderate to high but additionally consider a less emetic anaesthetic technique like TCA

Intraoperative
- Omit nitrous oxide
- Effective pain management
- Avoid dehydration
- Avoid hypotension
- Avoid excess air into the stomach

Postoperative
- Adequate hydration and oxygenation
- Adequate pain management
- Avoid sudden movement
- Consideration of non-pharmacological methods

IF:

An antiemetic has not been given prophylactically:
- Metoclopramide
- Ondansetron

IF:

An antiemetic has been given intraoperatively:
- Consider an antimetic with a different mode of action

IF:

A combination of antiemetics were given intraoperatively:
- Consider a different combination with different modes of action

Added to the above non-pharmacological treatments should also be considered.

Figure 6.4 PONV Algorithm (Adapted from Golembiewski and O'Brien, 2002)

supports the view that pain is subjective and unique to the individual experiencing it. The way we experience pain is influenced by social, cultural, physiological and psychological factors. The study of pain is vast and because of this, in this section the subject will only be examined on a surface level and applied to the recovery area.

Pain is a protective mechanism. We need to be able to feel pain in order to protect ourselves from injury. Melzack and Wall (1982) cite the example of a young woman who died at the age of 29 of injuries caused by her inability to feel pain. She did not shift her weight and thus strain was put on her joints. She developed something known as 'Charcot joint', meaning that her joints became inflamed and infected, eventually leading to osteomyelitis. This is an extreme example but it serves to demonstrate the importance of the ability to feel pain.

While it is a protective mechanism there is no reason why postoperative patients need to experience pain, indeed they should be managed in such a way that they do not feel pain throughout their surgical experience. However the reality is that this does not happen (Salomaki et al. 2000). In order for the practitioner to effectively treat the patient it is important they have an understanding of pain, the physiological principles underpinning it and the psychological influences that impact on the experience of pain. Although these will be examined separately one will influence the other. The way that pain is perceived is twofold. Firstly the physical pain, but that in turn will be influenced by anxiety or fear associated with the physical pain (Moline 2001).

Physiology of pain

Pain is experienced due to pain receptors in the tissue, known as nociceptors detecting a noxious stimuli. Each nociceptor is connected to a nerve, which when stimulated will fire an electrical impulse along its length. There are three types of nerves concerned with the transmission of pain, and dependent upon their diameter and whether or not they have a myelin sheath, the pain response is mediated. First, there are the A-beta fibres which have a large diameter and are myeli-

nated. Secondly, B-delta fibres which are myelinated and have a small diameter. These fibres conduct impulses quickly and are concerned with pinprick pain, pain that only lasts a short time. Finally, the C fibres; these are concerned with slower onset duller pain that lasts much longer and they are smaller and unmyelinated. These are termed as the first order neurones and carry the impulse to the posterior horn of the spinal cord activating cell layers, the most important of which is the substantia gelatinosa.

The information from the nociceptors reaches the brain by various pathways named from where they originate and end. The main one and best described is the spinothalamic pathway, known as the second order neurones. These pathways are afferent pathways. In the spinal cord they divide into the neospinothalamic tract which goes to the posterior thalamus and is implicated with the duration location and intensity of pain. The paleospinothalamic tract goes to the medial thalamus and is associated with emotional and autonomic aspects of pain. At this point pain is appreciated and messages are passed to the prefrontal lobes and the limbic lobes where the emotional response to pain is experienced. All messages are integrated at this point to elicit the appropriate response; these are known as the third order neurones (Hatfield and Tronson 2001).

The degree of pain sensation can be increased by substances such as prostaglandin, histamine, substance-P and bradykinin, and this is thought to explain why pain continues after the noxious stimulus has been removed (Barasi 1991).

The gate control theory of pain

Controversy still exists about how pain is mediated, and scientific study continues. From this theories have evolved, against which new facts can be tested and the theory evolves further. Over the years many theories of pain have been proposed, however one widely documented is the gate control theory of pain proposed by Melzack and Wall in 1965. The gate control theory is acceptable because it accounts for the many differences in the ways individuals experience pain.

The basis of the gate control theory is that the substantia gelatinosa is the essential site of control and this control mechanism is referred to as the 'gate'. Pain impulses can only pass through the 'gate' when it is opened. The opening and closing of the 'gate' is influenced by internal as well as external factors.

External influences

When the nociceptors are excited by noxious stimuli pain impulses travel along the A-beta, B-delta and C fibres, and the speed at which they travel is mediated by their thickness and myelination. The gate control theory proposes that if non-painful stimuli such as vibration reach the substantia gelatinosa before the painful stimuli the gate will be closed and the experience of pain may diminish or stop due to the action of inhibitory neurotransmitters. This could explain why gentle rubbing at the site of injury lessens the pain because the A-beta fibres have been simulated. It is thought this is why transcutaneous electrical nerve stimulation (TENS) and hot and cold therapies are successful.

Internal influences

Impulses can travel down from the brainstem, cerebral cortex and thalamus and affect whether the 'gate' is open or closed. If a patient feels confident and in control through receiving adequate information, inhibitory signals will close the 'gate'. This is one of the reasons why patient controlled analgesia (PCA) is thought to work because it empowers the patient to control their own pain. The reverse of this is if the patient is anxious, does not feel in control and lacks information the 'gate' will be opened and the patient may experience more pain or perhaps have problems controlling existing pain (Davies 1993).

Psychology of pain

As previously mentioned, the physiological and psychological factors involved in the experience of pain are not mutually exclusive. Previous experience of pain, socioeconomic dimensions, the meaning of pain and perception of pain also influence the pain experienced. Added to this patients will have preconceived ideas of how they should deal with their pain, and the practitioner will have preconceived ideas about what should be painful and what degree of pain a patient should be suffering.

Common assumptions

Practitioners tend to assume that:

- patients will tell them when they are in pain
- analgesia will eliminate the patient's pain
- patients react in a similar way to the same type of injury, operation or procedure.

Patients however may assume that:

- the practitioner knows about the pain they are experiencing
- practitioners are too busy dealing with more deserving or demanding patients
- pain is an inevitable and inescapable part of being in hospital.

Therefore we must question our assumptions. This requires self-awareness. We must look at our own attitudes. A patient being admitted for a hernia repair may elicit a different response to a patient being admitted for an orthopaedic operation due to a road traffic accident. We must work hard to prevent ourselves from ignoring the needs of the patient in pain whatever the cause.

The personal meaning of pain

Research under taken by Beecher (1956) compared pain in soldiers and civilians. The soldier's pain threshold was much higher when they were injured on the battlefield than comparable injuries in civilians who had surgery. To the soldier injury meant escape and survival. Beecher (1956) found that civilians on the other hand needed higher doses of analgesics, as surgery meant a catastrophic interruption to their daily lives.

The nature of pain

Acute pain may be transient and quickly forgotten, whereas chronic pain may signify loss of work, break-up of interpersonal relationships, handicap and severe disability, loss of self-esteem, vulnerability or impending death. Therefore recovery practitioners must understand the psychological significance of pain.

The influence of culture on the perception of pain

Culture plays an important part in the development of people's psychological makeup. Zborowski (1952) studied the relationship between pain and culture. He observed four cultural groups: Irish, Jewish, Italian and Old American stock. What he discovered was:

- The Jewish and Italians had a low tolerance to pain, and demonstrated an emotional and expressive response. They demanded rapid pain relief and were uninhibited in their reactions.
- The old American stock were more reserved. Their description of the pain was unemotional, they preferred to be alone when experiencing pain, and they only cried when they were alone.
- The Irish group were reluctant to discuss their pain, but admitted to family and friends that they did suffer.

Anxiety and pain

Pain can be heightened by anxiety (Coll *et al.* 1999; Thomas 1998). Considerable research data is available, which demonstrates the positive effects of providing supportive information to patients (de C Williams 1998). It is therefore essential to spend time with the patient and listen to what they have to say.

The benefits of treating pain

- **Humanitarian**. Patients in pain may be fatigued and demoralised and sleep patterns may be interrupted. Fear of pain makes people reluctant to undergo surgical intervention. Therefore treating pain is an essential element of good quality care.
- **Respiratory function**. General anaesthesia and surgery, especially abdominal and thoracic surgery, have a detrimental effect on respira-

tory function, which will last well into the postoperative period. Poor pain relief may exaggerate these changes and lead to chest infections, respiratory failure, hypoxia and a longer stay in hospital.
- **Cardiovascular system**. Pain is associated with tachycardia and hypertension. This is undesirable and may lead to myocardial ischaemia and infarction, particularly in patients with myocardial disease. Good analgesia may reduce the incidence of this.
- **Gastrointestinal system**. Nausea caused by inappropriate analgesia may decrease fluid intake leading to dehydration, and dietary intake may be restricted. Pain may slow the return of normal gut activity, leading to an intravenous infusion of fluids for a prolonged period of time.
- **The stress response to surgery**. Metabolic and endocrine changes are an inevitable response to surgery. The stress response to surgery is not abolished by good analgesia, but its severity may be reduced.
- **Cost effectiveness**. It is likely that good postoperative pain relief is associated with earlier discharge from hospital. Also a pain free patient may make fewer demands on time. Pain also impedes mobility leading to DVT and pressure sores, which may necessitate admission to ITU. Preventing even a small amount of these will make significant savings.

Pain assessment

Hatfield and Tronson (2001) suggest that any pain assessment should be carried out in five stages:

1 What is the cause of the pain?
2 Assess the amount of pain.
3 Reassure and comfort the patient.
4 Use appropriate and effective analgesia.
5 Reassess the patient to test the efficacy of the treatment given.

What is the cause of the pain?

Consideration must be given to the other factors, which may be causing discomfort. There are many procedures carried out on patients that will cause discomfort. If they have been intubated they may have a sore throat; this will mean they will have a tonsillitis type pain where it is painful to swallow; up to 80% of patients suffer from a sore throat following laryngoscopy (Aitkenhead 2001). They may have had suxemethonium where the fasciculation causes muscle pains and the patient may feel as if they have been exercising 24 hours non-stop; this can occur in up to 50% of patients who have had suxemethonium administered (Aitkenhead 2001). They may have a headache caused by their anxiety prior to surgery or lack of nutrition. A full bladder can cause discomfort. Pressure may have been put on peripheral nerves during surgery. If they have been badly positioned, ligaments may have been stretched. Any dressings which have been applied may be too tight and causing discomfort. Finally there may be some underlying cardiac problem such as myocardial ischaemia and this may be causing chest pain. Finding out the cause of the pain is important because it may not be due to the surgery.

Assess the amount of pain

The analgesic regime will be dependent to some degree upon the intensity of the pain being experienced by the patient (Bodian *et al.* 2001). The most commonly used scale for assessing pain intensity is the visual analogue scale, which comes in various forms. Essentially it is a horizontal line with 'no pain at all' at one end and the 'worst pain imaginable' at the other. It is simple, reliable and valid to use to describe pain intensity and severity.

Numerical rating scales are a variation on the visual analogue, where 0 = no pain and 10 = the worst pain imaginable. There appears to be general agreement as to what level analgesia should be given. In a study by Salomaki *et al.* (2000) they used a score of 3/10 as an indication of inadequate postoperative pain relief, as did Pouzeratte *et al.* (2001). Buss and Melderis (2002) continue that in order to assess the level of pain correctly the patient must be prepared prior to surgery and the rating scale explained to them. It should be assumed that a patient entering the recovery area

following surgery will be in pain and therefore assessment is important. The assessment will be more meaningful if the assessment tool has been explained to the patient prior to surgery.

Other pain scales include the familiar Wong–Baker smiley faces used on children usually above the age of three. There are also verbal rating scales, which are based upon the graduation of words, for example: bearable, tolerable, through to unbearable.

Reassure and comfort the patient

Anxiety must be treated separately from pain; there is little doubt that anxiety can enhance the experience of pain (Hatfield and Tronson 2001). By assessing why the patient is anxious and reassuring them, the pain can be reduced. Giving patients information prior to their surgery can reduce the pain experienced after surgery.

Use appropriate and effective analgesia

It is usual to use a multimodal approach to effective analgesia. In 1990 the Royal College of Surgeons and the Association of Anaesthetists published a report about the inadequacy of the treatment of postoperative pain, and made recommendations for change. The result of this report 14 years on is that a multimodal approach to pain management is used. The majority of patients are likely to have non-steroidal anti-inflammatory drugs (NSAIDs) prior to anaesthesia. Analgesia is given as part of the anaesthetic technique and this will include consideration of the postoperative period. Wound infiltration is common, added to this PCA is available to patients and if PCA is not available opioids will be administered intravenously in the immediate postoperative period.

Reassess

This is to test the efficacy of what has been given. Assessment and administration of analgesia are meaningless if reassessment does not take place to find out whether it has been effective. The patient should not be returned to the ward or discharged home if they are still in pain.

Acute pain service

To control pain effectively management should commence before the patient has had their surgery and this is where the role of the acute pain service should commence. The idea of an acute pain service is not new. In North America they were established in the mid-1980s. In the UK the inception of acute pain services started as a result of the pain report (Royal College of Surgeons and the College of Anaesthetists 1990). In the report it stated, 'that this service should be introduced in all major hospitals performing surgery in the UK' (p. 1).

The acute pain service is responsible for the day-to-day management of acute postoperative pain and obstetric pain (Werner *et al.* 2002). Primarily the acute pain service is a multidisciplinary team usually consisting of physicians, nurses and/or physiotherapists, pharmacists and psychologists.

The role of the acute pain service should commence prior to surgery. A member of the team should visit the patient, assess them and discuss how their pain is going to be managed. The patient should be encouraged to participate in this process and develop strategies that are appropriate for them.

THE TREATMENT OF PAIN

The treatment of pain can broadly fit into five categories: opioids; non-steroidal anti-inflammatory drugs (NSAIDs); local analgesia; oral analgesia; and non-pharmacological techniques. These categories will be examined broadly rather than looking at specific drugs.

Opioid analgesia

An example of this type of analgesic is morphine. It mainly works on the opioid receptors in the central nervous system. The main receptors are the Mu (μ) which produce superspinal analgesia, respiratory depression, physical dependence, euphoria and constipation and are located in the brain and spinal cord (Bennett *et al.* 2001). The kappa (κ) receptors produce spinal analgesia and sedation and the delta (δ) receptors are involved in affective behaviour. From this it can be seen that the μ receptor is the main mediator of pain relief, but is also involved with the side effects associated with opioids (Moline 2001).

Morphine has two metabolites, morphine-3-glucuronide (M3G), which is inactive, and Morphine-6-glucuronide (M6G), which is excreted in the kidneys and is active. This is clinically significant in patients with impaired renal function where high levels of M6G can result, leading to excessive sedation and respiratory depression (Pesero *et al.* 1999a).

Patient-controlled analgesia (PCA)

PCA has gained popularity since the Royal College of Surgeons and College of Anaesthetists (1990) report on pain after surgery. It has been widely accepted by staff working in the perioperative arena. It negates the need for frequent administration of intramuscular injections and thus saves time (Koh and Thomas 1994). The efficacy of PCA is further enhanced by a dedicated pain service whose role is one of education of patients and staff (Coleman and Booker-Milburn 1996). Leaflets can be given to supplement any information given to patients. Chumbley *et al.* (2002) examined the leaflet information given to patients prior to PCA administration. With the use of focus groups and questionnaires, they found that the information patients wanted to know about was the drug used in the PCA pump. They were also concerned to know what the side effects were, their anxiety being primarily that they could not overdose and become addicted to the drug. The research also highlighted the need for detailed diagrams.

It is acknowledged that when administering opioids intramuscularly there is normally a poor response to the analgesic. This is because of the inherent differences in patients of the sensitivity of the opioid receptors. Therefore equilibrium between the plasma concentration and the receptor drug concentration must be achieved. This is defined as the minimal effective analgesic concentration (MEAC), where the analgesic given produces a steady-state plasma concentration at which effective analgesia is achieved. However it is difficult to predict each patient's MEAC levels, as these will vary with age and psychological profile. With PCA the amount of analgesic given is determined by the patient providing feedback control (Power and Smith 2001).

The overriding principle of PCA is that an opioid, most commonly morphine, is administered intravenously by the patient. They are taught to use a demand button, which delivers a preset amount of the drug with a lock-out period of between five and ten minutes. Initially a background infusion was used in conjunction with the bolus dose, however it was found to be unsafe and most PCA is given as demand bolus dose only.

The advantages of PCA are that a MEAC can be achieved for the individual patient because they are in control of dose delivery and because smaller doses are given there is less fluctuation in plasma concentrations. It reduces workload and empowers the patient because they feel they can control their own pain.

The disadvantages are that the equipment is expensive and technical errors can be fatal. The patient must be able to cooperate and understand how to use the PCA. Gagliese *et al.* (2000) examined whether age was a barrier to the effective use of PCA and concluded that the use of PCA was not hindered by age differences. The final disadvantage of PCA is the category of patients it is used upon. Anecdotally it appears to be determined by the type of surgery rather than an assessment of individual patients' needs. In most hospitals in the UK there is a limited number of PCA pumps and this governs who will receive PCA.

Non-steroidal anti-inflammatory drugs (NSAIDs)

Analgesia from NSAIDs is primarily from a peripheral action. They produce antipyretic, anti-inflammatory and analgesic effects. Examples are ketorolac and diclofenac.

Primarily they inhibit prostaglandin synthesis. Prostaglandin is involved in potentiating the movement of the pain impulse from the periphery to the central nervous system. It facilitates the activation of the nociceptors and the inflammatory process to produce peripheral pain

(Pesero *et al.* 1999b). This is achieved by blocking cyclooxygenase (COX), which converts arachidonic acid to prostaglandin (Moline 2001). By inhibiting prostaglandin these responses are diminished and analgesia is achieved without the side effects of opioids.

Although widely used as postoperative analgesia, the side effects of NSAIDs are due to the inhibition of prostaglandin, which has numerous sites of action. For example prostaglandin has a protective action on the gastrointestinal system which is lost with the use of NSAIDs, and thus bleeding from injury and irritation to the gastrointestinal mucosa can be a problem. In certain groups of patients there can be reduced renal blood flow due to the vasoconstrictive effects of angiotensin II, usually inhibited by renal prostaglandins. Patients particularly at risk are hypovolaemic patients; patients with reduced renal function; the older patient; and patients with congestive heart failure. Ketorolac in particular inhibits platelet aggregation, although this is a reversible process, returning to normal values within 24–48 hours. This however may result in prolonged bleeding times (Fiedler 1997).

Local analgesia

Local analgesia is another adjunct to the overall management of the patient's pain. Broadly it fits into four groups:

- Topical
- Wound infiltration
- Regional blocks
- Central blocks.

Topical local analgesia

Primarily used in children with the use of EMLA™ cream to reduce the pain of venous cannulation (Thompson 2002). Also reported is the use of lidocaine gel topically to reduce pain following circumcision (Rudkin 1997a).

Wound infiltration

The practice of infiltrating the wound with local anaesthetic upon closure is well-established in day surgery and deemed effective (Rudkin

1997b). However the benefit is not clear after major surgery (Power and Smith 2001).

Regional blocks

The reasons for administering a regional block are twofold. Firstly they may be given for the purpose of the surgery. If the patient is not being anaesthetised, the regional block will promote loss of sensation and pain. Secondly it may be given specifically to provide postoperative analgesia. However unless a continuous catheter is used these blocks may be wearing off by the time the patient reaches recovery, and so supplemental analgesia has to be administered (Power and Smith 2001). They have additional benefits in vascular surgery of improving 'run off', improving vascular graft uptake and performance.

Central blocks

Included in this group are spinal and epidural analgesia, which are discussed in Chapter 4. The recovery practitioner must however be familiar with caring for patients who have received a central nerve blockade.

Spinal analgesia has the same problems associated with it as a regional block in that it is a single injection and supplemental analgesia may be required. The recovery practitioner must be aware that the patient may still be hypotensive due to the cardiovascular effects of the spinal anaesthetic. Thus fluid intake must be maintained and the patient observed for the attendant side effects of a lowered blood pressure such as nausea and vomiting. The main issue for the recovery practitioner is the avoidance of a spinal headache and this is accomplished by gradually sitting the patient up. Psychologically the patient will feel odd following spinal anaesthesia due to the complete loss of sensation in their legs, and reassurance must be given, plus care to protect the limbs from accidental damage.

When a patient enters the recovery unit having undergone epidural anaesthesia, there is the immediate advantage of the epidural catheter being in place, which can be used to top up the epidural or it can be used for continuous infu-

sion, and thus give excellent postoperative analgesia. The patient will be treated in the same way as for spinal analgesia, but additional issues have to be considered.

Continuous epidural infusion

The use of continuous epidural infusions is now well-established as one of the protocols for the management of postoperative pain, with the natural progression to patient-controlled epidural analgesia (Wootton 2000). This works on the same principle as patient-controlled analgesia in that it empowers the patient, allowing them to be in control of their analgesic regime. However after the initial loading dose there does need to be a high level of anaesthetic input (Russell 2001). This may be because there is a lack of sufficiently trained recovery practitioners in the use of this technology, but with wider use this problem will dissipate.

Continuous epidural anaesthesia is gaining popularity. It is now accepted that the use of epidural anaesthesia/analgesia reduces postoperative morbidity and mortality. The boundaries for use of continuous epidural anaesthesia are being pushed wider. The recent evidence highlights its use in cardiac surgery patients who are fully heparinised (Faccenda and Finucane 2002). Once this would have been an absolute contraindication because of the risk of a compressing vertebral canal haematoma. However the use of low molecular weight heparins has had a major impact in the use of epidurals in cardiac surgery patients (Vandermeulen 1999).

When using a continuous epidural infusion the following observations must be made.

- Respiratory rate, especially if an intrathecal opioid has been administered. Respiratory depression can be reversed by the use of naloxone. This is a competitive antagonist with the μ receptors. Repeated doses may need to be given because of its short duration of action (one hour) (Moline 2001). Naloxone should be given slowly because it can produce sympathetic stimulation leading to hypertension, tachycardia, pulmonary oedema, arrhythmias and culminating in cardiac arrest (Pesero *et al.* 1999a).

- Oxygen saturation.
- Motor sensation and function – a decrease in motor or sensory function may indicate an epidural haematoma, although this is extremely rare.
- Signs of local anaesthetic toxicity.
- Blood pressure – if the patient becomes very hypotensive additional fluids must be administered.

Oral analgesia

Oral analgesics are rarely used within main inpatient recovery, but they are the mainstay of day surgery recovery where avoidance of an opioid is indicated if at all possible. Usually oral analgesics are given as part of the multimodal approach, combining NSAIDs, wound infiltration and oral analgesics, which will be continued by the patients at home.

Non-pharmacological techniques

Recovery practitioners must never discount the use of non-pharmacological techniques. There is much the practitioner can do that is not prescribed. Simply talking to the patient and trying to make them less anxious may help some patients. Holding their hand and soothing their brow may sound old-fashioned in this high-tech world, but for some patients this can be exceedingly comforting.

Other forms of non-pharmacological treatments are distraction therapies and the application of heat or cold. Transcutaneous electrical nerve stimulation (TENS) is helpful to some patients (Rudkin 1997b).

In summary it can be seen that the management of pain in the postoperative period is complex. The recovery practitioner has a wide variety of analgesic strategies at their disposal. However these can only be effective if the practitioner is knowledgeable about the interface between the physiological and psychological components of pain.

FLUID MANAGEMENT IN THE POST-ANAESTHESIA PATIENT

All surgical patients will have fluid loss to a greater or lesser degree. This is in the form of sensible and insensible loss, which can be overt or covert. Insensible loss from the lung and skin increases in the presence of hyperventilation and fever. Loss of fluid from the gut is common. In order to appreciate the fluid replacement the patient may require in the recovery area, the practitioner must understand the normal composition and distribution of fluid within the body.

Total body water (TBW) is apportioned in the following way. One-third is contained in the extracellular fluid volume (ECFV) and two-thirds in the intracellular fluid volume (ICFV). The ECFV is further subdivided into interstitial and intravascular compartments (McVicar and Clancy 1997).

The main constituents of extracellular fluid (ECF) are sodium as the principle cation and chloride as the principle anion. The capillary endothelium is a freely permeable membrane to water, cations and anions, but not protein. Thus protein is in a higher concentration in the plasma. In the intracellular fluid (ICF) the principle cation is potassium and the anion is phosphate. Additionally there is a high protein content. The membrane is selectively permeable but water moves freely so that equalisation of osmotic forces occur continuously. Water has to be able to move freely from the ICF to the ECF to eliminate any osmolal gradient. Sodium is kept out of the ICF by means of the sodium pump. It follows therefore that any fluids infused that contain sodium remain in the ECF, so saline 0.9% expands the ECFV only. If an infusion with 5% glucose is given the glucose enters the cells and is metabolised. The water enters the ICF and ECF thus expanding the TBW (Turner 2001).

For the patient undergoing any surgical procedure there is additional 'third space' loss. This is not contained in an anatomical compartment; rather there is an expansion of the ECFV. This loss is from fluid, which comes from surgical tissue trauma and is proportional to the extent of surgery (Stark 1998).

The normal fit surgical patient will have lost fluid by fasting, blood loss, 'third space' loss and loss from the skin, gut and lungs. If a patient is critically ill, a child or an older person the losses are greater. Proportionally more care will be taken in these categories of patients, and if larger volumes of fluids need to be infused this will be carried out through a central line and should be guided by central venous pressure monitoring (Turner 2001).

Postoperative fluid management is guided by maintenance of normal fluid levels taking into account the losses during surgery. Additional fluid should be administered if there is excessive loss from drains greater than 500 millilitres or if there is continued gastrointestinal loss, for example from a nasogastric tube. Fluid will also be required if there is continuing 'third space' loss, for example in total gastrectomy and if the patient has become hypothermic during surgery and requires rewarming (Edwards 2001).

Essentially there are three types of fluid that can be administered to the patient: (i) crystalloids such as saline 0.9%; (ii) colloids which include human albumin solution or a synthetic substitute; and (iii) blood products such as fresh frozen plasma and packed blood cells (Krau 1998). Traditionally it was thought that when volume needed to be replaced it was generally agreed that a colloid solution was appropriate to re-establish haemodynamic stability (Krau 1998). However in a review of randomised trials looking at fluid resuscitation, it was concluded that the use of colloids should not be used for volume replacement in critically ill patients (Schierhout and Roberts 1998). This is an ongoing debate and the type of replacement used is still not universal; it is based on physician preference in the area they practice.

In conclusion, in order to care for the post-surgical patient, the recovery practitioner must be aware of how fluid is lost, and when replacing it which compartment it is affecting, what constituents are needed and the appropriate fluid to be infused.

MONITORING THE CARDIOVASCULAR STATUS OF THE PATIENT IN RECOVERY

Monitoring of the patient's cardiovascular status is essential once the patient leaves the comparative safety of the operating room with the attendance of the anaesthetist, other practitioners and the array of available monitoring equipment. Mandatory assessments of blood pressure, oxygen saturation and heart rate and rhythm should be instituted and maintained until the patient is ready to be discharged from the recovery area.

Many of the factors discussed earlier in this chapter can deleteriously affect the cardiovascular status, notably electrolyte or fluid imbalance, hypoxia, pain, nausea, vomiting and anxiety. A blood pressure recording using one of the methods described in Chapter 4 should be taken on the patient's arrival in the recovery room, pulse oximetry should be instituted and the patient attached to continuous cardiac monitoring for heart rate and rhythm.

Blood pressure

The significance of the blood pressure relates to the preoperative value recorded. Essentially, a change to the postoperative blood pressure needs investigation to find its cause in order that appropriate treatment can be initiated. Both hypertension and hypotension are common in postoperative recovery and are generally caused by factors relating to the anaesthetic, operation or cardiovascular factors and hence management is targeted at treating the cause.

Pre-existing hypertension

Postoperative hypertension is likely to occur in known hypertensive patients and it is important that the anaesthetist has conducted a preoperative assessment of the hypertensive patient to assess their postoperative risk (Shammash and Ghali 2003). The value of preoperative blood pressure control is recognised and the general guidance is to continue with antihypertensive medications during the perioperative period. It is particularly important to avoid withdrawal of beta-blockers because of the potential rebound tachycardia and hypertension which might occur. Concern has been expressed that angiotensin converting-enzyme (ACE) inhibitors, such as ramipril, and angiotensin 11 (A11) receptor antagonists, such as losartan, may augment the blood-pressure lowering effect during anaesthetic induction. These patients may require vasopressor or sympathomimetic drugs during induction, but there is no expert advice to withhold the dose of ACE, A11 or diuretics preoperatively (Shammash and Ghali 2003).

Hypertension

Acute hypertension is common in the recovery room and can be defined as a blood pressure which is 20% higher than the preoperative baseline blood pressure (Hatfield and Tronson 2001). Hypertension can be caused by numerous factors including those listed below:

- Pain
- Hypoxia
- Hypercapnia
- Emergence and arousal from anaesthesia
- Hypervolaemia
- Full bladder
- Ketamine anaesthesia
- Vasopressors
- Epidural or spinal anaesthesia that is wearing off
- Phaeochromocytoma.

The most common reasons for hypertension in the recovering patient are pain and fluid overload and usually swift recognition and management of the cause will result in a slow, steady lowering of the blood pressure to normal values. Uncontrolled hypertension, however, is associated with many risks, particularly for the elderly or patients with pre-existing cardiovascular problems. These risks include potential for myocardial ischaemia or even infarction, cardiac failure, stroke (haemorrhagic), cardiac arrhythmias and bleeding from the operative sites. Fulminant (malignant) hypertension can occur if the blood pressure rises above 220/120 mmHg.

It is rare, but it can be seen in undiagnosed phaeochromocytoma, tetanus or spinal cord damage. It manifests as rapid deterioration in neurological status due to cerebral oedema resulting in confusion, disorientation, drowsiness and headache. Malignant hypertension requires rapid investigation and treatment usually with vasodilatory drugs such as glyceryl trinitrate, sodium nitroprusside or hydralazine. During the treatment, careful observation of the neurological status, cardiac rhythm and operative wound sites will elicit any other complications.

Hypotension

Hypotension, defined as more than 20% reduction in preoperative blood pressure recordings, is also fairly common and once again, finding the cause will direct the practitioner to the appropriate treatment (Hatfield and Tronson 2001). Hypotension may be caused by:

- Cardiac arrhythmias – bradyarrhythmias, tachyarrhythmias
- Haemorrhage
- Extracellular fluid loss, e.g. burns
- Epidural or spinal anaesthesia
- Residual effects of general anaesthesia, e.g. thiopentone or propofol
- Myocardial ischaemia or infarction
- Cardiac failure
- Pulmonary or air embolus
- Pneumothorax
- Drugs, e.g. beta-blockers or neostigmine
- Sepsis
- Hypotensive anaesthetic technique such as used in cardiac, neuro and ear, nose and throat surgery.

This list is by no means exhaustive, but identifies the commonly encountered causes in the recovery room. Many patients will tolerate a low systolic blood pressure of 80–90 mmHg systolic, as a result of the residual effects of epidural, spinal or general anaesthetic. If however the patient is elderly or has pre-existing cardiac, cardiovascular or cerebrovascular disease the hypotension needs closer evaluation. Monitoring of the cardiac rhythm with particular emphasis on observing any deviation in the ST segment or ventricular extrasystoles is imperative as this may indicate myocardial ischaemia. Oxygen should be given by mask and the O_2 saturation monitored. If the problem is due to intravascular or extracellular fluid loss then fluid replacement will be necessary using the principles described in the section above (Krau 1998). Careful monitoring of the patient for evidence of early signs of shock – cool clammy skin, tachycardia and a poor urine output, should be maintained.

Cardiac monitoring

Cardiac arrhythmias are common in the perioperative period and are mostly clinically insignificant (Sloan and Weitz 2001). Arrhythmias are most likely to occur in patients with known cardiac disease. Preoperative assessment of the patient with known hypertension, heart failure, haemodynamically significant arrhythmias and valvular heart disease is imperative to establish the postoperative risk. Similarly, comorbid states that can affect cardiac function such as respiratory disease, diabetes and peripheral vascular disease should be noted. A standard 12-lead ECG is a basic clinical assessment tool which will give information about previous cardiac disease, conduction abnormalities and arrhythmias and will direct the clinician to the need for any further evaluation and management (Shammash and Ghali 2003). It is usual for a patient with a pre-morbid state to have a 12-lead ECG recorded during pre-assessment. During the perioperative period it is usually sufficient to monitor the patient's cardiac rhythm from a 3-lead system. Lead 11 is generally used for rhythm monitoring purposes, as it will record a predominantly positive deflection – a positive P wave and a tall positive R wave. However in rare situations it may be necessary to monitor the cardiac function from more than one view – i.e. a 5-lead monitor system. For example, if a patient is known to have myocardial ischaemia affecting the anterior wall of the heart, it may be helpful to record a V3 lead to view the anterior anatomy of the heart.

However, many arrhythmias can be triggered in healthy individuals by a variety of factors such as hypoxia, electrolyte or fluid imbalance, pain, nausea and anxiety. The anaesthetic or surgical insult may also initiate an arrhythmia; the physiological impact of the arrhythmia, its subsequent management and treatment, will be dependent upon the patient's clinical status and their cardiac function (Hollenberg and Dellinger 2000). Technological advances have led to sophisticated monitoring systems which can be used in recovery areas which incorporate rate and rhythm analysis with pulse oximetry; cardiac monitoring however is an essential element of recovery practice as it gives a continuous picture of the heart's electrical activity in real time (Jevon and Ewens 2002). It is important therefore that recovery practitioners can demonstrate rhythm interpretation as a core skill to maintain patient safety. As with any technical skill, it is only, however, an adjunct to your care and the old adage *'look at the patient, not just the monitor'* should always be borne in mind (Woodrow 1998).

The electrocardiogram (ECG)

The ECG is a graphic representation of the electrical activity generated by the cardiac conduction system. Monitoring electrodes placed on the body's surface detect this activity and transmit it via monitoring leads to either an oscilloscope or to recording paper where it is amplified and displayed as a series of waveforms.

Minding your Ps and Qs

The basic ECG waves are labelled alphabetically and begin arbitrarily at the P wave. The P wave represents atrial depolarisation (atrial stimulation); the QRS complex represents ventricular depolarisation (ventricular stimulation); the ST-segment, T wave and U wave if present, indicate ventricular repolarisation (recovery). The QT interval represents the complete electrical activity time of ventricular stimulation and recovery and it varies with heart rate. When there is no electrical activity present the ECG will show a straight line – the isoelectric line. It is normal for example for the line to be isoelectric in between the P

Table 6.1 Normal waveforms; amplitude, duration and shape

Waveform/interval	Amplitude	Duration	Shape
P wave	1.0–2.5 mm	40–100 ms	Pointed or rounded
PR-interval	Isoelectric	120–220 ms (varies with heart rate)	Isoelectric
QRS complex	8–25 mm	60–100 ms	Sharp and narrow
ST-segment	Isoelectric	N/A	Isoelectric
T wave	5 mm	N/A	Asymmetric, pointed
QT-interval	N/A	300–430 ms (varies with heart rate)	N/A

wave and the QRS complex (the PR-segment), and between the QRS complex and the T wave (the ST-segment). When waveforms deviate above the isoelectric line they are termed *positive deflections* and when they deviate below the line they are *negative deflections*.

ECG paper

The electrical events are recorded onto special ECG graph paper (Figure 6.5), which consists of boxes which are intersected with dark and light vertical and horizontal lines, thus forming small and large boxes (Huszar 2002). Each small box is 1 millimeter square (1 mm^2) and each large box is 5 millimeter square (5 mm^2). Conventionally the paper speed is 25 mm/second and the paper allows measurement of time (along the horizontal axis) and voltage or amplitude (along the vertical axis).

As the ECG uses standardised paper and paper speed, the ECG waveforms can be described in terms of both amplitude (voltage) and duration (time) and abnormalities of waveforms can be readily identified. The normal duration and amplitude for the ECG waveforms is given in Table 6.1.

Generally cardiac arrhythmias can be considered within three groups, determined by the site of origin of the arrhythmia: supraventricular (atrial); junctional (nodal); and ventricular. The rhythms which are most likely to occur within the recovery area will be discussed with regard to cause, recognition, clinical significance and treatment. The goal of management in any arrhythmia will be to establish haemodynamic stability as quickly as possible. In a tachyarrhythmia the aim will be to slow the heart rate and in a bradyarrhythmia the ventricular response must be restored. Arrhythmias which do not cause haemodynamic compromise may not require urgent intervention (Hollenberg and Dellinger 2000).

Sinus rhythm

Sinus rhythm is the normal rhythm of the heart, when all the component waveforms are present – P wave, PR-segment, QRS complex, ST-segment and T wave. Sinus rhythm originates from the sinoatrial node (hence *sinus rhythm*) and is defined as a heart rate between 60 and 100 beats per minute (bpm) in an adult (Spiers 2002).

Figure 6.6 identifies the supraventricular arrhythmias that are frequently seen in recovery.

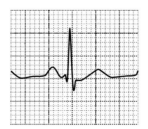

Figure 6.5 ECG paper

- Sinus tachycardia
- Sinus bradycardia
- Sinus arrhythmia
- Atrial fibrillation
- Narrow complex tachycardia

Figure 6.6 Supraventricular arrhythmias

Sinus tachycardia (Figure 6.7)
This is probably the most frequently observed arrhythmia in the recovery room. It can be defined as a normal sinus rhythm, but at a rate faster than 100 bpm (Riley 2002). In adults, the heart rate will be between 100 and 150 bpm, although in young, fit healthy individuals it may reach 180 bpm.

- **Recognition.** Figure 6.7 gives an example of sinus tachycardia. Note that all the component parts of P, QRS and T wave are present, but the intervals between each waveform is significantly reduced. Each QRS complex is preceded by a P wave, but at very fast rate, the P wave may merge with the preceding T wave making it difficult to distinguish the two waveforms. The QRS rate is fast (>100 bpm) and regular.
- **Causes.** Sinus tachycardia may be considered a physiological response to a variety of situations in which sympathetic tone is increased or vagal tone decreased including those listed in Figure 6.8.

Sinus tachycardia can be induced by drugs that increase sympathetic tone (e.g. epinephrine, dopamine, cocaine, atracurium, pancuronium and ketamine) and drugs that decrease vagal tone (e.g. atropine and other anticholinergic drugs). It is a frequent response to pain and anxiety and may often be seen in the recovery room as the patient regains consciousness. Sinus tachycardia may also occur as a compensatory response to reduced cardiac output in serious cardiorespiratory conditions such as left ventricular failure, acute myocardial infarction and pulmonary embolism. As sinus tachycardia will reduce car-

- Physiological – anxiety, nausea, pain, exercise
- Pathological – fever, anaemia, septic and hypovolaemic shock, thyrotoxicosis
- Fluid loss – vomiting, diarrhoea, bleeding, burns
- Pharmacological – epinephrine, atracurium, salbutamol, atropine, ketamine
- Cardiac ischaemia, infarction or failure

Figure 6.8 Causes of sinus tachycardia (adapted from Spiers 2002)

diac output and reduce myocardial oxygenation, it will exacerbate the existing pathology.

- **Clinical significance.** Sinus tachycardia is essentially a physiological response and hence its treatment depends upon eradicating or at least identifying and managing the cause. In the recovery room it may be an early indication of inadequate analgesia or hypovolaemia (Hatfield and Tronson 2001). As cardiac filling time is reduced at heart rates above 130 bpm, most patients cannot tolerate a sinus tachycardia for prolonged periods of time. Reduced cardiac filling time results in reduced cardiac output, hypotension and syncope, and the conscious patient may complain of significant symptoms. In addition myocardial perfusion will also be reduced during period of tachycardia and this may cause angina-type pain due to myocardial ischaemia. These symptoms will be exacerbated in the elderly and in patients with known cardiac or respiratory disease (Spiers 2002).
- **Management.** Clinical assessment of the patient should include: monitoring of the trends in BP, CVP, oxygen saturation and if possible ST-segment monitoring. A 12-lead

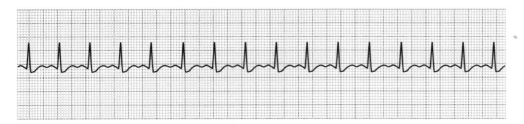

Figure 6.7 Sinus tachycardia

ECG may also reveal ST-segment depression due to myocardial ischaemia. In general no specific treatment is offered for sinus tachycardia, but considerable attention should be paid to finding and rectifying the underlying cause. Managing fluid replacement, pain and improving oxygenation will all reduce the heart rate.

Sinus bradycardia (Figure 6.9)

Sinus bradycardia is a commonly encountered *normal variant* and it is frequently seen in fit, healthy individuals with high vagal tone, during sleep and it is also seen in athletes (Da Costa *et al.* 2002).

- **Recognition.** In sinus bradycardia, sinus rhythm is present at a rate less than 60 bpm but usually more than 40 bpm. At slower rates the patient will become considerably compromised due to reduced cardiac output. During sinus bradycardia, the pauses between complexes are lengthened and hence the period for cardiac filling is enhanced. At rates between 40 and 60 bpm sinus bradycardia may actually enhance cardiac performance as cardiac output and myocardial perfusion will be optimised (Spiers 2002). Figure 6.9 indicates sinus bradycardia.

- **Causes.** Sinus bradycardia can occur in any situation that increases vagal tone or decreases sympathetic activity (Spiers 2002). It is a normal variant in fit, healthy individuals during sleep and in trained athletes who may have a resting or sleeping heart rate as low as 35 bpm (Goldberger 1999). Sinus bradycardia is seen frequently during the perioperative period and has many causes.

Drug therapy is frequently implicated in sinus bradycardia in the postoperative period. Narcotic agents used during surgery cause bradycardia due to central vagal stimulation. Anticholinesterases (such as neostigmine) used to antagonise the effect of non-depolarising neuromuscular relaxing agents, increase acetylcholine in the heart and may cause bradycardia. Timolol and pilocarpine eye drops used during ophthalmic surgery may be systemically absorbed and can cause bradycardia (Sloan and Weitz 2001).

Bradycardia is often caused by activation of a reflex arc involving the vagus nerve. Hence reflex bradycardia may occur during many surgical procedures, such as eye surgery particularly where enucleation is involved, abdominal surgery with mesenteric traction and manipulation of vagally innervated structures such as the oesophagus and rectum. Many anaesthetic agents can also activate this reflex arc and drugs such as atracurium, vecuronium, halothane and fentanyl are particularly implicated. The reflex can be prevented by incorporating an anticholinergic

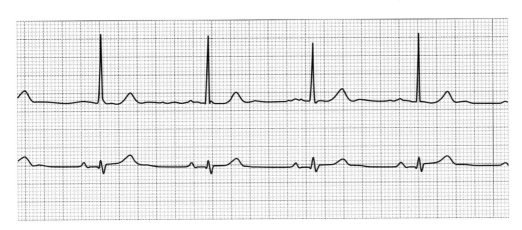

Figure 6.9 Sinus bradycardia

agent such as atropine into the premedication (Sloan and Weitz 2001).

- **Clinical significance.** As bradycardia is a frequently observed arrhythmia, postoperative clinical monitoring of blood pressure, O_2 saturation and peripheral perfusion are mandatory. At heart rates of 50–60 bpm, the cardiac output may be augmented and the patient may be clinically stable. Some patients however will not tolerate slow rates of sinus bradycardia and will complain of light-headedness and syncope. Syncope is often associated with collapse and the patient may describe this as a 'fainting attack'.

- **Management.** As with sinus tachycardia, no specific treatment is offered for sinus bradycardia, but in the compromised patient Atropine 1 mg IV will increase the heart rate quickly. During operative procedures which may initiate reflex bradycardia, extra care should be taken with patients who are already taking beta-blockers (atenolol), calcium channel blockers (diltiazem) or digoxin to ensure that their heart rates do not fall to precipitously low rates.

Sinus arrhythmia (Figure 6.10)

In healthy individuals, the sinus node does not always pace the heart at an entirely regular rate – a slight beat-to-beat variation is often seen. This cyclic variation in sinus rhythm is referred to as 'sinus arrhythmia' and it is considered *a normal variant* in young adults and the elderly (Goldberger 1999; Wiederhold 1999).

- **Recognition.** Sinus arrhythmia is a sinus rhythm with normal P, QRS, ST and T waves, but it manifests as a slightly irregular rhythm. This irregularity occurs in a healthy cycle and hence the rhythm is said to be *irregularly irregular* (Spiers 2002).

- **Causes.** The cyclic variation in sinus rhythm is commonly associated with respiration. *Respiratory sinus arrhythmia* occurs in response to changing thoracic pressures and is a normal result of changes in vagal tone that occurs during the different phases of respiration. Hence in sinus arrhythmia, the heart rate will increase slightly during inspiration and decrease during expiration. The effect on the heart rate can be quite marked (up to 10–20 bpm) in children and young adults (Riley 2002).

- **Clinical significance.** Sinus arrhythmia is generally considered to be a very benign arrhythmia, particularly when observed in young adults and in relation to respiratory cycles. It requires no clinical intervention in these circumstances.

- **Management.** *Respiratory sinus rhythm* and sinus arrhythmia seen in young adults is entirely benign and requires no clinical intervention. Occasionally sinus arrhythmia seen in elderly patients may herald early sinoatrial node disease known as *sick sinus syndrome* and extreme variations in heart rate may require a permanent pacemaker (Mangrum and DiMarco 2000).

Atrial fibrillation (Figure 6.11)

Atrial fibrillation is a ubiquitous and yet diverse cardiac arrhythmia, which for many years was considered a Cinderella arrhythmia. Until recently, the arrhythmia was rarely given much credence, poorly managed and inadequately

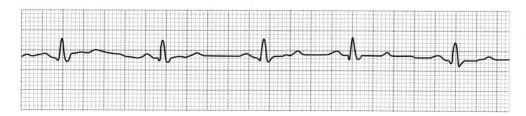

Figure 6.10 Sinus arrhythmia

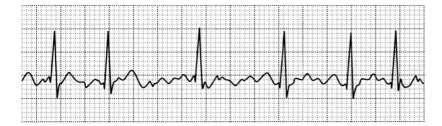

Figure 6.11 Atrial fibrillation

treated (Allesie *et al*. 2001; Pepper 2001). Atrial fibrillation is the most common sustained arrhythmia; its prevalence increases with age and it is frequently associated with structural heart disease. It may however be seen in patients with no known heart disease and its haemodynamic and thromboembolic consequences result in significant morbidity and mortality for affected individuals (Task Force Report 2001). The scope of this chapter does not allow extensive discussion of the management of this arrhythmia, therefore discussion will be focused upon the emergency management of paroxysmal atrial fibrillation in the postoperative patient.

- **Recognition.** Atrial fibrillation results from multiple ectopic foci forming throughout the atria. These ectopic foci override the sinus node function and cause the atria to *fibrillate*. The ectopic foci create electrical activity which are observed on the ECG as a wavy baseline or as *f waves*. These *f* waves may occur at a very fast rate (up to 600 bpm); the electrical activity generated 'bombards' the AV node with stimuli. Due to the physiological decremental activity of the AV node, not all impulses are conducted into the ventricles (which could prove disastrous) and the ventricular response is therefore fast and irregular. Conduction to the ventricles occurs at an irregular and fast rate, usually between 60 and 180 bpm, and is evident in the rhythm strip below as a fast *irregularly irregular rhythm*. There are no discernible P waves, a wavy baseline, 'f waves' and normal-shaped QRS complexes. Due to the fibrillatory waves,

the T waves may also become difficult to identify (Spiers 2002).

- **Causes.** Atrial fibrillation is commonly encountered in patients undergoing major surgical procedures and is frequently seen in the elderly population (Pepper 2001). It is particularly prevalent in patients undergoing abdominal and thoracic aortic aneurysm repair, thoracotomy for lung cancer and cardiac surgery. The causes of atrial fibrillation are numerous and are summarised in Figure 6.12. Essentially atrial fibrillation may occur in situations which cause atrial dilatation or stimulation – such as sympathetic stimulation or fluid overload (Spiers 2002).

- **Clinical significance.** Atrial fibrillation is by far the most common arrhythmia seen in the perioperative period and it also has the most potential for serious consequences. Fast ventricular rates in atrial fibrillation can cause significant haemodynamic compromise. Atrial fibrillation causes reduced cardiac output,

---

- Atrial enlargement – mitral or tricuspid stenosis, fluid overload, cardiac failure
- Coronary heart disease
- Cardiomyopathy, cardiac failure
- Thyrotoxicosis, phaeochromocytoma, major thoracic, cardiac or abdominal surgery
- Sympathetic stimulation – anxiety, stimulants, anaesthetic drugs, ethanol
- Hypoxia – asthma, COPD, acute pulmonary embolism
- Fluid or electrolyte imbalance – hypokalaemia, hypomagnesaemia, positive fluid balance

Figure 6.12 Causes of atrial fibrillation

decreased cardiac filling time and loss of atri-oventricular synchrony. Conscious patients may experience significant symptoms including palpitations, dyspnoea, syncope and chest pain; the symptoms can be both alarming and distressing. In the unconscious patient, a fall in blood pressure and oxygen saturation herald the need for urgent intervention (Bubien 2000).

- **Management.** The patient's haemodynamic status dictates the treatment plan; if the patient is unstable the goal is to restore sinus rhythm either pharmacologically or by direct current (DC) cardioversion (Sloan and Weitz 2001). If the patient is stable and uncompromised there is time to identify the rhythm and to confirm a diagnosis. The aim in this situation will be to establish ventricular rate control. This may be achieved by anti-arrhythmic therapy using drugs such as amiodarone, flecainide, esmolol or defetilide. Unfortunately, most anti-arrhythmic drugs have only a moderate efficacy in terminating atrial fibrillation and many of the drugs also have proarrhythmic tendencies; that is that they may induce other and more serious arrhythmias in certain situations. For example, Flecainide may induce serious ventricular arrhythmias particularly in the presence of poor left ventricular function (Opie and Gersh 2001). Assessment of the patient's medical history is therefore mandatory before pursuing this approach.

In a compromised patient with atrial fibrillation, particularly when the ventricular rate is fast (more than 150 bpm), and poor perfusion is evident, prompt electrical conversion under sedation may be indicated. The European Resuscitation Council (2002) recommends cardioversion using an algorithm of 100J, 200J, 360J or appropriate biphasic energy as indicated. If atrial fibrillation recurs it is recommended that intravenous amiodarone 300 mg is administered over a one-hour period before cardioversion is reattempted. Alternatively flecainide 100–150 mg IV over 30 minutes may be given.

In addition, because of the propensity for atrial fibrillation to cause thrombus formation in the atrial chambers, intravenous anticoagulation is recommended in conjunction with either anti-arrhythmic or electrical therapy. Systemic anticoagulation therapy should be continued several weeks after electrical or pharmacological cardioversion to prevent thromboembolic episodes (Opie and Gersh 2001).

Supraventricular tachycardias (Narrow complex tachycardia)

The term 'supraventricular tachycardia' (SVT) can really be considered an *umbrella term* to describe any arrhythmia which arises above the level of the ventricles (Goldberger 1999); they are also referred to as narrow-complex tachycardias (NCT). Commonly SVTs can be divided into two distinct groups of arrhythmias, dependent upon whether they arise from the atria or the atrioventricular node/junction (Goodacre and Irons 2002). Tachycardias which arise from the atrial tissue include:

- Atrial fibrillation
- Atrial flutter
- Atrial tachycardia.

Tachycardias that arise from the atrioventricular node or junction and are commonly associated with re-entry circuits as seen in patients with Wolff–Parkinson–White syndrome include:

- Atrioventricular re-entrant tachycardias (AVRT)
- Atrioventricular nodal re-entrant tachycardias (AVNRT)
- Junctional tachycardia.

It is generally accepted that the underlying electrophysiological abnormality or arrhythmia mechanism classifies arrhythmias. A careful clinical history, examination of the 12-lead ECG and occasionally an electrophysiological study will lead to the correct diagnosis. However in perioperative practice this is not always practical or possible and therefore the term *narrow-complex tachycardia* (NCT) is used to describe the paroxysmal SVTs which are frequently seen (Sloan and

Weitz 2001). The recognition, causes and treatment in an emergency situation is essentially the same for all narrow-complex tachycardias and is described below.

- **Recognition.** It is not always possible to determine the focus of the tachycardia which may be in the atrial tissue or AV nodal tissue. The P wave will therefore be abnormal in shape, not present at all or 'hidden' within the preceding T wave. The QRS complex will be normal as usually the impulse is conducted using the intraventricular pathways. It may however present as a broad QRS complex (>100 ms) if the rhythm is aberrantly conducted. In practice, however, most SVTs can be considered to be narrow-complex tachycardias. The ventricular rate will be fast, generally faster than 150 bpm and may even be as fast as 250 bpm (see Figure 6.13).

- **Causes.** SVT/NCT may be a benign arrhythmia and is seen in children, young adults and the elderly. It tends to be paroxysmal in nature and has an abrupt onset and cessation. It may be triggered by sympathetic activation and the stress response. It may therefore be the sequelae to pain, anxiety or fluid imbalance. Caffeine, tobacco and alcohol are common precipitators. While it is seen in normal, healthy individuals it is also seen with virtually any type of heart disease.

- **Clinical significance.** The rapid ventricular rate may induce hypotension, reduced cardiac output, cerebral and myocardial ischaemia, acute cardiac failure and syncope. For conscious patients it may be an extremely

unpleasant experience associated with palpitations, breathlessness and chest pain. Haemodynamically compromised patients require urgent intervention, while some patients can tolerate the tachycardia for a period of time. Spontaneous reversion to sinus rhythm occurs in some patients.

- **Management.** The European Resuscitation Council guidelines (2002) give clear guidance on the management of narrow-complex tachycardia. It is considered within the group of peri-arrest arrhythmias as it is a critical situation and may trigger ventricular fibrillation. Urgent intervention for persistent NCT is therefore recommended and includes vagal manoeuvres, antiarrhythmic therapy and electrical cardioversion (Jevon 2002).

In a conscious, relatively uncompromised patient vagal manoeuvres may be employed. Vagal stimulation by carotid sinus massage or Valsalva manoeuvre are the most commonly used approaches. Vagal manoeuvres stimulate the vagus nerve and slow the heart rate down. In narrow complex tachycardia, vagal manoeuvres will be effective in up to 25% of cases. Carotid sinus massage should only be undertaken by skilled personnel, assessing first for carotid bruit by auscultating of the carotid artery with a stethoscope. This reduces the risk of arterial embolisation which may result in a cerebral infarction (European Resuscitation Council 2002). Carotid sinus massage may also induce severe bradycardia and this may precipitate a ventricular escape rhythm.

If vagal maneouvres are unsuccessful Adenosine is the drug of choice, except when

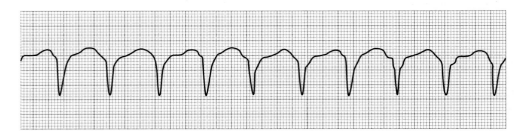

Figure 6.13 Supraventricular tachycardia

pre-excitation syndromes such as Wolff–Parkinson–White syndrome are suspected; in this case the clinician should proceed directly to cardioversion as outlined below. Adenosine inhibits AV nodal conduction and produces a transient AV nodal block when administered. It has an extremely short half-life (1–6 seconds) and is therefore very safe to administer, but needs to be given by fast bolus injection for effect. Adenosine 6 mg is given as a rapid bolus followed by a saline flush. If unsuccessful three more does of up to 12 mg may be administered, once every 2–3 minutes (Resuscitation Council 2000). The patient should be advised that adenosine may cause chest pain, facial flushing and bronchospasm and it should therefore not be given to asthmatics. It is otherwise a relatively safe drug to use except in the presence of pre-excitation syndromes (Opie and Gersh 2001).

If the patient is severely compromised by the SVT then synchronised cardioversion under sedation should be performed (100J, 200J, 360J). The patient needs reassurance and consent should be gained if possible. If cardioversion is unsuccessful then Amiodarone 150mg may be administered IV over 10 minutes, followed by a further 300 mg in the following hour if needed. Further cardioversion may then be attempted (Resuscitation Council 2000). At this point a cardiology consultation should be sought.

Ventricular arrhythmias

Ventricular arrhythmias arise from the cells in the ventricles or the Purkinje fibres and are potentially the most dangerous arrhythmias that can occur. However, haemodynamically significant ventricular arrhythmias are rare in the perioperative period (Shammash and Ghali 2003), but due to the serious nature of these arrhythmias the recovery room practitioner should be familiar with their recognition and management. In patients without structural heart disease, ventricular arrhythmias are usually benign and the risk of haemodynamic derangement is minimal. In patients with a previous history of coronary artery disease (previous myocardial infarction, known angina, cardiomyopathy) these arrhythmias may be harbingers of potential doom and require comprehensive assessment and management (Hollenberg and Dellinger 2000).

Ventricular arrhythmias include:

- Ventricular ectopics (extrasystoles)
- Ventricular tachycardia (pulseless or with a pulse)
- Ventricular fibrillation
- Pulseless electrical activity
- Ventricular asystole
- Ventricular standstill.

Ventricular arrhythmias therefore include the cardiac arrest rhythms, which require prompt recognition and urgent management.

Ventricular ectopics (extrasystoles)

Ventricular ectopics may occur in fit healthy individuals as well as those with structural or organic heart disease and result from early depolarisation of ventricular cells outside of the normally expected sinus rhythm.

- **Recognition.** The abnormal ventricular impulse is conducted aberrantly throughout the ventricles leading to a broad, bizarre QRS complex, no P wave will be apparent and the T wave will generally demonstrate an abnormal shape. The ventricular ectopic beat will usually be followed by a compensatory pause before the next sinus beat and hence the rhythm will become irregular. Ventricular ectopics may be unifocal (from one focal site in the ventricles) (Figure 6.14) or multifocal (multiple sites) (Figure 6.15) and may be infrequent or occur in a regular pattern. For example, when an ectopic occurs every other sinus beat it is referred to as *bigeminy*, and when the ectopic arises every third beat this is named *ventricular trigeminy*.
- **Causes.** Ventricular ectopics may occur in healthy individuals as well as those with coronary artery disease. In patients with known cardiac disease they are considered to be more

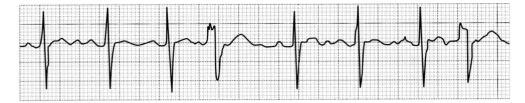

Figure 6.14 Unifocal ventricular ectopics

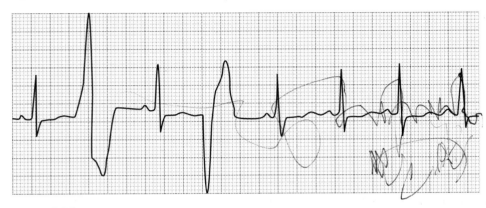

Figure 6.15 Multifocal ventricular ectopics

significant. Ventricular ectopics may arise in various situations and the possible causes are listed in Figure 6.16.

- **Clinical significance.** In the absence of known cardiac disease, ventricular ectopics are usually benign. However, if the number of ectopics is frequent (more than 10–15 per minute), if the ectopics are multifocal or occur in salvoes or occur close to the T wave of the preceding sinus beat (*the R on T phenomenon*) they require more urgent attention. Similarly if the patient is compromised by the ectopics (hypotension, syncope) then urgent investigation of the cause should be instigated.
- **Management.** Ventricular ectopics rarely need treatment as such, however identifying the cause of the ectopics may lead to an appropriate treatment plan. For example, if the patient is hypoxic this should be corrected with oxygen therapy, if the patient is stressed or in pain, reassurance and pain relief will reduce the frequency of the ectopics. It is wise to investigate the patient's blood chemistry as a

notable cause is a relative reduction in potassium and magnesium levels; these are readily correctable with intravenous therapy. It is unlikely that antiarrhythmic therapy will be used, as many of the available antiarrhythmic drugs have proarrhythmic potential (Opie and Gersh 2001). However, occasionally an intravenous bolus of Lidocaine (50 mg) may terminate the arrhythmia and a maintenance infusion may be used. Lidocaine is most effective in the presence of high potassium levels and hence hypokalaemia must be corrected for maximum effect (Opie and Gersh 2001).

- Increased catecholamines – stress, pain
- Stimulants – caffeine, alcohol, nicotine
- Drugs – anaesthetic agents, inotropes
- Hypoxia
- Electrolyte imbalance – hypokalaemia, hypomagnesaemia
- Cardiac disease – coronary artery disease, cardiac failure, cardiomyopathy

Figure 6.16 Causes of ventricular ectopics

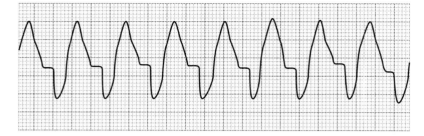

Figure 6.17 Ventricular tachycardia

Ventricular tachycardia (Figure 6.17)

Ventricular tachycardia (VT) is a life-threatening arrhythmia, which may be classified as benign or malignant, sustained or non-sustained, pulseless or with a pulse. Essentially these classifications relate to the patient's response to the arrhythmia and the management of the arrhythmia relates to the haemodynamic status of the patient.

- **Recognition.** VT is described as a broad complex tachycardia. The rhythm is hence fast (>130 bpm), there is no easily discernible P wave as the rhythm originates in the ventricles, the QRS is bizarre in shape and broad in width (>120 ms) and the rhythm is regular.
- **Causes.** VT results from either ectopic foci in the ventricles or rapidly firing macro re-entry circuits which cause fast impulse propagation in the ventricles (Riley 2002). There are numerous precipitating factors and the cause of the arrhythmia should be determined and provoking factors corrected where possible (Sloan and Weitz 2001). The predominant cause of sustained VT is the presence of structural heart disease (coronary artery disease, valvular heart disease and cardiomyopathy). Common causes of non-sustained VT in the perioperative period are given in Figure 6.18.
- **Clinical significance.** In patients without known structural heart disease, the risk of sudden death is minimal (Hollenberg and Dellinger 2000), but the rhythm can have serious haemodynamic consequences nevertheless. VT causes a reduction in cardiac filling and coronary artery perfusion and hence results in hypotension, syncope, chest pain and palpitations. In a patient with systolic dysfunction, the haemodynamic result can be devastating and urgent intervention may be necessary.
- **Management.** The European Resuscitation Council (2002) recommends three simple treatment options for VT. If the patient has no pulse, treatment should follow the protocol for ventricular fibrillation/ventricular tachycardia/cardiac arrest. If the patient has a pulse but displays adverse signs, seek expert help and cardioversion is the indicated treatment (Figure 6.19). Adverse signs include:
  - Systolic blood pressure <90 mmHg
  - Chest pain
  - Heart failure
  - Heart rate >150 bpm.

If the patient has no adverse signs, the arrhythmia can be managed with antiarrhythmic therapy (Figure 6.19). If this fails to control the arrhythmia then expert help and cardioversion is indicated. (European Resuscitation Council 2002). Correcting simple causes such as low potassium, magnesium and oxygen imbalances will also augment treatment and management.

- Electrolyte imbalance (potassium, magnesium and calcium)
- Myocardial ischaemia, injury or infarction (coronary artery disease)
- Mechanical or traumatic irritation (central venous catheters, valvular prolapse)
- Hypotension
- Fluid overload
- Drug toxicity (digoxin)
- Arrhythmia (bradycardia, ventricular ectopics)

Figure 6.18 Causes of ventricular tachycardia

If the patient is haemodynamically compromised then urgent cardioversion is required. This is a relatively reliable way of converting VT to sinus rhythm, but it is important that the shock is carried out on the R wave of the ECG rather than with the T wave. This is called synchronised cardioversion and it is safe as it avoids the relative refractory period of the cardiac action potential, reducing the risk of inducing ventricular fibrillation. In a conscious patient it is imperative that the patient is either anaesthetised or well sedated. If the synchro-

nised shock is not effective, Amiodarone 150 mg IV is given over 10 minutes followed by further cardioversion if necessary (European Resuscitation Council 2002).

If the patient is haemodynamically stable, antiarrhythmic therapy may be tried first using either amiodarone 150 mg IV over 10 minutes or lidocaine 50 mg over 2 minutes repeated every 5 minutes to a maximum dosage of 200 mg. If the antiarrhythmic therapy is unsuccessful, expert advice should be sought and it is likely that the patient will proceed to synchronised DC shock.

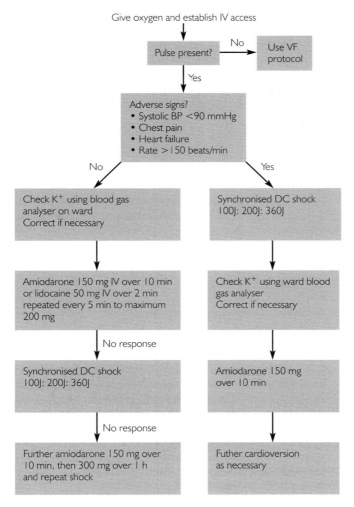

Figure 6.19 Management of broad complex tachycardia (adapted from ERC 2002)

Ventricular fibrillation (Figure 6.20)

Sustained ventricular tachycardia in the perioperative period should be stabilised as quickly as possible as it may rapidly lead on to ventricular fibrillation (VF). VF is one of the three cardiac arrest rhythms, the other two being asystole and pulseless electrical activity (previously called electromechanical dissociation). All perioperative practitioners should be able to recognise and articulate its management. Ventricular fibrillation arises from chaotic fibrillatory waveforms within the ventricles, the ventricles do not beat in any coordinated fashion but instead quiver or fibrillate ineffectively (Goldberger 1999). No cardiac output is generated by this rhythm and if left untreated it is a fatal arrhythmia.

- **Recognition.** Recognition of VF is relatively easy as there are no discernible atrial or ventricular depolarisations and hence it manifests as an undulating baseline with a jagged, irregular waveform on the cardiac monitor. It may display as either a *coarse* or a *fine* rhythm depending upon the length of time it has been present. Coarse VF is far more amenable to treatment (defibrillation).
- **Causes.** Essentially the causes of VF are the same as those identified for VT and ventricular ectopics. It is most likely to occur in patients with known cardiac disease and is the most common cause of sudden cardiac death in patients with acute myocardial infarction. It may however occur in normal hearts when it may be precipitated by electrolyte imbalance or drugs (see Figure 6.18) and it may also be precipitated by the previously described ventricular arrhythmias and even supraventricular tachycardia (NCT).
- **Clinical significance.** If VF is untreated permanent brain damage and death can occur within 5 minutes. On the other hand VF is an eminently treatable rhythm and the majority of people who survive a cardiac arrest present with this arrhythmia. The patient will have no pulse, blood pressure or spontaneous respirations and will demonstrate all the signs of peripheral and cerebral anoxia.
- **Management.** Treatment of VF should be immediate. If the cardiac arrest is witnessed or monitored (as it is likely to be in the recovery area), and a defibrillator is not immediately available, then a precordial thump should be delivered (European Resuscitation Council 2002). The precordial thump effectively acts as a low energy defibrillator and may be effective in the first 30 seconds of a VF cardiac arrest.

  The immediate treatment for VF is defibrillation, with up to three shocks given initially with energies of 200J, 200J and 360J. Gel pads should be applied to the patient's chest to protect against skin burns. If VF persists after the first three shocks, the patient's airway should be secured and intravenous access checked. Success in managing this rhythm still remains with defibrillation, but in order to ensure myocardial and cerebral viability, chest compressions and ventilation are maintained for one minute before defibrillation is attempted again. During this minute reversible causes should be considered and treated, gel pads, electrodes and other ECG connections checked for viability (European Resuscitation Council 2002) (Figure 6.19).

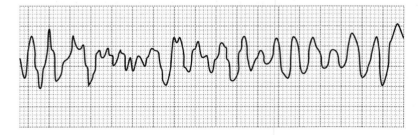

Figure 6.20 Ventricular fibrillation

Intravenous access may be gained either via the central or peripheral route. While central venous access is the optimal route to deliver any drugs, peripheral access is generally perfectly adequate, although drugs administered via the peripheral route should be followed by a flush of 20 ml of 0.9% saline. Epinephrine is given every 3 minutes throughout the cardiac arrest and while the evidence for the use of antiarrhythmic therapy is weak, intravenous amiodarone or lidocaine may be given in cases of refractory VF (European Resuscitation Council 2002).

If the patient remains in VF after the first minute, three further shocks each at 360J are given and then a further 1 minute of CPR is continued. This loop of three shocks followed by CPR for 1 minute is continued and a continual search for reversible causes is undertaken. Sodium bicarbonate (50 mmol) is considered if the arterial pH is less than 7.1 and in persistent VF, defibrillator paddle positions may be changed to anterior-posterior positions. At some point a decision to stop resuscitation might need to be made, although this is a matter of clinical judgement related to the individual patient's circumstances and chances of a successful outcome (European Resuscitation Council 2002).

Pulseless electrical activity (Figure 6.21)
Pulseless electrical activity (PEA) is a form of cardiac arrest, whereby a normal or near normal electrical trace is observed on the cardiac monitor in the absence of any cardiac output.

- **Recognition and clinical significance.** Pulseless electrical activity appears on the monitor as a form of sinus rhythm or bradycardia, although generally the rhythm is considerably slower than the patient's normal heart rate. The QRS complexes may also be wider than the normal duration (>120 ms) and the QT interval may also be lengthened. It is, however, a difficult rhythm to recognise, as it appears to be 'normal sinus rhythm' on the monitor, it carries a very grave prognosis and requires prompt supportive management as well as investigation of possible causes (European Resuscitation Council 2002).

- **Causes and management.** Resuscitation should be actively commenced while the causes are considered and airway and ventilation is maintained, CPR is continued and epinephrine is given every 3 minutes. If the PEA is associated with a bradycardia atropine 3 mg intravenously should be given.

  This rhythm carries an extremely grave prognosis and the patient's best chance of survival lies in the prompt recognition and treatment of potential reversible causes. These causes or aggravating factors are conveniently grouped into the 4 'H's and the 4 'T's for ease of memory (Figures 6.22 and 6.23) and potentially all of these causes apply to patients in the recovery area.

Hypoxia
Hypoxia can be avoided by ensuring that the patient's lungs are adequately ventilated, using 100% oxygen and ensuring that there is effective chest rise and bilateral breath sounds. The site of the endotracheal tube should be checked to ensure that it is not in the oesophagus or misplaced in either bronchus.

Hypovolaemia
PEA commonly arises in situations where there has been excessive haemorrhage or other fluid

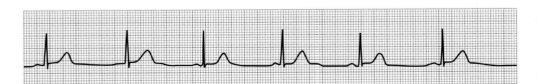

Figure 6.21 Pulseless electrical activity

losses. Catastrophic haemorrhage may occur from trauma, ruptured aortic aneurysm or oesophageal varices. Intravascular fluid losses should be replaced and urgent surgery is necessary to prevent further blood loss.

Hyperkalaemia, hypocalcaemia, acidaemia

These metabolic disorders may be investigated by requesting urgent blood biochemistry. A 12-lead ECG may help the diagnosis as may any indications in the patient's previous history (possible overdose of calcium channel blockers or renal disease are commonly implicated).

Hypothermia

This may occur if the patient has received non-warmed fluids during the surgery, or has had large surface areas exposed during the surgery. The elderly and the very young are particularly vulnerable.

Tension pneumothorax

This may result following a severe asthmatic attack, chest trauma or following repeated attempts at central venous cannulation. Urgent needle thoracocentesis should be performed (second intercostal space, mid clavicular line) followed by insertion of a chest drain.

Cardiac tamponade

Tamponade arises when blood accumulates in the pericardial space constricting the heart and preventing it from filling adequately. This may result from blunt or penetrating chest trauma, dissecting aortic aneurysm or following cardiac surgery where the pericardial sac has been opened. Emergency treatment includes needle pericardiocentesis.

Therapeutic or toxic substances

Unless a specific overdosage or use of a toxic substance is suspected, then the diagnosis can only be made by investigative laboratory tests. It is therefore difficult to diagnose, although supportive treatments and antidotes may be available.

Thromboembolic or mechanical circulatory obstruction

This usually means massive pulmonary embolus and the definitive treatment is either thrombolysis or transfer to a cardiothoracic surgical unit for pulmonary embolectomy.

Ventricular asystole (Figure 6.24)

Asystole is a very rare cardiac arrest presentation in adults. It is the absence of all electrical activity in the ventricles and is hence sometimes referred to as cardiac standstill (Huszar 2002).

- **Recognition.** As there is no electrical activity recordable from the ventricles, the rhythm generally manifests as a straight, slightly undulating line on the monitor. Occasionally electrical activity from the atria may be present as P waves on the monitor.
- **Causes and clinical significance.** The causes are as for those listed for PEA. It may also occur as a primary event in a patient with advanced cardiac disease where the dominant pacemaker (SA node) or escape pacemakers fail to generate electrical activity (Huszar 2002). In addition it should be borne in mind that asystole is the final rhythm seen in a dying heart following VT, VF or PEA.
- **Management.** Asystole is essentially managed in the same manner as PEA, with an active search being made for possible reversible causes (Figures 6.22 and 6.23). It is always prudent to

---

- Hypoxia
- Hypovolaemia
- Hyperkalaemia, hypocalcaemia, acidaemia
- Hypothermia

Figure 6.22 The 4 Hs – potential reversible causes of cardiac arrest

---

- Tension pneumothorax
- Cardiac tamponade
- Therapeutic or toxic substances
- Thromboembolic or mechanical circulatory obstruction

Figure 6.23 The 4 Ts – potential reversible causes of cardiac arrest

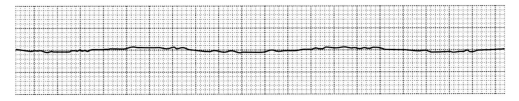

Figure 6.24 Asystole

ensure that the correct diagnosis has been made and that VT/VF is not mistaken for asystole (Jevon 2002). The European Resuscitation Council (2002) therefore advise that the ECG leads are correctly attached, that the ECG gain (size) is correctly set and that the rhythm is viewed through at least two ECG leads (i.e. lead 1 and lead 11). Spurious asystole may be observed on the monitor when using the defibrillator paddles for rhythm interpretation – this is not therefore recommended. It is also worth bearing in mind that myocardial stunning may result in asystole, which can occur for up to one minute following defibrillation.

Pacing

The rhythm should be carefully checked for evidence of atrial activity (P waves) on the monitor (Figure 6.25) as this is amenable to treatment with cardiac pacing. Emergency cardiac pacing can be delivered as percussion pacing, or via the oesophageal, transthoracic or transvenous route. Percussion pacing using repeated precordial blows can be used to stimulate the myocardium prior to mechanical pacing being instituted. In percussion pacing, a blow is delivered to the lateral lower left sternal edge using less force than a precordial thump at a rate of about 70 beats per minute (European Resuscitation Council 2002).

Summary

Practitioners working in the recovery area care for a variety of patients. Many patients may have underlying cardiac disease and this can readily contribute to the development of arrhythmias. In some patients, however, there may be no known cardiac disease, but the stress and trauma associated with the surgery, anaesthetic agents and disruption of fluid and electrolyte balance may contribute to the onset of an arrhythmia. Some arrhythmias are potentially very dangerous and may herald other associated problems, such as cardiac failure or myocardial infarction. While arrhythmias are common in the perioperative period, most are however clinically benign and do not require urgent intervention. It is vital however that recovery area practitioners can recognise the variety of arrhythmias previously discussed and understand the underlying rationales for treatment.

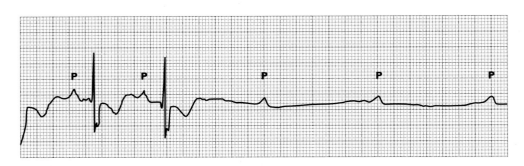

Figure 6.25 Asystole with P waves

DISCHARGING THE PATIENT FROM THE RECOVERY UNIT

Discharge of the patient from the recovery unit is as important as admission of the patient into the unit. Each unit will have its own criteria for the time the patient will spend within the unit and this will vary depending on whether they have had a general anaesthetic or a local anaesthetic. Broadly speaking if a patient has had a general anaesthetic they will be not be discharged for at least an hour. If they have had a local anaesthetic it will be at least half an hour. Once that time has elapsed there are general criteria that the patient has to fulfill. From a physiological perspective the scoring system illustrated in Figure 6.26 can be

	Activity 0–2	Respiration 0–2	Circulation 0–2	Consciousness 0–2	Colour 0–2	Total
Arrival in the recovery unit						
1 hour						
2 hours						
3 hours						

Scoring criteria

Activity

☐ Able to move 4 extremities voluntarily or on command = 2
☐ Able to move 2 extremities voluntarily or on command = 1
☐ Able to move 0 extremities voluntarily or on command = 0

Respiration

☐ Able to breathe deeply and cough freely = 2
☐ Difficult or limited breathing = 1
☐ No breathing = 0

Circulation

☐ Blood pressure +/– 20% of pre-anaesthetic level = 2
☐ Blood pressure +/– 20–50% of pre-anaesthetic level = 1
☐ Blood pressure +/– 50% of pre-anaesthetic level = 0

Consciousness

☐ Fully awake = 2
☐ Arousable on voice command = 1
☐ Not responding = 0

Colour

☐ Pink = 2
☐ Pale, dusky, blotchy, jaundiced, other = 1
☐ Cyanosed = 0

A score of 10 means the patient is ready to be discharged from the recovery unit

Figure 6.26 A scoring system for discharging the patient from the recovery unit (adapted from Aldrete 1970)

used. This is adapted from Aldrete (1970) who developed a scoring system for discharging patients from the recovery unit. He based this system on the APGAR scoring used when babies are first delivered. The Aldrete scoring system has been widely used and adapted (White and Song 1999; Aldrete 1998); however it does not take account of other criteria that are essential for the safe discharge of patients from the recovery unit.

One of the most important criteria to be met before the patient is discharged from the recovery unit is that they are pain free and have received or are receiving adequate analgesia. Furthermore they must be free from PONV. If these two criteria have not been met the recovery practitioner has not attended to the patient's needs, as they should do.

Added to this the patient must be fully orientated; this is covered in the Aldrete scoring system but is not elaborated upon. It has been suggested that the patient should be able to tell you things like their date of birth and the date and year currently (Hatfield and Tronson 2001). However these can be difficult questions normally without adding in having just had a general anaesthetic! So perhaps these questions are unrealistic to ask the post-anaesthetic patient.

General housekeeping duties should have been performed prior to the patient's discharge such as removal of all ECG stickers and cannulae that are no longer required. All documentation should be up to date, intravenous fluids, further analgesia and antiemetics written up so that the ward staff can follow these without further recourse to the anaesthetist. In day surgery, issues such as who will be accompanying the patient home and any discharge instructions should be taken into account. A contact number should be given in case there are any problems they wish to discuss once they are at home.

Discharge from the recovery unit is often a neglected area with a minimal evidence base. In current practice it must be remembered that patients discharged to the ward will be entering an environment where the ratio of staff to patients is significantly less than in the recovery unit.

Conclusion

In conclusion, the development of recovery practice has evolved significantly in the past 20 years. Practitioners who work in this area are highly skilled and highly motivated. There is no doubt that this is an area of rapid expansion with many opportunities for the recovery practitioner to develop their practice and give a high standard of care to patients recovering from anaesthesia and surgery.

References

Addei A (2003) Treatment of laryngospasm. *Anaesthesia* 58(2): 188.

Aitkenhead AR (2001) Post operative care. In: Aitkenhead AR, Rowbotham DJ and Smith G (eds) *Textbook of Anaesthesia*, 4th edn. London: Churchill Livingstone.

Aldrete JA (1998) Modification to the postanesthesia score for use in ambulatory surgery. *Journal of Perianesthesia Nursing* 13(3): 148–155.

Aldrete JA (1970) A postanesthetic recovery score. *Anesthesia and Analgesia* 49(6): 924–933.

Allesie MA, Boyden PP, Camm AJ *et al.* (2001) Pathophysiology and prevention of atrial fibrillation. *Circulation* 103(5): 769–777.

Andrews PLR (1992) Physiology of nausea and vomiting. *British Journal of Anaesthesia* 69(suppl 1): 2s–19s.

Arnold A (2002) Postoperative nausea and vomiting in the perioperative setting. *British Journal of Perioperative Nursing* 12(1): 24–32.

Association of Anaesthetists of Great Britain and Ireland (2002) *Immediate Post-anaesthetic Recovery*. London: Association of Anaesthetists of Great Britain and Ireland.

Baltimore JJ (1999) Postlaryngospasm pulmonary edema in adults. *AORN* 70(3): 468–479.

Barasi S (1991) The physiology of pain. *Surgical Nurse* 1–8.

Beattie WS, Lindblad T, Buckley DN and Forrest JB (1991) The incidence of postoperative nausea and vomiting in women undergoing laparoscopy is influenced by the day of menstrual cycle. *Canadian Journal of Anaesthesia* 38(3): 298–302.

Beecher HK (1956) Relationship of significance of wound to pain experienced. *JAMA* 161: 1609–1613.

Bennett J, Wren KR and Haas R (2001) Opioid use during the perianesthesia period: nursing implications. *Journal of Perianesthesia Nursing* 16(4): 255–258.

Bodian CA, Freedman G, Hossain S, Eisenkraft JB and Beilin Y (2001) the visual analogue scale for pain. *Anesthesiology* 95(6): 1356–1361.

Broomhead CJ (1995) Physiology of postoperative nausea and vomiting. *British Journal of Hospital Medicine* 53(7): 327–330.

Bubien R (2000) A new beat on an old rhythm. *American Journal of Nursing* 100(1): 42–51.

Buss HE and Melderis K (2002) PACU pain management algorithm. *Journal of Perianesthesia Nursing* 17(1): 11–20.

Chia YY, Kuo MC, Liu K, Sun GC, Hsieh SW and Chow LH (2002) Does postoperative pain induce emesis? *The Clinical Journal of Pain* 18(5): 317–323.

Chumbley GM, Hall GM and Salmon P (2002) Patient-controlled analgesia: what information does the patient want? *Journal of Advanced Nursing* 39(5): 459–471.

Chung DC and Rowbottom SJ (1993) A very small dose of suxemethonium relieves laryngospasm. *Anaesthesia* 48(3): 229–230.

Coleman SA and Booker-Milburn J (1996) Audit of postoperative pain control. Influence of a dedicated acute pain nurse. *Anaesthesia* 51(12): 1093–1096.

Coll AM, Moseley L and Torrance C (1999) Fine tuning the day surgery process. *Nursing Standard* 14(4): 39–41.

Da Costa D, Brady WJ and Edhouse J (2002) ABC of clinical electrocardiography: bradycardias and atrioventricular conduction block. *British Medical Journal* 324(7336): 535.

Davies P (1993) Opening up the gate control theory. *Nursing standard* 7(45): 25–27.

de C Williams AC (1998) Psychological techniques in the management of pain. In: Thomas VJ (ed.) *Pain, Its Nature and Management*, Chapter 7. London: Bailliere Tindall.

Diemunsch P, Korttila K and Kovac A (1999) Current therapy for management of postoperative nausea and vomiting: the 5-HT3 receptor and antagonists. *Ambulatory Surgery* 7(2): 111–122.

Edwards S (2001) Regulation of water, sodium and potassium: implications for practice. *Nursing Standard* 15(22): 36–42.

Ernst E and Pittler MH (2000) Efficacy of ginger for nausea and vomiting: a systematic review of randomized clinical trials. *British Journal of Anaesthesia* 84(3): 367–371.

European Resuscitation Council (2002) *Advanced life support course provider manual*, 4th edn. London: Resuscitation Council (UK) and European Resuscitation Council.

Faccenda KA and Finucane BT (2002) Epidural block: technical aspects and complications. *Current Opinion in Anesthesiology* 15(5): 519–523.

Fiedler MA (1997) Clinical implications of Ketorolac for postoperative analgesia. *Journal of Perianesthesia Nursing* 12(6): 426–433.

Gagliese L, Jackson M, Ritvo P, Wowk A and Katz J (2000) Age is not an impediment to effective use of patient-controlled analgesia by surgical patients. *Anesthesiology* 93(3): 601–610.

Golden SE (1997) The management and treatment of recurrent postoperative laryngospasm. *Anesthesia Analgesia* 84(6): 1392.

Goldberger AL (1999) *Clinical Electrocardiography: A Simplified Approach*, 6th edn. St Louis: Mosby.

Golembiewski JA and O'Brien D (2002) A systematic approach to the management of postoperative nausea and vomiting. *Journal of Perianesthesia Nursing* 17(6): 364–376.

Goodacre S and Irons R (2002) ABC of clinical electrocardiography: atrial arrhythmias. *British Medical Journal* 324(7337): 594–597.

Greif R, Laciny S, Rapf B, Hickie RS and Sessler DI (1999) Supplemental oxygen reduces the incidence of postoperative nausea and vomiting. *Anesthesiology* 91(5): 1246–1252.

Hatfield A and Tronson M (2001) *The Complete Recovery Room Book*, 3rd edn. Oxford: Oxford University Press.

Hawthorne J (1995) *Understanding the Management of Nausea and Vomiting*. Oxford: Blackwell Science.

Hitchcock M (1997) Postoperative nausea and vomiting (PONV). In: Millar JM, Rudkin GE and Hitchcock M (eds) *Practical Anaesthesia and Analgesia for Day Surgery*, Chapter 8. Oxford: Bios Scientific.

Hollenberg SM and Dellinger RP (2000) Noncardiac surgery: postoperative arrhythmias. *Critical Care Medicine* 28(10): Suppl. N145–N150.

Huszar RJ (2002) *Basic Dysrhythmias: Interpretation and Management*, 3rd edn. London: Mosby.

Jevon P (2002) *Advanced Life Support. A Practical Guide*. Oxford: Butterworth Heinemann.

Jevon P and Ewens B (2002) *Monitoring the Critically Ill Patient*. Oxford: Blackwell Science.

Johnstone R E (1999) Laryngospasm treatment – an explanation. *Anesthesiology* 91(2): 581–582.

Jolley S (2001) Managing postoperative nausea and vomiting. *Nursing Standard* 15(40): 47–52.

Kenny G and Rowbotham D (eds) (1992) *Postoperative Nausea and Vomiting*. London: Synergy Medical Education.

Kervin MW (2002) Residual neuromuscular blockade in the immediate postoperative period. *Journal of Perianesthesia Nursing* 17(3): 152–158.

Koh P and Thomas VJ (1994) Patient controlled analgesia (PCA): does time saved by PCA improve patient satisfaction with nursing care? *Journal of Advanced Nursing* 20(1): 61–70.

Krau SD (1998) Selecting and managing fluid therapy. Colloids versus crystalloids. *Critical Care Nursing Clinics of North America* 10(4): 401–410.

Larson CP (1998) Laryngospasm – the best treatment. *Anesthesiology* 89(5): 1293–1294.

Lerman J (1992) Surgical and patient factors involved in post operative nausea and vomiting. *British Journal of Anaesthesia* 69(suppl 1): 24s–32s.

Mangrum JM and DiMarco JP (2000) The evaluation and management of bradycardia. *New England Journal of Medicine* 342(10): 703–709.

McCaffery M and Pesero C (eds) (1999) *Pain: Clinical Manual*, 2nd edn. St Louis: Mosby.

McConkey PP (2000) Postobstructive pulmonary oedema – a case series and review. *Anaesthesia and Intensive Care* 28(1): 72–76.

McVicar A and Clancy J (1997) Principles of intravenous fluid replacement. *Professional Nurse Supplement* 12(8): 56–59.

Melzack R and Wall P (1982) *The Challenge of Pain*. Middlesex: Penguin.

Merritt BA, Okyere CP and Jasinski M (2002) Isopropyl alcohol inhalation: alternative treatment of postoperative nausea and vomiting. *Nursing Research* 51(2): 125–128.

Mevorach DL (1996) The management and treatment of recurrent postoperative laryngospasm. *Anesthesia Analgesia* 83(5): 1110–1111.

Millar JM, Rudkin GE and Hitchcock M (eds) (1997) *Practical Anaesthesia and Analgesia for Day Surgery*. Oxford: Bios.

Ming JI, Kuo BIT, Lin JG and Lin L (2002) The efficacy of acupressure to prevent nausea and vomiting in postoperative patients. *Journal of Advanced Nursing* 39(4): 343–351.

Moline BM (2001) Pain management in the ambulatory surgical population. *Journal of Perianesthesia Nursing* 16(6): 388–398.

Murray-Calderon P and Connolly MA (1997) Laryngospasm and non-cardiogenic pulmonary edema. *Journal of Perianesthesia Nursing* 12(2): 89–94.

Nawful M and Baraka A (2002) Propofol for the relief of extubation laryngospasm. *Anaesthesia* 57(10): 1036.

Odom JL (1993) Airway emergencies in the post anesthesia care unit. *Nursing Clinics of North America* 28(3): 483–491.

Opie LH and Gersh BJ (2001) *Drugs for the Heart*, 5th edn. Philadelphia: WB Saunders.

Pepper C (2001) Atrial fibrillation: recent developments in anti-arrhythmic therapy. *Cardiology News* 4(5): 6–10.

Pesero C, Pertenoy RK and McCaffery M (1999a) Opioid analgesics. In: McCaffery M and Pesero C (eds) *Pain: Clinical Manual*, 2nd edn. St Louis: Mosby.

Pesero C, Paice JA and McCaffery M (1999b) Basic mechanisms underlying the causes and effects of pain. In: McCaffery M and Pesero C (eds) *Pain: Clinical Manual*, 2nd edn. St Louis: Mosby.

Pouzeratte Y, Delay JM, Brunat G, Boccara G, Vergue C, Jaber S, Fabre JM, Colson P and Mann C (2001) Patient-controlled epidural analgesia after abdominal surgery: ropivacaine versus bupivacaine. *Anesthesia Analgesia* 93(6): 1587–1592.

Power I and Smith G (2001) Post operative pain. In: Aitkenhead AR, Rowbotham DJ and Smith G (eds) (2001) *Textbook of Anaesthesia*, 4th edn. London: Churchill Livingstone.

Prowse M (1999) Airway complications in the post-anaesthetic unit. *Anaesthetic and Recovery Nurse* 5(3): 10–13.

Rajan GRC (1999) Supraglottic obstruction versus true laryngospasm: the best treatment. *Anesthesiology* 91(2): 581.

Resuscitation Council (UK) (2000) *Advanced Life Support Provider Manual*, 4th edn. London: Resuscitation Council.

Riley J (2002) The ECG: its role and practical application In: Hatchett R and Thompson D (eds) *Cardiac Nursing: A Comprehensive Guide*, Chapter 6. London: Churchill Livingstone.

Royal College of Surgeons of England and The College of Anaesthetists (1990) *Pain after Surgery*.

London: The Royal College of Surgeons of England and The College of Anaesthetists.

Rudkin GE (1997a) Local and regional anaesthesia in the adult day surgery patient. In: Millar JM Rudkin GE and Hitchcock M (eds) *Practical Anaesthesia and Analgesia for Day Surgery*. Oxford: Bios.

Rudkin GE (1997b) Pain management in the adult day surgery patient. In: Millar JM, Rudkin GE and Hitchcock M (eds) *Practical Anaesthesia and Analgesia for Day Surgery*. Oxford: Bios.

Russell R (2001) Pain relief in labour: regional, epidural and patient controlled analgesia. *Anaesthesia and Intensive Care Medicine* 2(5): 185–189.

Salomaki TE, Hokajavi TM, Rauta P and Alahuhta S (2000) Improving the quality of post operative pain relief. *European Journal of Pain* 4(4): 367–372.

Schierhout G and Roberts I (1998) Fluid resuscitation with colloid or crystalloid solutions in critically ill patients: a systematic review of randomised trials. *British Medical Journal* 313(7136): 961–964.

Shammash JB and Ghali WA (2003) Preoperative assessment and perioperative management of the patient with nonischaemic heart disease. *Medical Clinics of North America* 87(1): 137–152.

Sinclair DR, Chang F and Meizei G (1999) Can postoperative nausea and vomiting be predicted? *Anesthesiology* 91(1): 109–118.

Sloan SB and Weitz HH (2001) Postoperative arrhythmias and conduction disorders. *Medical Clinics of North America* 85(5): 1171–1189.

Spiers CM (2002) Arrhythmia interpretation in the perioperative arena. *British Journal of Anaesthetic and Recovery Nursing* 3(3): 12–18.

Stark J (1998) A comprehensive analysis of the fluid and electrolyte system. *Critical Care Nursing Clinics of North America* 10(4): 471–475.

Sukhani R, Barclay J and Chow J (1993) Paradoxical vocal cord motion: an unusual cause of stridor in the recovery room. *Anesthesiology* 79(1): 177–180.

Task Force Report (2001) ACC/AHA Guidelines for the management of patients with atrial fibrillation. *European Heart Journal* 22(20): 1852–1923.

Tate S (1997) Peppermint oil: a treatment for postoperative nausea. *Journal of Advanced Nursing* 26(3): 543–549.

Tate S and Cook H (1996) Postoperative nausea and vomiting 1: physiology and aetiology. *British Journal of Nursing* 5(16): 962–973.

Thomas VJ (1998) (ed) *Pain, Its Nature and Management*. London: Bailliere Tindall.

Thompson AM (2002) Anaesthesia. In: Sheilds L and Werder H (eds) *Perioperative Nursing*. London: Greenwich Medical Media.

Thompson H (1999) The management of postoperative nausea and vomiting. *Journal of Advanced Nursing* 29(5): 1130–1136.

Turner DAB (2001) Fluid, electrolyte and acid–base balance. In: Aitkenhead AR, Rowbotham DJ and Smith G (eds) *Textbook of Anaesthesia*, 4th edn. London: Churchill Livingstone.

Vandermeulen E (1999) Is anticoagulation and central neural blockade a safe combination? *Current Opinion in Anesthesiology* 12(5): 539–543.

Werner MU, Soholm L, Rotboll-Nielson P and Kehlet H (2002) Does an acute pain service improve postoperative outcome? *Anesthesia and Analgesia* 95(5): 1361–1372.

White PF and Song D (1999) New criteria for fast-tracking after outpatient anesthesia: a comparison with the modified Aldrete's scoring system. *Anesthesia and Analgesia* 88(5): 1069–1072.

Wiederhold R (1999) *Electrocardiography: The Monitoring and Diagnostic Leads*, 2nd edn. Philadelphia: WB Saunders.

Woodrow P (1998) An introduction to the reading of electrocardiograms. *British Journal of Nursing* 7(3): 135–142.

Wooton H (2000) A nurse led innovation in the administration of epidural infusions. *British Journal of Anaesthetic and Recovery Nursing* 1(4): 7–10.

Zborowski M (1952) Cultural components in responses to pain. *Journal of Social Issues* 8: 16–30.

7 MANAGEMENT ISSUES IN THE OPERATING DEPARTMENT

J Howard Shelley

CHAPTER AIMS

- To outline the role of the Operating Department Manager
- To explore problem solving and how to develop a management vision
- To demonstrate how improved personal effectiveness can be the key to gaining room to manoeuvre
- To examine specific problems of Operating Department management
- To compare and contrast the roles of manager and leader.

INTRODUCTION

This is not a management tome. Neither is it a learned treatise, extensively based on research, with a proliferation of references and dropped names. It will employ a slightly different style to the other chapters in this book in that, while references will, of course, be used they will be headline references for further reading rather than detailed justification of the text. Neither is this an in-depth discussion of the various tasks and roles of management with a comprehensive tool kit to enable the manager to meet every challenge. There is neither the space here nor is it desirable within the context of this book. This then begs the question, what is it? The text draws on a number of different themes to sketch out for the reader the practical challenges that an operating department manager is likely to face during the early days of their career and to highlight those areas where the skill base required is different to that in other nursing disciplines.

There would appear to be no definitive source on the subject of operating department manage-

ment. Since this is the case, a choice has had to be made over which areas should be discussed and which should be left out. Over 15 years of personal experience of clinical management have been drawn on to decide which areas are most likely to be of use. In defence of those choices, careful consideration has been given firstly, to those topics on which other staff just starting out on the management or supervisory ladder have sought advice and have perceived most difficult, and secondly, those areas which senior management have identified as key priorities.

Nevertheless, it is hoped the student will be sufficiently interested in the topic to investigate it further and there is no better primer in management than Professor Charles B. Handy's (1993) *Understanding Organisations*. Many of the issues addressed in this chapter are discussed there in greater depth and in a very readable manner. Some of the techniques he uses, such as the use of stories taken from real life and used to illustrate a point, have been directly lifted, with thanks, from his book.

Clearly, it behoves the manager to make as many right decisions as possible and to minimise the potential for wrong ones. The purpose of this chapter is to try to provide some guidelines that may help the new manager to maximise their effectiveness. Three distinct areas of management practice will be examined in some detail. Firstly, we will attempt to propose a structure that will allow the individual manager to develop an approach to the daily business of management. This will include the process of problem solving and the development of the manager's vision. Secondly, some aspects of personal effectiveness within the operating department environment will be discussed and some possibilities offered for developing a power base. Thirdly, and finally, some of the key areas of responsibility for the manager within the operating department will be examined and some possible solutions offered to commonly occurring problems.

Throughout the chapter suggestions for further reading will be offered. They will obviously be those authors who it is believed represent the clearest and most cogent approach to the subject under discussion. No apology is made for the texts chosen. This whole chapter is just operating department management viewed through one set of spectacles; the reader may choose another pair. They will be as good, just different.

THE ROLE OF THE MANAGER

Before approaching specific problems, however, it is necessary to place some structure to the role of manager. The first point is obvious, but still worth mentioning: *managers are judged by the output of others*. In other words, to succeed, the operating department manager must provide an environment that enables others to deliver effective, efficient and patient-centred care. This is the key difference between the role of the clinical practitioner and that of clinical manager.

This may sound like a small, almost semantic, difference but it requires a profound change in outlook.

A subject often debated in a clinical forum is the effectiveness or otherwise of managers who have no clinical background. Most professionals,

perhaps not unreasonably, believe that clinical environments are best managed by people with clinical skills. How can, the argument runs, an individual who does not understand what we do possibly make informed decisions? The counter approach is to assert that management is a discipline on its own, independent of the function being managed. A good manager will therefore be successful irrespective of the environment.

It is clear that if the role is *primarily* management the ability to manage effectively is the more important skill and the fact that the manager lacks a clinical background, while undoubtedly making the job more difficult, is not critical to success.

However, in operating department management there should be no need to compromise. As long ago as 1980 Sue Pembrey identified that a clinical manager was the 'key to nursing' and there are many individuals who can demonstrate a record of success in the clinical environment and who have the necessary skill base, or the ability and drive to learn, and the motivation to manage a department. While it is obviously important that a managerial post-holder can manage it is also highly desirable that they understand the process that they are managing

The second point is less obvious. An effective clinician, while maintaining a sufficiently broad perspective to provide effective care for a patient group, must also have a sufficiently narrow focus to ensure that the patient who is being cared for at

PRACTICE EXEMPLAR 7.1:

A very highly regarded staff nurse was appointed to the post of junior sister in charge of the orthopaedic service. After six months she was exhausted. She was working flat out as a clinical practitioner during the day and taking piles of work home in the evening. In addition she had created a great deal of resentment among previously supportive colleagues who felt that she was taking all the best clinical jobs for herself and justifying this by pointing out that she was the most experienced. The orthopaedic surgeons were complaining that however good she was 'at the

table' she frequently forgot to order equipment and any changes that they requested took much longer than necessary.

Her manager took her aside and pointed out that her responsibility was to make the service run, not to do all the work herself. In desperation (and not with any great enthusiasm) she took his advice and to her surprise discovered that by doing less she became much more effective. By letting her staff do their job her own performance improved.

PRACTICE EXEMPLAR 7.2:

A group of staff who had been very poorly managed in the recent past, and who had acknowledged this, discovered that the person appointed to manage the department had no clinical background. They were in uproar. Petitions were raised and official protests through the unions made to senior management. The chief executive came to meet the staff and he posed the following question:

'By whom would you rather be managed? An ineffective manager with a record of success as a clinician or a person with a record of success in management, who knows what he doesn't know and when to seek advice, who can deliver your agenda, but who has no clinical background?'

that moment receives the care that is needed. The manager, in contrast, must maintain a wide focus most of the time. The question to address is: how can I provide the best care for my patients? There is an essential difference in emphasis. The clinical practitioner has a one patient focus, the manager has many patients. Furthermore the clinician has a direct link with the patient and thus a direct focus, managers on the other hand may consider their input to patient care in terms of creating space within the budget or creatively deploying staff in such a manner as to improve availability at peak workloads.

The manager's perspective is not only different in breadth but it is also different in time. The present time may not be under current consideration at all. The manager may be thinking about tomorrow's service or working on a long-term plan to improve quality. The clinician, in contrast, focuses almost exclusively on the present or the near future.

This may explain why many excellent clinical practitioners fail to make the transition into management. They cannot reconcile the need to broaden their perspective with the immediate need to care for the patient in front of them at that moment. It may also explain why some practitioners who, while being perfectly satisfactory, but mediocre, clinical practitioners suddenly start to shine when promoted into a management role. As clinical practitioners they have had problems narrowing their focus sufficiently to give adequate attention to the patient in hand.

A graphic demonstration of this effect can be

seen among some consultant medical staff. Medical education and training directs the doctor to concentrate on one patient at a time and to ignore all side issues. All the equipment required and the drugs prescribed are somebody else's problem to procure. Once the doctor has examined the patient and made the diagnosis, treatment is prescribed and the doctor then passes on to the next patient. Doctors are often genuinely puzzled at other professions' frustration at their inability to see the side issues and understand the difficulties faced by other groups involved in the patient's care.

A further point, often missed by those not actively participating in a management role, is that managers have a much greater potential for creating a disaster than do their subordinates. If a clinical practitioner makes a mistake then, in general, although the mistake may imply a disaster for the patient under the practitioner's care at that moment, the problem will be restricted to one individual. In contrast, if a manager makes a mistake, the consequences may affect many patients and cover an extended time period.

A further difference between the role of clinician and manager is the level of responsibility the individual is expected to carry. The classic statement of, 'the buck stops here!' is an example of this. All professionals carry responsibility, but managing clinicians are not only expected to take responsibility for clinical and managerial decisions and practice, but also the decisions and actions of those staff responsible to them. Often the first time the manager will know that one of

PRACTICE EXEMPLAR 7.3:

Due to manufacturing problems, the supplier of sutures failed, over a period of months, to deliver a specific item required for arterial surgery. The operating department manager, once he realised that there was going to be a supply problem, alerted the arterial surgeons and asked them whether there was a possibility that an alternative product might be used. One of the surgeons, popular with the operating department staff and in general regarded as very amenable, replied that he was not prepared to use any other product than the one he was used to and further, that it was the operating department manager's job to ensure that it was available. When the operating department manager tried to explain the difficulty, he wouldn't even listen, merely restating his original point in respect of the manager's job.

Realising that he had failed to get through and that it was essential, given that there was no immediate prospect of the situation improving, that the surgeon understood the situation, the manager went to see his business manager. He explained the situation and requested him to address the matter. The surgeon was genuinely puzzled when the matter was brought to his attention, stating that he couldn't understand why the operating department manager hadn't brought the matter to his attention directly and had felt the need to take the matter higher.

---

the staff has made a bad call is when the letter of complaint arrives, yet they cannot argue that they knew nothing about it. Unless the decision was so outrageous as to be in defiance of all logic and accepted reasoning, management will still bear ultimate responsibility.

Managerial responsibility implies that on occasion an unpopular call will have to be made. Few managers like to make these decisions but none would deny that it is part of the job. Perversely, it is the ability to make the unpopular decisions under pressure that often brings the most respect

PRACTICE EXEMPLAR 7.4:

A manager in a hospital facing a financial crisis was instructed to reduce the costs of her department immediately and by any means at her disposal. On investigation she discovered that many areas in the hospital had developed the habit of using the operating department as an unofficial store and that, as a consequence, she was subsidising their budgets. Having given two weeks' notice of her intentions in writing to all the areas she instructed her staff that under no circumstances were they to give anything out to other areas.

It caused uproar. Some areas complained that they had never been informed. Two patients complained to the local press after having been told the name of the manager responsible. One consultant wrote in the patient's notes that she (the manager) had put the patient at risk over a matter of a few pounds. The local MP phoned the hospital and then contacted the Minister of Health.

A decision that seemed perfectly sensible to a manager under pressure to deliver a balanced budget compromised the care of a number of patients. Her staff, who had to implement the policy and were the ones faced by angry surgeons and patients' relatives, completely lost confidence in her and demanded her removal. As a consequence her position became untenable, and she decided to resign. The hospital suffered some extremely undesirable press attention and senior hospital managers had to explain themselves to the Health Minister in person.

One ill-considered management decision caused an effect on a much wider scale than a poor clinical one could possibly have done.

from subordinate colleagues. This is not as strange as it sounds; if the employees know that under the same circumstances they would have made a decision of a lower quality, then irrespective of any personal difficulty as a result of the decision, and although they may not like it, they will, in general, respect it.

PROBLEM SOLVING AND VISION DEVELOPMENT

Problem solving

Among the many skills that practitioners are expected to master is the art of clinical problem solving. In the early days when the practitioner has little experience, this is a difficult activity and one which produces much anxiety. However, with experience, it becomes much easier and the practitioner is able to make decisions and know that they are right. New managers have the same experience, often experiencing self-doubt and anxiety over the quality of their decisions. Yet the management problem solving process is exactly the same as the clinical one and requiring the same disciplines and approach.

A clinical practitioner, confronted by a clinical problem, studies the problem to make sure she understands it, plans a strategy to deal with it, executes the plan and evaluates the result to ensure that it matches the desired outcome. We call this decision methodology, 'The nursing process'.

Pedler, Bugoyne and Boydell (2001) suggest that a manager uses two distinct decision making methodologies, the 'rational' approach and following a 'hunch.' Sometimes everyone needs to make a judgment call based on what they think is the right thing to do but clearly a rational, argued approach is preferable. A manager making a 'rational' decision follows the same process of analysis, planning, execution and evaluation as the clinical practitioner but applies it to a much wider range of potential situations. In the early days this may be a useful process to follow every time the manager is confronted with a new problem since the problem may, while not being totally unfamiliar, have a different context. Some problems will be totally new and outside the experience of the practitioner. As confidence and experience grow the manager will be able to make decisions instantly, without recourse to in-depth analysis and still be reasonably sure that the outcome will be a positive one.

Yet it is never possible to leave the above strategy behind entirely. There will always be knotty problems requiring a careful and thoughtful approach and many of the issues with which a manager must deal will be much more complicated and cover a longer term than clinical problems. Few patients are in hospital for more than a few days, but a manager's plans can often be measured in years. Long-term objectives often require many interim steps that also require careful planning and execution before the eventual goal is realised. The only safe way to proceed is through careful examination of the problem, a detailed and robust plan, thorough execution and a constant process of evaluation.

In Practice Examplar 7.5 a single decision was clearly impossible. Delivery of the objective – a functioning information system – required an ongoing process of planning, implementation and evaluation of every step throughout the project. The complexity of the project was such that unless the managerial planning process was employed the project would have been almost certainly doomed to failure.

Vision development

Why does anyone want to become a manager? It is an important point. Although in industry or other parts of the public sector there may be an attractive salary package, clinical managers' salaries are little better than their clinical practitioner colleagues, and because they work office hours they tend to lose unsocial hours enhancements. As any clinical manager will tell you there is a lot of extra stress involved in management and much of it often seems so unnecessary. So why do it? It is submitted that it is probably something to do with 'vision'. The individuals with the power and the authority to direct care to their own agenda are managers.

PRACTICE EXEMPLAR 7.5:

A senior practitioner was asked to manage the introduction of an information technology system within the operating departments at his hospital. When asked how long this would take his response was 'at least a year'. This startled his manager who was expecting a reply in the order of weeks and he then requested an explanation of the extended timescale.

Prior to purchasing an IT system it is necessary to develop a specification. This consists of detailed performance criteria and technical information which any proposed system must meet in order to be considered. It is a rather large document and all interested parties (medical, nursing, management, financial, personnel, etc.) must be given the opportunity to contribute. Once this is complete the systems available in the marketplace have to be examined to see whether they comply with the specification and a shortlist is then drawn up. Given that the purchase will cost in excess of £100,000, an extended and carefully managed tender exercise must be undertaken and a recommendation to purchase made which must be considered and ratified by the hospital board.

Once a supplier of the system has been agreed it is necessary to install the hardware on which it will run. Cables need to be run in to allow network access and extra power points supplied. In some cases shelves will need to be constructed. The software will have to be installed on the network and all users will need to be trained. Finally, the process will have to be evaluated to ensure that the original aims have been met.

The student practitioner, throughout her training, watches the activities of the trained staff and takes those parts of their practice of which the practitioner approves and assimilates them into the individual's own model of practice. On completion of training it is discovered that life is not as simple as it might have seemed from the protected environment of the university. In the first place, the ward manager may have an agenda that is at variance with that of the practitioner and there are always organisational constraints that limit freedom of action. It is only when a level is reached where the employer places the responsibility for the total care of the patients in a particular ward or departmental area in the practitioner's hands, together with the requisite staff and financial resources, that practitioners are in a position to implement their own vision.

The clinical manager's vision is an intensely personal perspective on the way care should be delivered to a particular client group. The vision is not just restricted to care approaches. It will include, among other things, the manager's attitude to staff, feelings about the employing organisation, the priorities over the tasks that need to be carried out and the use of the financial resources. There may be a wide agreement over what constitutes good practice and the manager may have to function within strict organisational

PRACTICE EXEMPLAR 7.6:

A tall male manager and a short female manager were discussing their own management styles. The female manager was known in her department as a tyrant, a manager whose word was law and someone with whom you 'didn't mess'. During the discussion it became clear that she had adopted this style because otherwise people tended to patronise her. In contrast the male manager had a very laid-back style and rarely had to raise his voice or resort to an authoritarian style. If he had used her style staff would conclude that he was using his sex and size to bully and overbear his subordinates.

guidelines but nonetheless all managers have their own style and agenda.

The thrill of management is the opportunity to put that individual perspective into practice, and make it work. The next question is therefore obvious. Is a vision necessary? Is it not possible to borrow a vision from another source, such as a respected clinical colleague or a good book? It is submitted that the successful manager must have a personal, unique and workable vision that can be articulated to others. If there is no vision the manager does not have any real sense of direction and will have grave difficulties in leading the staff anywhere.

Without a clear vision of the path ahead the manager cannot set goals because there will be no sense of what the manager is trying to achieve. Appraisal and individual performance review become dry and uninspiring because no challenging or interesting objectives will be developed.

But the individual manager is far more than just the sum of professional education and experience. Cultural influences will be just as important. Just as sex and race, religious beliefs and personal sense of ethics and all the years' accumulated personal experience render the manager's personality individual and unique, so will they also, in part, define the managerial style, agenda and vision. A workable vision, while bits of it may be borrowed, *must* therefore as a whole unit, be unique. It is the answer to the question, 'what do *I* believe in?'

Communicating the vision

Having a vision is one thing, understanding it and being able to articulate it is another thing entirely. The successful manager needs to have a clear view of good practice. As stated above, this does not stop at clinical practice but includes other parts of the manager's job as well. The individual manager must understand their own motivation for believing in a particular path. A manager might say 'I believe in discipline'. On its own this is insufficient; the manager must understand why. A better statement would be 'I believe in discipline because then everybody knows

exactly where they stand'. Motive endows the vision with a measurable outcome.

Developing and communicating a vision requires work. Most people have a hazy view of their personal philosophy but few can articulate it with sufficient clarity so that others can understand it. Many add too much detail so that the vision becomes unclear and confused and others make bold statements with little justification and alienate their staff. Another common mistake is to give a long list of disjunctive statements that are not linked together by any common theme. While of course a vision needs detail, the manager should be able to encapsulate it in a few well-argued and consistent points which chart the course for the department and yet leave sufficient room for other members of staff to pad it out and add their own touches so that they feel a part of the whole process.

The vision must be communicated in such a way that it allows the staff to understand how the manager thinks. It is not possible to communicate all of the responses the manager might have to every single situation or problem that might present so the staff need to have some idea of what the response might be. The manager is not present all the time and the department needs to be consistent. It is the staff (*not* the manager) who have to deliver the vision; in order to do this they have to understand it. This is not achieved by the manager standing up at a staff meeting and grandly proclaiming the vision for the future and imperiously demanding the staff come on board. It is done in discussion and informal meetings and in dealing with problems. It is done when supporting junior managers and explaining the changes that are proposed. Above all it is achieved by being consistent. The same question must have the same answers week after week. Staff learn their manager's priorities very rapidly and providing they are clearly and consistently articulated, produce results, and are conducive to good patient care, the staff will generally fall into line.

In conclusion, it is submitted that the two essential tools of the manager are the ability to solve complex problems in an ordered and structured manner, and the possession of a clear personal vision of the route ahead coupled with the ability to communicate it. The first, the competent practitioner will already possess, although in the past it will have been applied in a different context. The manager will therefore have to discipline herself to the requirements of the new problem set. The second, the practitioner will also already have in her possession, although as a manager it may require work to ensure it is clear, logical and articulated in a meaningful fashion.

PERSONAL EFFECTIVENESS

Power

A question few managers ask when going about their daily duties is, 'why do my staff do what I ask them to?' It is not such a silly question as it sounds. Since managers often have to request staff to do jobs that those staff might not themselves choose to do, why do the staff not simply turn round to the manager and say 'no.' The answer is about power. French and Raven (1959), in their seminal work on the sources of power, detail six basic types:

- **Physical power.** This is the power of superior force, the power of the bully. Only in organisations such as prisons and the armed forces would the use of this power on a routine basis be regarded as ethical.
- **Resource power.** This is the power to grant or withhold resources or rewards.
- **Position power.** This derives from an individual's position or role within the organisation or group. If he is perceived as having a senior role that then endows him with some legitimacy.
- **Expert power.** This is self-explanatory. An individual is perceived to have power in a particular field or endeavour if he has special skills or knowledge that render him an expert.
- **Personal power.** This is the power of the charismatic individual. He is the leader who is instinctively trusted by his followers.
- **Negative power.** This is generally regarded as a disruptive force because it is the power to delay, filter or inhibit.

It will be seen from a brief review of the above list that there are few sources of power to which the operating department manager can immediately lay claim. Only in rare or extreme circumstances would it be appropriate for the manager to use physical power. Perhaps in a disciplinary setting or to prevent the immediate abuse of a patient, but even then other strategies could be used. In an organisation like a hospital it is rare that an individual manager has the ability to reward, or withdraw privileges from, a member of the staff. These are issues that are decided at a corporate level. It is true that managers may have some position power but it is weak compared to the power vested in surgical and anaesthetic consultants, and while they may be experts in their field, with today's hyper-specialisation there will be members of staff who can lay claim to greater expertise. If lucky they may have a certain degree of charisma, but in an environment where an individual is judged by professional competence there will be few opportunities to 'exercise charm' on colleagues. While most managers have occasionally used negative power, and it can be a useful tactic to delay or stall, in general its use is counterproductive because it tends to reduce the credibility of the individual using it.

If most sources of power are either unavailable or ethically unacceptable, and those that are available are weak, how is the manager to create sufficient room to implement plans and achieve the vision? All groups and individuals will have an agenda which may, in some parts, conflict with the manager's, and furthermore, one of the main user groups, i.e. doctors, has far more power than the manager. They have a major input into the function of the department and are responsible for most of the expenditure. It is no use at all to rail against the unfairness of the power balance within a hospital; this is unlikely to change in the near future and the situation will have to be managed as it stands.

Credibility

The answer is 'credibility'. If the staff perceive that the manager is willing and able to help them achieve their objectives, to provide an environment conducive to good patient care and has a clearly articulated vision to which they can 'sign up' then they will 'give' the necessary power to do the job. The opposite is also true. A manager who is perceived to lack credibility will find little room to move because of staff mistrust; they will consider the manager powerless and irrelevant. This is also true in respect of the attitudes taken by senior management. A manager who is perceived to be competent and trustworthy, who delivers to deadlines and who contributes positively to the corporate objectives will be given more freedom to act and less active supervision than less credible colleagues.

As implied in the previous paragraph credibility is largely about perception. A manager who is perceived to be effective will also be credible. The reverse is also true.

Practice Exemplar 7.7 illustrates that although the manager wasn't doing anything wrong in the first place, his staff *perceived* that he was. That perception, because it was shared by all staff, became the received truth. The manager had to manage the perception not the fact.

This example demonstrates that credibility can be lost very easily and with a total absence of malice on the part of the manager. Credibility is

based on the record of performance. The manager should consider the following questions:

1 How well do I represent the views of my staff?
2 How well do I represent the views of the medical staff?
3 How well do I understand the policies and procedures of the organisation for which I work?
4 Do I give good advice?
5 Do I take every step possible to ensure that my staff and clinicians are made aware of all the information that they need to know? Are the methods of communication suitable to the information to be communicated?
6 Am I aware of the needs of my staff?
7 Do I understand my manager's agenda?
8 Do I keep my promises?
9 Can I do 'that bit more?'

In Practice Exemplar 7.8 the manager could just have furnished the consultant with the requisite telephone number as requested and nobody could have criticised his performance.

Being a credible manager is not the same as keeping everybody happy. In the words of the proverb 'you can keep all the people happy some of the time ...' On many occasions man-

PRACTICE EXEMPLAR 7.7:

A manager took up a post involving management of a small operating department and sundry other responsibilities on a project basis. The project part of the manager's job involved him leaving the department on a regular basis and he developed the habit, on the way out, of informing two or three people where he was going and how long he was likely to be.

It therefore came as something of a surprise when he was informed by one of his sisters that he kept leaving the department without telling anybody where he was going. Since he knew this not to be true he investigated a little farther and discovered that this was a general view. It soon became clear

that what was happening was that, although he was informing a selection of the staff every time he left the department, an individual only knew where he was about 20% of the times he left.

Each individual perceived that since they knew where he was 20% of the time, 80% of the time he wasn't telling anybody at all. This caused considerable resentment and so he changed his practice. He had a white board fixed to the outside of his office door and wrote on it where he was going when he left the department. He also made a point of going into every room and announcing that he was leaving.

PRACTICE EXEMPLAR 7.8:

A consultant surgeon asked the operating department manager if he had the telephone number for a particular company. He wanted a modification made to a custom set of instrumentation and he needed to discuss the matter with a representative. The manager suggested that the matter be left to him and he arranged for the representative to call on the day when the surgeon next had an operating list. In between cases he worked with the representative and the surgeon to ensure each understood the others needs and then agreed with the representative a timescale for making it happen.

The outlay in time and effort on the part of the manager was minimal but the surgeon now perceived the manager as someone on whom he could rely to get things done. As a result the manager had given himself room to move and had created a valuable ally.

---

agers will gain more credibility for saying 'no' *more* than they would have done for saying 'yes.' Staff do not have a right to expect you to agree with them all the time but they emphatically do have the right to expect justice, truth, honesty and fairness and to be kept well informed. In addition, most staff respect the manager who is able to make the tough call even if the decision does not suit them personally.

To conclude, successful managers have a good understanding of their own and other sources of power within the department. They will know how to increase power when it is necessary in order to achieve a given end. Managers also understand the importance of personal credibility, and the relationship between it and the perception of those with whom they must interact.

SPECIFIC PROBLEMS OF OPERATING DEPARTMENT MANAGEMENT

Introduction

What are the special challenges with which the operating department manager must deal? It is clear that every area will present the manager with a different problem set and it cannot be denied that operating departments differ from hospital to hospital. But the similarities are greater than the differences and it is possible to state with some certainty the major issues that are likely to confront the clinical manager.

How does any manager decide which issues need to be addressed? To some extent this depends on the priorities of the manager and indeed those of the organisation, but one way to approach the problem is to examine in detail the salient features of the area to be managed. There is insufficient space here to do a detailed analysis of the management environment of the operating department. For simplicity a number of tasks that the manager in any department will have to accomplish have been selected and then described in a somewhat mechanistic fashion. No attempt has been made to structure them in an 'operating department management process', rather they will be discussed as discrete entities. Most managers, once they have mastered the basic skills will be able to integrate them into their personal model of management.

Inevitably, choosing the subjects to be examined is a subjective judgement and it may be that someone else would choose a different list, yet a choice has to be made and it is suggested that the major challenges facing the newly promoted operating department manager will be mastering skills in the following areas:

1 Managing the team structure
2 Controlling expenditure
3 Managing the inventory
4 Delivering quality care.

Managing the team structure

All operating department staff are aware, at some level, that they belong to a very special type of team. This is not to decry other teams; rather it is recognition that while teams do exist in other areas they do not tend to have the same cohesiveness and interdependency. In order to manage an operating department team, the leader must examine the functions of the team and understand, not only how, but why it functions in the manner it does.

As far as I am aware, no-one has tried to define precisely the dynamics of an operating department team and it is thus hard to recommend further reading. Nevertheless there are few books which present the subject of team dynamics better than *Effective Team Building* by John Adair (1986). Regrettably Adair is out of print, although its influence was such that it is available in most libraries. An alternative source may be found in Forsyth (1999) *Group Dynamics*, although this does take a much more academic view of the subject.

In order to have achieved of the post of clinical manager in an operating department the practitioner will have learned how to function within the team and will hopefully understand its power and dynamics. It should therefore only be a small step to managing a number of teams.

The function of a manager in this 'tight team' situation is to ensure that the direction and goals of the team are always focused on the right issues. It is submitted that, in the vast majority of cases, practitioners are motivated to deliver good care. The manager can harness this motivation by ensuring that he keeps issues of patient care constantly top of the agenda. This ensures a patient focussed team constantly moving in the same direction.

Another good tactic, and one rendered much easier if the manager is possessed of a clear vision, is to give the team and its individual members clear objectives and responsibilities. Most hospitals have a programme of individual performance review during which objectives and targets can be discussed, but there is nothing to stop the manager developing them for teams as well. Many changes in the operating room are complex and difficult to plan and can only be achieved by a group of people working together so there is no need to be artificial about the process.

PRACTICE EXEMPLAR 7.9:

I went to a symposium entitled 'Managing the Work Team'. During the day there was a group discussion where each member had to describe the team environment in which they, as individuals, had to function. I described a multidisciplinary team of specialists, each absolutely dependent on each other, where every member of the team had to function correctly all of the time and where it was very difficult to escape from interpersonal conflict. Each member of the team had their own function and while there was a nominal team leadership structure the individual actually 'in charge' at any one moment would depend on the job in hand. The team leader was absolutely dependent for his success on the smooth functioning of the team and the individuals who made it up, and as a result there was a legitimate power-base independent of the organisation's management structure.

Most of the other managers in the symposium found this a very difficult structure to relate to, perceiving their team and its members as a basic and simple structure allowing group effort towards a defined goal, but all directly and constantly responsible to themselves.

There were only two individuals who recognised the structure described. They were firstly, a manager of a small research laboratory in the pharmaceutical industry staffed by technical experts in their own field who had to work together to a common aim respecting the specialist skills and knowledge of their colleagues. The other was a manager in the motor industry who also happened to be an officer in a Territorial (part-time) 'special forces unit' specialising in 'demolition'.

Managing the operating department team is a challenge for any manager, especially since, as discussed in Practice Exemplar 7.9, the team has a power base of its own. A cohesive team can, if its members act as a unit, effectively resist management action and it is a balancing act to ensure that it has enough power and freedom to achieve the job in hand but is still controllable if it shows signs of becoming too independent. It will take some time to get the balance right; interfere too much and the team will put up barriers, interfere too little and it will go its own way. Nevertheless, the importance of the manager's ability to take his team with him cannot be overstated since without it the department will stand still, go off at a tangent or worse, move backwards.

Controlling expenditure

Finance and financial management are 'dirty words' to many practitioners. Partly, this is because the finance department has much power and tends to make unpopular decisions; partly it is due to the fact that they (the accountants) are not very good at explaining their decisions and partly it has to do with the fact that few teachers of nursing take the time to make a clear link between the financial and clinical functions.

Yet the link is clear: if there is no money, there is no health care. Rich countries by and large have good health care and in poor countries it varies between indifferent and non-existent. If there is no money staff receive no pay and there is no money to train them. There is no money to buy consumables or capital items and no money to build hospitals. This is, it is suggested, blindingly obvious and yet the point is often missed. Given that finance is critical it has to be managed. If managed well then the resource goes further and the patients benefit and conversely if managed badly the patients suffer.

Money is the currency of society, and in general (and whether we like it or not) the ultimate standard by which an activity in an economic society, including its hospitals, is measured. Budgets, financial targets, spending limits and pressure to reduce costs are therefore facts of life. In order to maintain credibility in the eyes of the hospital's management the operating department manager needs to ensure that costs are controlled and that care is delivered in a demonstrably efficient manner.

The question is therefore raised. How can we, given that there is little choice in spending available, manage the finances in the most effective manner to the benefit of patients?

Good care

It is perhaps surprising that, arguably, the most effective way to make the money spread further is to deliver good care. This runs counter to the received wisdom among many health-care staff on this issue, who in general believe that improving care *costs* money. It is suggested that, in contrast, good care almost always equals cost-effective care. This is not to say that no expenditure is involved, as often a considerable outlay is required, but when the *total cost* of caring for the patient is considered the initial expenditure is usually outweighed by the benefits.

Consider the following: if we raise the standards of care for surgical patients they should be less anxious, suffer less pain, contract fewer infections, suffer from less tissue viability problems and have fewer complications from surgery and anaesthesia. If the above assumption is correct, then the inevitable corollary is that they will stay in hospital for less time, consume fewer drugs, need fewer investigations and require less follow-up. They will need less staff attention, reduced administration support, generate fewer complaints and are less likely to have accidents or be the victims of negligence.

In addition, patients who are treated well are likely to be more satisfied with their treatment, the staff who administer it and the organisation responsible. This enhances their view of the professions and develops good press for the hospital.

The Center for Disease Control (CDC) in the USA reported in March 2000 that the then cost of hospital-acquired infections was running at $5 billion a year (www.cdc.gov). Against this kind of backdrop it is clear that almost any effective programme for infection control, no matter how expensive it was to implement, would be cost-effective. Good care saves money.

PRACTICE EXEMPLAR 7.10:

A hospital which was performing many joint replacements every year calculated that the total cost of treating one patient who contracted a postoperative wound infection was £77,000. In any one year they expected to see around six such infections costing them in the region of £385,000.

The cost of systematically examining and reducing these infections was estimated to be around £50,000, a large sum in itself, but one which would show a return if only one patient who would otherwise have contracted an infection, did not.

One of the best ways, therefore, that the clinical manager can control costs is to ensure that the highest standards of care are delivered to the patient at the lowest clinical risk. It is submitted that no practitioner, manager or not, can argue that the above is not the absolute duty of the clinician anyway.

Other costs

Operating departments are expensive places to run. Staff/patient ratios are very high, probably higher than any other clinical environment. In addition consumable costs, in most areas a relatively small proportion of the total expenditure, often make up 40% of the manager's budget. In extreme circumstances, consumable and implant costs can be the single most expensive item over the whole patient stay. A custom-made prosthesis for revision arthroplasty can cost in excess of £5000 against a total cost for the whole care episode of £7500.

The practitioner starting out in management and wanting to get a handle on budgetary management should, as a first step, look for the hospital's 'Standing Orders and Standing Financial Instructions'. Every hospital has a set and each department within that hospital should have access to them. These are the basic rules the hospital uses to conduct its business. As light reading they cannot be recommended, but they do contain some very useful information. Furthermore every employee responsible for spending money is expected to know what they say and failure to follow the rules is generally regarded as a serious matter.

For example, they will tell you how much money can be spent with a particular supplier before the order must be approved by the board.

More importantly, they lay out in detail the responsibilities of employees and the procedures to be followed in the management of hospital assets.

In addition there are a number of other issues that it is worth being aware of. A basic knowledge of the law of contract is helpful (unfortunately outside the scope of this chapter), and an understanding of the public procurement rules. Your supplies department will be only too pleased to help you; indeed, if you show an interest they will probably greet you with open arms. It is rare to find a clinician with more than a passing interest in procurement matters. For the present it is enough to say that if a contract with a supplier exceeds £93,896 over the term of the contract then a whole raft of European legislation comes into play.

Before discussing costs in further detail, it is necessary to describe the difference between 'fixed' and 'variable' costs. This is a simple concept but it must be understood before effective strategies for the management of expenditure can be developed.

Fixed costs will be incurred irrespective of the activity level of the department. Examples of this type of cost include the basic salaries of the staff, the costs involved in driving the operating department plant, cleaning and domestic costs and equipment maintenance contracts. The only way fixed costs can be reduced is by reducing capacity. Clearly, if a particular hospital closes two of its operating rooms then it can shed the cost of keeping them open. One of the arguments for having bigger centralised operating departments is that because of fixed costs they cost less to run. A very simple demonstration of this is that the domestic, clerical and portering staff required for one suite of ten operating rooms is significantly less than that required for two suites of five.

Variable cost is that portion of the cost incurred which varies with activity levels. Examples of variable cost are staff overtime payments, surgeon's gloves, rubbish bags, prostheses, sutures and piped medical gases. Reducing variable cost involves finding cheaper products, negotiating better deals with suppliers, changing clinical practice to a more cost-effective method and managing the inventory to free up cash.

Readers should bear in mind the above distinction when considering the following paragraphs since it is critical to understanding the actions described.

A further strategy, and one which will not be discussed in any detail, is to reduce or re-profile activity. If fewer procedures are performed, fewer gloves are used. Sometimes hospitals are judged not on what procedures are done but on how many. It is common sense that it costs less to repair 20 inguinal hernias than it does to replace 20 knee joints. While attractive and simple, against a national background of increasing activity and patient dependency, this strategy is unlikely to be a feasible option.

Staff cost

Where can the manager's intervention make a difference? The majority of staff costs may be regarded as fixed in that they do not vary with activity levels. There is however a proportion of variable cost in the staff bill. This is made up of the costs of overtime, enhanced rates for 'out of hours' working and locum, agency and bank staff wages. The most significant part of the variable section of the staff cost is usually the cost of locum staff. Typically the cost of employing a member of staff from a locum agency is *at least* twice the cost of having somebody in post to do the work.

A number of strategies can be successful in reducing this. Possibilities include moving to a system where 'time back' is offered in lieu of overtime payment, employing bank staff and trying to move activity from expensive times (i.e. weekends and evenings) to daytime hours. None

of these are particularly easy; anything that affects staff earnings is likely to be opposed by the staff and their Unions so it may be necessary to enter into a period of negotiation and consultation.

The cost of locum staff can also be reduced, but again some effort is required. One strategy involves employing more staff than are strictly needed to do the work. The logic of this approach is that if the department is only staffed to the number required to do the job there will be times when peak holidays and sickness coincide and locum staff will be required to maintain the service. If over the year the total amount of staff needed is three whole time equivalents (WTE) (a whole time equivalent is the number of hours equal to one full time worker) it will cost at least the equivalent of six WTEs in locum fees. Simple maths leads to the conclusion that employing two more people than are needed may actually save the cost of four WTEs.

A further effective strategy is to reduce labour turnover by investing in staff development and education. This last strategy is particularly effective because it gives staff a reason to remain with a particular employer, thereby reducing the costs involved in replacing them. Typically it can take up to 4 months or longer to recruit to a vacancy which must be covered in the interim by locum staff. In the operating room a further six months of training may be required before the practitioner is able to function as a member of the team. In the case described above one person leaving will create a 10-month requirement for locum staff.

Tackling the fixed proportion of staff costs is more difficult. The manager must ensure that there is the correct skill mix and a balanced staff profile with clear lines of command and control. This can only be done after careful consideration of the roles and requirements of each staff grade. Skill mix analysis is not something to be undertaken lightly. If, following the exercise, it turns out that the skill mix is incorrect and requires revision the result may be that staff suffer a downgrading of their grade or status. Such an upheaval, however necessary for the long-term success of the organisation, produces, in the short term, major disruption and de-motivates staff.

One of the common mistakes made by managers looking at skill and grade mix is to confuse reward, in terms of the payment for the job, with responsibility. The structure, the type of activity and its timing, the level of activity and the level of performance required of the staff all have a bearing on the number at each grade required for the department. While it is undeniable that nursing staff are, in general, paid little for the commitment they deliver, and it is natural that managers wish to take every opportunity to reward that commitment, upgrading staff on that basis tends to become counter-productive. In the first place it produces an extremely expensive staff structure and secondly, and more importantly, it reduces the number of grades through which staff may progress, cheapening the value of higher grades in the process.

Consumables cost

The first requirement before even considering trying to save on consumables is accurate information. Many practitioners do not even realise that the information is there if only it were organised in a usable fashion.

A good example of the inability to use available information may be found in the common practice of filing purchase orders in date order in a box. Every time managers wish to look at previous orders they have to sort through piles of back orders until the right sheet of paper is located. If it is necessary to take this process further and look at all purchase orders placed with one company over time, it becomes even more difficult and the process may be abandoned on the basis that the returns will not be worth the effort.

In contrast, if copies of purchase orders are filed in date order but also by supplier, then all the information relating to one supplier is in one place and can be readily accessed. In addition, since on most occasions the manager will know the source of supply of a particular product, locating the previous order becomes extremely simple. As we will discuss later the ability to access demand histories and to isolate areas of spend is absolutely critical to the ability to not only control consumables expenditure but to the generation of a properly structured inventory.

Once the clerical routines described in the paragraphs above are in place then there are a number of questions to be asked:

1 Which are my biggest accounts?
2 Can I develop a good business relationship?
3 Are there any opportunities for introducing competition into the portfolio?
4 Can I reduce the number of suppliers with which I deal?

Major suppliers

There is an old 'rule' (whose origins are now lost in antiquity) called the 'pareto' rule (the 80/20 rule). The rule states that 80% of the expenditure will be with only 20% of the suppliers. In most operating departments the biggest areas of spend will be sutures, implants, drugs and with the primary supplier of volume consumables. It is a matter of basic mathematics that making a one per cent saving on a very large account will generate more cash than a 10% saving on a very small account. The shrewd manager will therefore always target the big accounts first.

Business relationships

Before considering more detailed strategies for managing the non-pay budget it is necessary to discuss the concept of 'the business relationship'. In a very real sense the operating department manager and the staff who work within the department are dependent on the ability of the supplier company to deliver the requisite goods. And while in many instances it is possible to 'second source' items, jumping around from supplier to supplier on a regular basis is undesirable and makes for hard work. It is therefore incumbent on the manager to develop working relationships with the representatives and customer services departments of their main suppliers.

In order to generate a better deal it is necessary to understand those things on which supplier companies place a value. If the manager is prepared to offer an exclusive contract for a time period it is likely that improved discounts will be forthcoming. Exclusivity is something of a prize for suppliers. This is often in the form of a legal contract which, in theory, would provide grounds for legal action on the part of the supplier were the hospital to purchase the goods elsewhere. In addition, it allows the company to set up systems which would make it at least difficult and at worst expensive to consider switching to another company at the end of the term of the agreement.

Supplier companies also place a value on standing orders (an order which requires the supplier to deliver a fixed amount at fixed intervals for a fixed duration); blanket orders (an order for goods to a value to be delivered when required over a given period); and an increased level of business. The value of increased business is obvious and requires little explanation, however standing and blanket orders are a little more complex. Suppliers regard this type of order in the light of a commitment to spend. If a blanket order is placed for a given volume of goods to value over a period of time then the hospital is in general undertaking to spend at least that amount. The same argument is true of standing orders. Not only does this represent some exclusivity, but it also allows them to predict much more accurately future demands and likely profits. It introduces an element of certainty into an unpredictable business environment.

It is simplistic to regard the relationship of supplier and the operating department as a simple customer/supplier transaction-based relationship. The manager who takes the time to understand the market in which the supplier is operating and develops relationships that are mutually beneficial will find that costs will reduce.

Competition

Is there any opportunity to introduce competition? Very often, goods have been obtained from a particular supplier for no better reason than they have always been obtained from that source. There are very few products that cannot be obtained from more than one source, and, even where this is the case, equivalent products (i.e. ones that do the same job) are usually available. Quite often, the mere threat of losing an established customer is sufficient to induce a supplier to improve its pricing.

It is important to note here that no care organisation will expect its operating department manager to have to deal with the complexities of competitive tendering and the placing of exclusive contracts without expert advice. The usual arrangement is that the clerical, legal and professional purchasing services are managed by the buying department with the operating department manager providing specialist clinical advice.

Reducing suppliers

There are many companies around that offer warehousing and distribution services. It is usually possible to consolidate goods obtained in small quantity, from a number of different suppliers down to a single source. Not only does this save on order processing cost and staff time but, because of the extra volume of business, improved discounts may be obtained.

Many departments, in the belief that they are being efficient, buy goods from many sources at the lowest available prices. It is often the case that one supplier, if offered a contract for all of the products (for example a vascular products contract) will reduce the total cost even if some of the individual products could be purchased cheaper elsewhere. The value of the *whole* contract is less than all of the component parts added together and there is once again a reduction in processing costs by reducing suppliers and consolidating orders and invoicing.

PRACTICE EXEMPLAR 7.11:

The supplies manager at the hospital where I work estimates the cost of processing orders at £60 each. Reducing the number of suppliers so that more goods can be ordered from one source at the same time clearly represents the possibility of a significant saving.

Managing the inventory

Inextricably linked with the management of consumables cost is the management task of managing the inventory. Practitioners tend to be 'risk averse' and, as a result, keep much higher stocks that are actually necessary to ensure the availability of essential products. While, as a general rule, it is accepted that 'over stocking' is preferable to 'under stocking' there are a number of problems inherent in this practice:

1 The organisation has a great deal of money tied up in stock that is not moving. This is in effect 'dead' money.
2 Stock rotation is difficult and goods tend to go out of date and have to be thrown away. This is wasted money.
3 The cost of holding stock (storage, racking, and the hours necessary to maintain it) is higher than necessary.
4 Changes in clinical practice are more difficult to achieve and take longer because of the need to use up old stocks.

The management information necessary to ensure expenditure is properly controlled on purchases can also be used to manage the inventory. Factors which need to be considered when deciding on an appropriate stock level are the criticality of the item under consideration, the length of time required to obtain a replacement, the possibility of using substitute products, the volume of the item (i.e. its physical size) and the demand history. (Note that a demand history is a record of consumption *not* a record of orders.)

Stock volume

The size of the stock can be viewed in two ways: the most obvious is to state it in terms of the number of items held, but it is often more helpful to look at it in terms of the length of time it will last. Instead of stating that there are six items on the shelf it might be said that there was three weeks stock. Where items are used in volume, such that any weekly variations in consumption can be averaged over a period, considering the stock in this way can have a number of advantages.

Imagine that over a period the demand history reveals that on average 50 items are consumed per week. It is decided that, after due consideration of the risk involved in holding the stock and lead time involved in replenishing it, it is necessary to carry a six-week' stock of the items. In order to maintain the stock level it is only necessary for the individual whose job it is to check the shelves to requisition the difference between what is there and 300.

After a while it might become clear that there is never less than three weeks' stock on the shelf. It will then be possible to reduce the stock by 150 units generating a one-off cost saving by not purchasing for three weeks and still maintaining a safe stock level.

High value items

Unfortunately many of the most critical items (such as arterial prostheses) do not have a predictable usage pattern. To complicate the matter, they are usually the more expensive items and it is often necessary to carry the full range before any operative procedure can commence. In addition, if clinical practice changes the hospital can be left with significant amounts of obsolete stock for which it has no use and which has no resale value. All that can be done is to discard the items and accept the cost involved in doing so. This is an example of a type of cost usually known as 'exit cost'.

In recent years a way of avoiding wastage such as that described above has developed in the form of a device known as 'consignment stock'. This approach shifts the burden of stock costs onto the supplier because they retain ownership of the stock even though it is held within the hospital. Payment is only made once an item is withdrawn from the stock and used, and a replacement requisitioned from the company. It is usual for a blanket order to go with the consignment stock to reduce the lead time to the order of 48 working hours. If it is then decided at some stage in the future that this range of products is no longer required then the company can be asked to remove it at no cost to the hospital.

PRACTICE EXEMPLAR 7.12:

The orthopaedic surgeons at one hospital decided that, on clinical grounds, they were going to switch to a different type of knee prosthesis. The stock was the property of the hospital and they agreed to use up what was left on the shelf.

Soon however the most popular sizes had all been used and the surgeons pointed out that they never knew for certain what size they needed until they had commenced operating. Under these circumstances they could not use the remaining stock. The hospital was left with £45,000 worth of useless prostheses that had, in the end, to be 'written off'.

Given the total volume and value of the inventory commonly stocked in operating departments, and the sheer range of items, it makes good economic sense to ensure that it is properly structured because, given proper thought and some little work, significant financial benefits can be generated.

Delivering quality care

Few would argue with the proposition that the prime responsibility of the clinical manager is to develop and ensure high-quality care is delivered within the area of responsibility. The other chapters of this book are devoted to providing practitioners with the necessary information to ensure this end. Of course, clinical managers are expected to have a clinical input and need to be well-informed in order to deliver quality care themselves. But this chapter is about management and the question we are addressing here is: how can the manager ensure that others are delivering quality care and how would we recognise good quality clinical care in the first place?

The starting point for any discussion about a particular subject is usually to define it. Where quality is concerned there is, unfortunately, no such agreed definition. Writers on quality inevitably frame the essence of quality in their own terms and there have been many authors on the subject. Quality has been defined as 'conformance to requirements' (Crosby 1979); as being about 'care, people, passion, consistency, eyeball contact and gut reaction' (Peters and Waterman 1982); 'fitness for function or purpose' (Lochyer, Muhlemann and Oakland 1988) and many other things besides.

A moment's thought and it becomes clear that these definitions are of little use when applied to the health-care environment. How can the requirements of the health-care delivery process be specified with any certainty especially if it is one particular patient under consideration? We can, perhaps, specify the *desired* outcome but we know that no matter how well our care is delivered there will be significant deviation in a proportion of our patients. An example might be a patient who was admitted to hospital for repair of his inguinal hernia. Possible outcomes would include the patient discharged home with no treatment, the patient dying after a prolonged stay in hospital and all stops in between. None of the outcomes necessarily imply that the patient received poor quality care.

PRACTICE EXEMPLAR 7.13:

An operating department manager agreed with a supplier company for a consignment stock of arterial prostheses to be placed within his department. Although there was no significant price differential between the previous supplier and the new supplier, the value of stock already held and owned by the hospital was of the order of £25,000. It was possible, therefore, to use up the old stock at no risk since the new supplier had already delivered. This produced a one-off saving of £25,000.

Detailed discussion of this is the subject of a book in itself but some guidance is clearly appropriate. Recognising quality care is fairly simple; there are a number of reliable sources including the experience of the manager and other senior staff with the department, current research, policy statements, guidelines from the various professional bodies and statements of good practice from the employing organisation. In addition, comparison is possible against 'benchmarks' with the various auditing tools currently available.

So the 'what' of quality may take some time and work to find, but most of the information is available somewhere. The real challenge is in managing the department staff so that they are motivated to deliver quality.

Most staff reading this book would probably admit to not having always delivered 'best' care to all of their patients. If asked to justify this, some of the reasons offered would be cogent and be to do with resources or other issues outside the sphere of influence of the individual practitioner; others would be subjective and less able to stand rigorous examination. A similar situation exists in respect of change. Most practitioners would readily admit that care is a dynamic thing that cannot possibly stand still and thus change is a fact of life. Yet the experience of most practitioners will be that change is difficult, slow, often produces anxiety and on occasions totally fails.

The logical conclusion reached from reading the above paragraph is that practitioners are reluctant to change and are consequently unconsciously committed to delivering poor care to their patients. All practitioners, it is suggested, while perhaps being prepared to admit that they do not always deliver 'best' care and sometimes do not fall over themselves to change practice would refute, with more haste than civility, this suggestion. Is there, therefore, an alternative solution?

It is submitted that, faced with a complex, dynamic and often frightening situation in which practitioners have a personal involvement with both their colleagues and their patients, and where exact communication between colleagues who may not always agree with each other is difficult and restricted by organisational constraints, staff take refuge in certainty and keep doing that which they have always done. This at least means that they are doing no worse than they have done previously and are taking no further risks with their practice and their patients.

Many practitioners do not have time to reflect. Their day is spent chasing their tail and trying desperately to keep up with an ever-increasing workload of ever increasingly dependent patients. Under such circumstances getting them to think constructively about change and new practices is perhaps a little unreasonable. The message is that managers must create the space for change to occur allowing staff time to assimilate new working practices and to overcome the novel problems caused by them. However desirable the change might be, if this is not done the staff are entirely justified in taking the view that management did not really want them to change because they (i.e. the managers) have not demonstrated the requisite commitment.

The problem is that the manager is also under pressure to deliver both the change and increasing activity and as a result the temptation is to try

PRACTICE EXEMPLAR 7.14:

Many readers may have seen the following spoof notice on office walls:

We aim to deliver a planned, organised service, meeting customer needs at minimal cost and in an environment characterised by tranquillity and good humour.

However:

When you are up to your waist in alligators and you have a nibbling sensation in your toes it is extremely difficult to remember that the object of the exercise was to drain the swamp!

Anon

PRACTICE EXEMPLAR 7.15:

I was recently walking past a well-known department store. There was a sign on the door which stated 'This store will not open until 09:30 on Thursdays to allow for staff training'.

The store had decided that the possibility of some loss of profit caused by reduced opening hours would be more than made up for by the increased revenue generated by having well-informed staff.

---

to cut corners. Properly managed change and maintaining activity are, to some extent, mutually exclusive. Sometimes the department manager will have to say to senior management that you can have change or you can have activity but without investment you cannot have both.

It is not proposed to enter into a discussion on the principles and practice of change management. This can be learned in much greater detail from a book on the subject. I would recommend two sources, neither of which are, strictly speaking, change management textbooks, but they do demonstrate key issues in developing an innovative quality driven culture. The first, *The Change Masters* by Rosabeth Kanter (1983), describes some of the best change managers and the strategies they use. The second book, *In Search Of Excellence* by Tom Peters and Bob Waterman (1982), although a little dated, is still an object lesson in innovative management.

Nonetheless it is appropriate to lay out for the reader some of the more important aspects of ensuring that staff have the opportunity and the motivation to deliver the care of which they are able.

- Communication
- Clarity of purpose
- Managerial commitment.

Communication

Staff cannot deliver best care in any co-ordinated fashion if they do not understand the environment in which they work. On a basic level they need to understand what is expected of them and what is going on around them. These are functions of communication.

It is submitted that it is almost a universal truth that hospitals do not communicate as well as they

should, or as well as the staff who work in them *think* they should. OK, but what is good communication? How is it done? Communication takes a number of forms, the most obvious one being a conversation. Other forms of conveying information, and this is by no means an exclusive list, are staff meetings, information files, memos, letters and appraisal meetings.

One of the most common mistakes made by new managers is not choosing the correct medium of information transfer. The list below provides some guidance:

- **Conversations** – This is an appropriate way of communicating where the information is required by only a limited number of people *and* where it is vital the manager has the opportunity to ensure that the message has been received correctly or where information needs to be exchanged. The conversation is also the only method to use when information needs to be conveyed urgently.
- **Staff meetings** – Staff meetings are excellent for generating ideas. In addition they have the benefit of allowing the development of consensus. Managers need to ensure that they retain control of the meeting however, since if there is a burning issue which the staff want to discuss, and especially where it is clear that the manager and the staff have a difference of opinion, the agenda can be hijacked and it can become a 'slanging match'.
- **Information files** – A loose-leaf file containing such items as team briefs, memos to the department, discussion documents, minutes and notes of meetings and other written information which, while not being urgent, need to be brought to staff attention. These can be left in sitting rooms and other ancillary areas so they

can be read whenever staff have a few spare minutes. It needs to be made clear that it is a staff responsibility to read the file or the manager will still get complaints that they were not informed.

- **Notice boards** – Notice boards have a tendency to become cluttered and the information on them rapidly out-of-date. As such they have limited use as a communication medium and, where they are used they need to be actively managed. There are two types of notice board: those with standing notices on them and those where, while the theme remains static, the actual information and the way it is laid out changes on a regular basis:
  - Notice boards where the information is held in a standard form, such as the board that holds the staff off-duty and the on-call rosters, should be laid out on a standardised form with a labelled place marked off for each document. No other notices should be permitted on this board because the information is important and staff need to be aware where they can find it at a moment's notice.
  - Notice boards which have a theme should have a member of staff responsible for ensuring that they are kept tidy and all 'out-of-date' notices are removed. Examples might include the health and safety notice board or the one dedicated to staff further education and development opportunities.

From the above discussion it is clear that the factors to be taken into account when communicating with staff are: (i) the information to be conveyed; (ii) the urgency of the information; (iii) the size of the audience; (iv) the level of certainty that the information has been understood; and (v) whether the manager is seeking to generate ideas from the staff.

Clarity of purpose

Lack of clarity can be fatal to the process of change. If there is confusion over what is expected or why it is expected then it is not reasonable to expect the staff to follow the process through. A frequent remark from staff undergoing a process of change is that, while they have a general understanding of the need to progress and change, they are unclear why it is that the specific change they are being expected to make is better than that which they currently practice. This is especially the case if the change is one to improve efficiency or management. This represents a failure of communication. Staff must understand not only the reasons for the change but the process of making it happen or they will conclude that it is a 'change for change's sake'.

If the staff perceive that this is the situation in the department then the manager has failed to communicate why change is required.

PRACTICE EXEMPLAR 7.16:

A manager had a new notice board fixed to the wall in his department. At the top of the notice board he fixed a laminated sign which said 'general information notice board'. For a while it worked very well, all notes of departmental meetings and relevant memos and notices were put on the board and staff knew where to find them. After a while however other notices started to appear: 'evening out at local restaurant', 'sale at church hall', 'RCN annual general meeting', 'collection for Julie', 'first meeting of the journal club in the social club', etc.

Not surprisingly, the notice board became cluttered and staff found it very difficult to obtain any useful information. After a while, it became ignored and thus irrelevant. One day in a departmental meeting the manager brought up a topic mentioned in a memo which he had pinned to the notice board some three weeks previously. All the staff emphatically denied any knowledge of the memo and became extremely angry that their manager had not had the courtesy to tell them about it.

The manager became angry himself at this point and stalked out of the meeting with the intention of removing the memo from the notice board and bringing it back into the meeting to show them. It took him five minutes to locate the right piece of paper!

PRACTICE EXEMPLAR 7.17:

We trained hard, but it seemed that every time we were beginning to form up into teams, we would be reorganised. I was to learn later in life that we tend to meet any new situation by reorganising; and a wonderful method it can be for creating the illusion of progress while producing confusion, inefficiency and demoralisation.

Gaius Petronius Aribiter 210 BC

PRACTICE EXEMPLAR 7.18:

Most children will have played 'Chinese whispers'. A group of people sit around in a circle and one member whispers a message to the person on his left. Each member in turn whispers the message to the rest until the message returns to the person who originated it. The originator then compares what he received with what he sent. The result can be hilarious.

The key is therefore to do with perception. Even if the manager has a dedicated notice board for guiding through the change, even if they have personally informed everybody who is involved in it, even if a project plan has been drawn up so that staff have the opportunity to understand the timetable, things can still go badly wrong. Communication is about that which is received *not* that which is sent.

The point is that the managers cannot do all the communication themselves and even if they personally brief all the members of the team they will still pick up different messages. Staff will talk to each other during breaks and often the message that comes back to the manager is entirely different to the one sent out. Effective managers ensure that communications received by staff are

the same as those which they intended to send.

This issue often confronts managers with their greatest difficulties in their daily working life and is one that managers also find very stressful. 'How could practitioner "X" possibly have thought that this was what I meant?' It may even seem that staff are being deliberately obstructive, though if confronted with this suggestion nearly everyone would be grossly insulted. However, the wise manager keeps his or her perspective and realises that whether it is 'fair' or not is really irrelevant since it is still the manager's responsibility to ensure that the message gets through and that the end result is that which is desired.

The easiest technique for ensuring the staff have the same perception of a particular process or required change as the manager is to issue the

PRACTICE EXEMPLAR 7.19:

An experienced practitioner came on duty one lunchtime to discover that a patient having an emergency aortic aneurysm repair was on the operating table in the designated emergency operating room. Such had been the urgency in the case that the anaesthetic room was in a terrible state and required cleaning and tidying. Although this particular practitioner did not routinely work in anaesthetics she had nothing else to do at that moment and decided to help out her colleague by clearing up after her.

Some five minutes after she had started, the anaesthetic services manager walked into the

anaesthetic room and, surprised to see her there, asked 'what are you doing here?' The service manager meant to send the message 'you do not have to do this work; it is the duty of the anaesthetic practitioner working this room'. What the practitioner heard however was, 'what are you doing in my anaesthetic room, you don't work in anaesthetics?' The practitioner stripped off her gloves, put down the piece of equipment she was cleaning on a trolley and stalked out of the room.

It took some time for the manager to retrieve his position.

message and a few days later question a sample of staff as to their understanding. There will usually be something that the manager thought was obvious and did not require stating that staff have missed and, if it is critical to the understanding of the whole process, then the message will usually have missed the target. The manager can take this opportunity to correct the misconception and remedy the situation before it becomes more difficult to deal with.

Sometimes the received message is so far away from what was actually said that it is worth running through the entire conversation again to clear up the misunderstanding. This is a particularly useful technique where a member of staff has latched on to a particular statement that is perceived as threatening and has completely ignored the remainder of the points the manager made. The manager must focus the staff member's mind on the whole issue and not just that which is threatening.

Managerial commitment

It has been stated before in this chapter, and it bears stating again, that in order for staff to achieve the aims of the department, a clear vision needs to be laid out before them. They need leadership. Leadership is not just about clear communication and clarity of purpose, it is also about personal managerial commitment. A common theme among clinical staff, medical and

nursing, is that all managers seem to care about is the budget.

Even a cursory examination of this belief will show it to be fundamentally incorrect. In the first place many managers still have a personal clinical responsibility or have come from a clinical background. It is unreasonable to suppose that merely because they no longer have a primarily clinical role they no longer care about quality or patient based issues. Secondly, this belief presupposes that all managers have little integrity. There can be few jobs in health care management where the possession of a sense of integrity and ethics would not be a primary qualification for the post.

Yet the belief persists. Many, if not most, staff have a rather cynical view of their managers, preferring, at least if their spoken words accurately reflect the way they feel, to disbelieve and doubt the commitment of their managers. Indeed, if the reverse attitudes were demonstrated by the managers to their staff there would be, and justifiably, a horde of complaints in respect of the manager's behaviour.

So where does this belief come from? It is submitted that staff in general will take their cues from the totality of their manager's behaviour: what he says *and* what he does. It will do little good to hold a meeting every fortnight to discuss the subject of quality if the manager spends all the time in between discussing how to save money and stay within the budget. It should be

PRACTICE EXEMPLAR 7.20:

A manager conducted an individual performance review interview with a practitioner generally thought to be very good at her job if a little lacking in confidence. He spent some considerable time working through her (praiseworthy) achievements over the year and then worked out with her personal development plan for the following three years which included an assertiveness course and some opportunities to develop her leadership skills.

Some two hours after the interview concluded the practitioner returned to the manager accompanied by her union representative accusing the manager

of telling her that she was totally incompetent. Since the manager knew he hadn't said that at all he invited them in and ran through the interview again referring to his notes. It became clear that the practitioner found the prospect of having to confront her lack of confidence so threatening that she had completely ignored everything else that the manager had said and had left the meeting only conscious of the one issue which required improvement. The commendations she had received had passed totally unnoticed.

obvious that the staff will come to the conclusion that the manager's real agenda is to save money and that he is only paying lipservice to the subject of quality.

Philip Crosby (1986), the man many people credit as being the 'father of quality management', emphasises in *Quality Without Tears* time and time again that in order to get quality managers have to live and breath it. Quality improvement has to be top of every agenda, it is never the subject of compromise and managers have to demonstrate their determination to deliver quality by constant effort and commitment. He says 'Trying, is not enough ... dedication, determination, drive are necessary if something is to happen'.

Few stories on the subject of quality have a clearer message than the following story from Tom Peters' and Bob Waterman's (1982) *In Search of Excellence*, which, it is submitted, is a simple but dramatic demonstration of probably the easiest way to ensure quality. For brevity it has been paraphrased:

A car worker, just having been made redundant from a factory in Detroit, was being interviewed as he left the plant for the last time: 'I made bad cars for 20 years', he said, 'Nobody ever asked me how to make a good one'.

Leadership

Some readers will have noticed that only cursory reference has been made to the topic of 'leadership' and may be wondering why. A glib answer could be that the chapter is on management and not on leadership but that is not really an answer. It is a common mistake that leadership and management are, if not exactly the same then certainly two sides of the same coin. This is not the case. A moment's thought will serve to confirm this. Many managerial jobs are not concerned with leadership at all. An example of this might be the stores manager. Increasingly the reverse is also true. Look, for example at the development of 'Modern Matron' and 'Nurse Consultant' type roles. The salient feature of these posts is one of clinical *leadership*.

In reality of course, many jobs presume that the post-holder is both clinical manager and clinical leader. This will almost always be the case with the clinical operating room manager. A review of this chapter will reveal that we have talked about leadership, we have discussed vision development and communication, and we have looked at the manager's personal credibility. These are issues central to leadership too. But, and here is the crux, managers have to make sure it happens, *they do not have to do it themselves*.

The key here is knowing yourself. Over the years most practitioners will have come across inspirational leaders who were perhaps not wonderful managers and great managers who could not lead. The clinical manager needs to know what their own personal strengths are, and how to work to them.

Managerial and leadership skills can be learned, if they could not there would be no point in this book, but even after diligent study and a few years' experience an individual may be better at some things than at others. Yet the department needs to be both managed and led. What then does the individual do? Probably the most effective solution is to use pre-existing expertise in the department staff.

The good manager always knows when to take advice and the staff within the managed depart-

---

PRACTICE EXEMPLAR 7.21:

A manager of an operating department, while generally regarded as a very good manager who was able to get things done, when faced with difficult staffing matters which required leadership skills greater than he could claim occasionally struggled.

After some time he discovered that one of the senior sisters seemed to have an instinctual understanding of what made the staff tick. Faced with difficult situations the manager simply asked her what he should do.

ment are very often the best resource. In addition it has the side benefit that the staff know that their views are valued and taken into account.

There is one small caveat here: when taking advice make sure that the person giving it knows that in the end it is your decision. You are, after all, the person who will answer for it.

CONCLUSION

It is hoped that this chapter has not been a boring litany of management theory. If it is, then it has failed. The references cited have been chosen on the basis that they interested me when I read them and inspired me to improve my own skill-base and techniques as a manager. It is undeniable that they are a subjective selection that another author might reject. There has been no attempt to generate a 'pocket guide to management theory', but it is hoped that the reader will have some idea of the challenges the new manager will have to face in the operating department. As above, it is true that other writers might fundamentally disagree with the choice of topics discussed here, but in the last analysis it is the reader who is the ultimate critic.

With a chapter this short it is inevitable that there are gaps and that some subjects are explained with less than thoroughness. With more space a wider discussion of the academic background to management theory and practice could have been attempted. It would also have been possible to have examined in much greater detail the rather eclectic selection of topics which have been discussed. These must be left up to the reader to investigate further for themselves in their own reading and perhaps at a professional manager's course.

REFERENCES

Adair J (1986) *Effective Team Building*. London: Pan.
Crosby P (1979) *Quality is Free; The Art of Making Quality Certain*. New York: McGraw Hill.
Crosby P (1986) *Quality without Tears*. New York: McGraw-Hill.
Forsyth DR (1999) *Group Dynamics*, 3rd edn. California: Brooks Cole.
French JRP and Raven B (1959) *The Bases of Social Power*. In: Cartwright D (ed) Studies in Social Power. Ann Arbor MI: Institute for Social Research.
Handy C (1985) *Understanding Organisations*, 3rd edn. London: Penguin.
Kanter R (1983) *The Change Masters – Corporate Entrepreneurs at Work*. London: Unwin.
Lochyer K, Muhlemann A and Oakland J (1988) *Production and Operations Management*, 5th edn. London: Pitman.
Pedler M, Bugoyne J and Boydell T (2001) *A Manager's Guide to Self Development*, 4th edn. London: McGraw-Hill.
Pembrey S (1980) *Ward Sister – Key To Nursing*. London: RCN.
Peters T and Waterman R (1982) *In Search of Excellence*. London: Harper and Row.

Website addresses
www.cdc.gov
http://simap.eu.int

8 CONSENT AND ASSOCIATED LEGAL ISSUES FOR PERIOPERATIVE PRACTITIONERS

J Howard Shelley

CHAPTER AIMS

- To discuss the legal necessity of obtaining consent and the concept of a 'defence'
- To examine who can give consent to surgery and explain the legal situation
- To answer the question: What is consent?
- To provide some examples of real-life consent problems and outline the correct responses

INTRODUCTION

This chapter is something of a strange beast. It is, at least as far as possible, a chapter on legal issues without any law in it.

In England, legal frameworks are an often taught element of many perioperative courses. They include a basic introduction to the structure of English law, issues such as the legal framework of the NHS, the rules controlling the administration of medicines and the legal structures of the professions. However, many perioperative practitioners suggest that they 'don't want to know the law', they 'want to know what to do'. A discussion on the origins of English Common Law may be useful and interesting if you are a lawyer, but as a perioperative practitioner you are interested in the mechanics of safeguarding the interests of patients and fellow professionals and remaining within the law. Therefore there will be little in-depth discussion of legal concepts in this chapter.

When discussing the content of this chapter with colleagues, my thoughts were that this book is concerned with perioperative practice, not nursing in general. Topics such as the rules con-trolling the administration of medicines and the legal structures of the professions should have been covered in basic training. Therefore, an obvious question to ask is 'what do perioperative practitioners want to know about?' The almost universal response from my colleagues was 'consent'. I suggested that covering the 1967 Abortion Act might be relevant; my colleagues felt that as perioperative practitioners you would know all that was necessary. Well then, how about the law surrounding human organ trans-plantation, organ harvesting and the legal meaning of death? Too specialised, my colleagues said, and anyway, when those events happen there is always plenty of advice available.

The point is, I was told, consent to surgery is a problem faced by perioperative practitioners on a daily basis. It is a complex and poorly under-stood concept and one which is central to your practice. So here it is, an introduction to the legal concept of consent.

Three other points are worth stating at this juncture. Firstly, this chapter deals with the law in England and Wales only; the law in Scotland and Northern Ireland, while similar in structure, is different in detail. Secondly, law changes very rapidly and while correct at the time of writing one significant judicial decision could alter the situation such that the chapter would need total re-drafting. Finally, lawyers use a different refer-encing system to the rest of the world (and to the conventions applied elsewhere in this book), and so where I have referred to case law I have included the citation in the text and not in a con-ventional bibliography. In order to allow the reader to explore the topic more fully I have included a reading list at the end of the chapter.

WHY CONSENT?

Why do we need to obtain consent prior to surgery? There are a number of perfectly valid answers to this question. You can argue that treating someone without their consent is unethical and dehumanising and reminiscent of the treatment meted out to inmates of concentration camps by their Nazi hosts. You can point to evidence that suggests patients do better if involved in their care (Greenfield *et al.* 1985). You can suggest that caring professions should obtain consent because it is obviously the 'right thing to do'. The lawyer's answer is that consent is required because consent by the patient is a defence to a later action in negligence or assault brought by that patient. It is this last reason that forms the subject matter for this chapter.

The lawyer's answer requires a little analysis. We need to understand what 'consent' means, who can give it and under what circumstances. We need to understand what the meaning of 'defence' is and we should understand the meaning of negligence and assault.

Negligence and assault

Negligence occurs when a duty of care arises, this duty is breached and damage occurs as a result. An in-depth discussion is beyond the scope of this chapter but suffice it to say that a duty will almost always arise between nurse and patient and if the standard of care is below that of the 'reasonably competent' nurse, and the patient comes to some harm as a result, then the practitioner will be negligent if the facts can be proved.

Assault is a word which is used to denote two separate legal issues: assault and battery. Battery is 'the direct and intentional application of force to another person' and assault is causing 'reasonable apprehension of the infliction of a battery' (Rogers 1998).

If a practitioner were to approach from behind and jab a needle into the patient without any warning, then a battery may have occurred. If that practitioner warned the patient but went ahead irrespective of any refusal of consent, the patient could bring an action in both assault and battery.

Negligence, assault and battery are examples of a type of law called 'tort'. Torts are characterised by the fact that generally an action is brought by one individual, the claimant, against another, the defendant. If the case is proven on the 'balance of probability,' the defendant is 'liable' (not 'guilty') and will have to pay damages. These are calculated on the basis of the losses suffered by the plaintiff, and any costs likely to be incurred in the future as a result of the defendant's action.

Defence

In legal terms a 'defence' is an argument which can be raised by a defendant to counter the claimant's position. In the situation described above, if the practitioner explained to the patient why it was necessary to give the patient an injection, and the patient consented to it, then the fact of the consent is a defence to facts which would otherwise constitute a battery. Consent is regarded as an 'absolute' defence since if consent to the alleged battery can be demonstrated by the defendant, the action will completely fail.

Consent

Almost every discussion on the Law of Consent starts with the seminal words of Mr Justice Benjamin Cardozo in the United States Supreme Court in 1914. He said:

> *Every human being of adult years and sound mind has a right to determine what shall be done with his own body; and a surgeon who performs an operation without his patient's consent commits an assault.*
>
> Schloendorff v Society of New York Hospital, 105 N.E. 92.

Few would argue with this. As a statement of principle it cannot be faulted, but once you have read it once or twice a number of questions spring to mind:

- What does 'adult years' mean?
- What do you do if the patient is not of 'adult years?'

- What is 'sound mind?'
- What is the position with a patient who lacks capacity?
- How can we define consent?
- How can we tell when a patient has consented?

AGE AND THE ISSUE OF CONSENT

Few would argue with the proposition that an adult should be able to decide what treatment or care they are prepared to accept, and that a baby is in no position to make any decisions at all. But adulthood is not an overnight phenomenon. The individual does not go to sleep a child and wake up the following morning an adult so how does the law, a discipline which favours absolute concepts, deal with this?

In respect of consent, the law recognises three categories of individuals:

1 Adults, i.e. those who are 18 years or older.
2 Individuals who are aged 16 or 17 years.
3 Minors aged less than 16.

Children under 16 years

At one time children had no rights in law to consent to treatment until their sixteenth birthday; however, following the 'Gillick' case (*Gillick v West Norfolk and Wisbeech Area Health Authority* (1985) 3 All ER 402), it was accepted that children under 16 could and should have a say in their health care. If a child is competent to understand the issues involved in treatment then it should be their decision whether to go ahead or not. Since the case concerned the right of children to receive contraceptive advice without parental consent this did not at the time seem to be too radical a decision.

Since then there have been a number of instances where children, who were, at least on the face of it, competent to consent, have refused treatment in circumstances where the refusal, if accepted, meant that that they would die. A recent example of this was the widely reported case of a 15-year-old girl with a deteriorating heart condition who refused transplant surgery,

(Re M [child: refusal of medical treatment] (1999) 2 FCR 577.) The libertarian stance taken in Gillick has therefore been 'revised'. The courts have decided that although children can consent to treatment, refusal of consent needs to be taken in the context of the gravity of the decision. Where a refusal will lead to the death of the child it is unlikely that the court will accept that the child will be sufficiently competent to refuse.

16 and 17 year olds

The Family Law Reform Act 1969 specifically mentioned the child of 16 or 17 years stating that they could give consent for treatment. The Act seemed clear. Any person who had reached the age of 16 could consent and was to be treated like an adult. Unfortunately Parliament had not foreseen the situation where a 16-year-old might want to make treatment choices which were likely to lead to her death (*Re W. [A Minor] [Medical treatment: Court's jurisdiction]* (1992) 4 All ER 627). The Court decided that since the Act only mentioned consent and not 'refusal of consent,' a child of 16 or 17 could only consent. Refusal was subject to being overruled. The situation is therefore very similar to children under 16.

Adults: 18 years or older

As strange as it may seem, the position of adults refusing to consent was only finally resolved in 1998. A succession of cases in the late 20th century had led to the situation where a pregnant woman who refused a caesarean section against medical advice was on very shaky ground. The courts tended to overrule the woman. Finally, however, it was accepted that the right to consent or to refuse consent by an adult was absolute and no-one, not even the court, could overrule them. Lord Justice Judge said:

> *Even when his or her own life depends on receiving medical treatment, an adult of sound mind is entitled to refuse it. This reflects the autonomy of the individual ...*
>
> St Georges Hospital NHS Trust v S (1998) 3 All ER 673

CAPACITY AND THE ABILITY TO CONSENT

Most people would agree that in order to consent the ability to understand is a prerequisite. It would not be reasonable to expect someone with advanced senile dementia to consent to surgery. But what happens if the required understanding is lacking and treatment is still required?

We need to consider a number of related issues:

- What are the medical staff obligations?
- What level of understanding is necessary?
- What happens in emergencies?
- What about advance directives? (living wills).

Treatment obligations

The basic requirement of health-care professionals is that patients should be treated as necessary in their best interests. This is a professional obligation as well as a legal one and it is central to the issue of dealing with incapacity. We have already discussed the fact that adults of sound mind are treated as autonomous, and that only the patient can give consent for medical treatment on themselves. This is also, unfortunately, true of the incapacitated. No-one can consent on their behalf. *Any suggestions that a relative, the court, or someone with a power of attorney, can give consent on behalf of an adult patient, incapacitated or not, are totally false.*

But it is obvious that occasionally a person who is incapacitated will require treatment, so, if consent cannot be obtained what should happen? The answer is that the patient must be treated 'in their best interests'. While doctors can consult with others, in the end the decision is theirs. We will return to this later.

Incapacity and understanding

Removing an individual's right to consent or refuse consent to medical treatment involves removing a basic right. As a consequence, the law sets a low standard that the patient must reach in order to be regarded as competent to make treatment decisions. In order to demonstrate capacity the patient must pass a three-part test:

First, comprehending and retaining treatment information, second believing it and, third, weighing it in the balance to arrive at a choice.

Mr Justice Thorpe in Re C (adult: refusal of medical treatment) (1994) 1WLR 290

This case is the leading authority on consent and capacity. 'C', the patient, was an elderly gentleman with a long history of psychotic illness featuring a fixed delusion that he was a surgeon of international renown, being treated as an inpatient in a secure mental hospital. It was noted that he suffered from 'an all pervasive illness' and yet the Court decided that he had capacity to consent to treatment decisions. The balance is very much weighted in favour of the patient.

Emergencies

In the case above the patient in question had a chronic condition which was not likely to change much in the near future. What about the acute condition? If a patient, under normal circumstances possessing capacity, is suddenly and temporarily deprived of it (e.g. the patient brought in unconscious following a road traffic accident), what then? In fact the answer is simple: the patient must be treated as necessary in his best interests. The emphasis here is on 'necessary'.

Imagine a woman in a collapsed state following a rupture of her ectopic pregnancy. It is clearly both 'necessary' and in her 'best interests' that surgery should be undertaken to stop the bleeding. Suppose at the time of surgery it is noted that the other fallopian tube is badly scarred and it is considered likely that a further pregnancy would result in a second ectopic. Is the surgeon justified in excising the second fallopian tube?

While it may be in her best interests to proceed, and indeed, it may be that the patient will require further surgery and a second anaesthetic to do it, it is not, at that time, *necessary*. The patient has the right to be consulted prior to being sterilised.

Advance directives

This is the lawyer's term for the situation where a patient has previously indicated that if a particular set of circumstances happens then a defined set of actions must take place. They are commonly called 'living wills'. The question is: are they valid? Unfortunately the best answer is 'maybe'.

Consider the case of *AK (Re AK (Medical Treatment: Consent) (2000) Fam 885)*. The patient had motorneurone disease and had indicated that two weeks after the first day on which he could no longer communicate with the world his ventilator was to be turned off and he was to be left to die. The court stated that not only were his wishes a valid statement of consent, but indeed to continue to treat him in the face of his express withdrawal of consent would constitute a battery.

The point here is that the advance directive was made with impending events in mind, at a time reasonably close to the events that the directive covered, and it covered the circumstances exactly. If there had been any doubt over whether the directive covered the situation in which AK found himself then the directive would not have been effective.

THE NATURE OF CONSENT

We have discussed who can consent and under what conditions but we also have to understand what consent is. Most people would have a common sense view of what they understand by the term 'consent', but for operating room practitioners this is not enough. We need to understand the legal definition.

At a basic level common sense operates in that it is obvious that in order for a patient to consent they must acquiesce to the treatment they are receiving. But this is not enough for legal consent. They must understand that to which they are acquiescing and the risks involved in it. Some issues arise out of this:

1 How much information should patients be given?
2 When may consent be given?
3 When and how can it be withdrawn?
4 How do we know when consent has been given?
5 Must consent be written?

Information

To be valid consent must be 'informed'; that is the patient must understand what he is consenting to. Unless patients have had the opportunity to discuss risk and outcome how will they know whether they want to proceed? So how much information should patients be told? There are two answers to this question. In order to satisfy the basic information requirement a health-care professional must have acted in 'accordance with the standard accepted by a responsible body of opinion' (Kennedy and Grubb 2000). So as long as the information provided was the same as another group of health-care professionals would have provided, then the practitioner is safe.

But suppose our patient then asks a specific question: 'Is there anything that can go wrong?' 'Will I be paralysed?' How should he be answered? The answer is that a specific question should be answered:

> *... truthfully and as the questioner requires.*
> Lord Bridge in *Sidaway v Board of Governors of the Bethlem Royal Hospital* (1985) AC 871

Timing of consent

In theory consent may be given by the patient at any time up to the event for which he is being asked to consent. A moment's thought will show that there a limits on this. A patient cannot be asked on their 18th birthday to consent to a hernia repair just in case at some time in their life they should be unfortunate enough to develop one. This is clearly a ridiculous example, but consider the opposite extreme. It is common practice in some hospitals to obtain consent to surgery and anaesthesia from a patient who has already arrived in the anaesthetic room. While most practitioners would frown on this as being less than ideal practice, it also effectively gives the patient no time to reflect and consider whether they have further questions. Since it is usually clear that if the patient refuses to sign, surgery cannot go ahead, there is the possibility that the patient might legitimately claim duress. Consent not given freely is no consent at all.

Clearly then, the time window for obtaining the patient's consent will vary from patient to patient. In some, with stable and chronic conditions, it may be appropriate to obtain it (say) two months in advance, although it would still be good practice to revisit it on the morning of surgery. In other patients whose condition changes from day to day, consent obtained only a week in advance of surgery might be invalid.

Withdrawal

Consent is not a contract. There is no penalty for the patient in changing their mind and so consent may be withdrawn at any time. The patient is not limited to the method of withdrawing it either. They can politely decline the procedure or they can get up and leave the hospital without a word. Withdrawal must be respected and any attempt to physically restrain a patient would be a battery and possibly false imprisonment. So the question is, can the practitioner intervene at all? As an advocate for the patient, health-care professionals have a duty to act in the patient's best interests. It would therefore be entirely reasonable for the professional faced with a patient who is scared witless but who has an operable cancer to talk through the issues with the patient. At some stage though, education and persuasion become duress and so it would be unwise to 'talk the patient into it'.

Evidence of consent

At some stage a practitioner may be asked to give evidence that a patient consented to a particular procedure. Suppose there is no consent form – is the case lost? If practitioners take nothing else away from this chapter but this, then you must understand: *Consent is not a signed consent form. The form is only evidence that consent has occurred.*

Consent may be express or implied. A patient who, fully informed of the risks of a procedure, comes into hospital, complies with all the requests of the hospital staff, climbs onto a trolley, goes down to the operating room and holds his arm out for the anaesthetist to perform intravenous cannulation, will be taken to have consented by implication. Patients are not allowed to be compliant and then claim that they did not consent because no-one asked them to sign a form.

Express consent is much more cut and dried. Any form of clearly indicating consent to a procedure will do, from a simple 'yes' or 'go ahead' in response to a direct question, to a signature on a properly completed form.

The problem for health-care professionals is that they deal with many people and a small event, although it may loom large in the mind of the patients, quickly becomes forgotten by the practitioner. Unfortunately some years down the line practitioners may be asked to account for their actions in a court. In this case it is obviously better to have a signed nursing note or consent form to refer to. If such a document can be offered in evidence it produces a presumption (albeit a rebuttable one) that the circumstances described in it actually happened. On the other hand if there is no consent form, the patient can claim that, since it is normal practice for one to be completed, in their case it never happened. Without evidence it is very difficult to argue your case.

Even if a consent form can be produced it is always open to the patient to argue that they signed following a 'pre-med' and were therefore drugged. Or that someone thrust a pen in their hand as they came through the theatre door and told them to 'sign this'. Or that although they signed it in advance of the operation the procedure and its attendant risks were never discussed with them and therefore they did not understand that to which they were consenting. *A consent form is not consent; it is only EVIDENCE of consent and it may not be conclusive.*

CONSENT IN PRACTICE

PRACTICE EXEMPLAR 8.1:

A patient, an elderly lady, arrived in the operating department for surgery on her fractured neck of femur with a completed consent form signed by the patient's nearest relative and the orthopaedic registrar. She had no previous history of confusion, although it was now very difficult to communicate with her and the orthopaedic registrar had diagnosed that she lacked the capacity to consent.

Practice Exemplar 8.1 demonstrates a frequent problem encountered in practice and raises a number of questions:

Can a relative sign a consent form for an adult?
The answer to this question is absolutely 'No'. It is obviously wise and good practice to seek the relative's agreement to the treatment plan, but from a legal perspective their consent or refusal carries no weight.

Is a short history of confusion sufficient to mean that the patient can be taken to lack capacity?
It would obviously depend on the circumstances. If the patient can be treated under the 'emergency rules' then it will be safe to proceed, but in this case the patient's condition is not immediately life-threatening and it could be argued that treatment *now* is not *necessary* in her best interests. A better course of action would be to delay and check to see if the history is accurate. If the patient is found to actually have a 5-year history of Alzheimer's disease, then treatment can proceed because the patient will never regain capacity, but if the problem is a combination of acute pain, dehydration and electrolyte imbalance the patient may have something to say about the hospital staff not taking the time to obtain her consent.

Is the orthopaedic registrar able to certify that the patient lacks capacity?
Unless the registrar is an expert in gerontology or psychiatry he is unlikely to be qualified to make

this clinical judgement. Again, if the patient has a history of Alzheimer's then that diagnosis has already been made, but where there is no history he will be on shaky ground. Whoever makes the judgement on the patient's capacity should therefore be qualified to assess the patient's mental state and have a working knowledge of the test in Re C.

Is the orthopaedic registrar able to state that treatment is necessary in the patient's best interests?
He may well be so qualified, but the question is really is he qualified to make the judgement on his own? As a basic precaution it is good practice for two professionals in a speciality to make the judgement and it is submitted that one of them should be the responsible consultant. Should the matter ever be litigated it will look a lot better if the consultant is able to testify to involvement at every stage.

What evidence would we expect to see?
The key here is documentation. It should be possible to see by reading the notes the entire decision making process. There should be an entry from the admitting doctor and one from the registrar stating that a specialist opinion is needed to verify the patient's capacity. Then there should be a note from the specialist stating that the patient lacks the necessary capacity and finally one from the consultant and the registrar, both stating that they have examined the patient and that they believe surgery is necessary in the patient's best interests.

PRACTICE EXEMPLAR 8.2:

A 17-year-old profoundly deaf woman came to the operating department for a termination of pregnancy accompanied by her mother who was acting as interpreter. The senior theatre nurse having discovered this patient was coming had arranged for a sign language interpreter to be available. Once the patient had completed admission formalities the mother returned somewhat reluctantly to the ward, and the patient was taken into the anaesthetic room. The anaesthetic room practitioner left the room with the interpreter for

about 30 seconds and when she returned she found the patient in floods of tears.

On discussion with the patient through the interpreter, it was discovered that this was the first time the patient had ever been able to talk to health-care professionals without her strong minded and very religious mother 'censoring' what she said. What she really wanted was to keep the baby and to obtain some good contraceptive advice.

Practice Exemplar 8.2 demonstrates that health-care professionals have an obligation to obtain the patient's consent and not someone else's view of it. Had the theatre nurse not intervened the patient would have had a termination she did not want and not have received the advice she so badly needed. Suppose the patient had complained, what would have happened? It is possible that the hospital could argue the patient should have had the courage to stand up for herself, but it is submitted that it is equally true that good practice states that it is the professionals' responsibility to ensure that patients are provided with the necessary support to allow them to communicate effectively.

The same arguments would apply equally to people who do not speak English. Are these patients to be deprived of the right to giving informed consent to surgery merely because of a language difficulty? Of course not, and any court would give such a suggestion short shrift. It is clearly inappropriate to use an interpreter who is unable to translate professionally or who has an interest in the subject matter of the discussion. The moral of the story is, always use a professional interpreter.

In Practice Exemplar 8.3 both the practitioner and the surgeon were wrong. In fact, more than adequate consent had been obtained. The surgeon had spent some time with the patient explaining what was to happen and the patient had given his authority to proceed.

The issue here is that there was no way that the patient could record the fact of his consent. This is a problem of evidence. It was easily

PRACTICE EXEMPLAR 8.3:

A patient who had some years previously suffered a stroke which had deprived him of the use of one hand was brought up to theatre with a crush injury to the other one. The practitioner admitting the patient became quite concerned that no consent had been obtained and the surgeon responded by pointing out that consent wasn't possible because he couldn't write.

solved by the surgeon writing in the patient's notes a description of the discussion he had had with the patient and inviting the patient to agree that that was in fact what had occurred. This agreement was then witnessed by a third party.

CONCLUSION

Some readers may have read this chapter and come to the conclusion that consent is about what the doctors have to do. Most of the cases are about medicine and only involve nursing on the periphery, if at all. This misses the point. Duties which apply to medical staff apply equally to all health-care professionals and while consent for surgery is generally regarded as the responsibility of the surgeon, perioperative practitioners are required to obtain consent for their actions, invasive or not. Would you just slap ECG stickers on a patient's chest without having gained their consent first? Of course not! We all have a legal and professional duty to obtain the patient's consent for proposed care and treatment.

Even where obtaining consent is the duty of someone else it is usually within the role of the perioperative practitioner to check it. As an advocate we ensure that patients understand their operation and its attendant risks. If the patient does not understand or expresses doubts then we should ensure the operation is delayed until the patient is satisfied. There is a great deal of confusion and ignorance about consent and its legal ramifications even among doctors. If a mistaken decision on (for example) capacity is made, not only does this mean that a patient has one of their basic civil rights removed, but it exposes both the hospital and the doctor to the risk of an action for battery.

A final point concerns the commonly held belief among both medical and other practitioners that a doctor can 'take responsibility' for the actions of another. Sadly in respect of unlawful acts, this is a misconception. No-one can 'take responsibility' for the unlawful acts of another. If negligent treatment or a battery has occurred, it is no defence for a perioperative practitioner to say, 'The doctor said it would be OK'. All of the people involved and their employer would be jointly and severally liable. In theory the patient could just sue the practitioner and ignore the doctors and the employer completely. In respect of the validity of consent it is in your own interests to check!

FURTHER READING

Unfortunately many of the texts on medical law are written by lawyers with the expectation that it is lawyers who will be reading them. The language tends to be turgid and written in a style which seems unnecessarily detailed and hard to follow. It is therefore not easy to offer suggestions to the student who wishes to examine the topic further. But there are a number of good sources available which can be used.

As a starter Margaret Brazier (1992) is worth a look. Although somewhat dated now, she does explain many of the problems of consent and capacity in a very readable manner.

There are also a number of web resources available which provide good commonsense advice on the subject of consent. The Department of Health Website describes good practice in consent, going so far as to provide a downloadable model consent policy. Similar guidance with a much more professional and ethical slant is provided by the General Medical Council and in addition the Nursing and Midwifery Council provides specific guidance for nurses.

Consent is not just a legal problem, it is also one of professional ethics. It might be legal to drag a reluctant 12-year-old kicking and screaming to the operating room to have an operation they do not want; case law suggests that it is lawful to use 'reasonable force', but is such a course of action ethical? The subject of ethics in consent is outside the remit (and word limit) of

this chapter but, without an understanding of ethics, the law is a rather blunt tool. John Harris (1985) discusses the ethical dimension of consent in a very readable way and places it in the context of a discussion on patient autonomy.

I hesitate to recommend a 'law book' but there will be some readers who wish to explore the topic in greater depth. There is a wealth of texts available but it is submitted that Michael Davies' (1998) *Medical Law* covers the subject in an understandable but structured manner. This text is also particularly strong on the ethical and Human Rights Law dimensions.

REFERENCES

Brazier M (1992) *Medicine, Patients and the Law*, 2nd edn. London: Penguin.

Davies M (1998) *Medical Law*, 2nd edn. London: Blackstone.

Greenfield S, Kaplan S and Ware JE Jr (1985) Expanding patient involvement in care. Effects on patient outcomes. *Ann Intern Med* 102(4): 520–528.

Harris J (1985) *The Value of Life: An Introduction to Medical Ethics*. London: Routledge.

Kennedy L and Grubb A (2000) *Medical Law*, 3rd edn. London: Butterworths.

Rogers WVH (1998) *Winfield and Jolwicz on Tort*, 15th edn. London: Sweet and Maxwell.

Turner NJ, Brown AR and Baxter KF (1999) Consent to treatment and the mentally incapacitated adult. *Journal of the Royal Society of Medicine* 92(6): 290–292.

Website addresses
http://www.doh.gov.uk/consent/06/08/2003.
http://www.gmc-uk.org/standards/CONSENT.HTM 06/08/2003
http://www.nmc-uk.org/cms/content/Advice/Consent%20.asp

9 ACHIEVING PERSONAL AND PROFESSIONAL DEVELOPMENT

Bernie County

CHAPTER AIMS

- An identification of what development is
- Clarification of key terms
- The factors that enable practitioners to develop
- The various support mechanisms and their relevance at different points in a career
- The role of appraisal, personal development plans and career planning in shaping development.

INTRODUCTION

In order to ensure the care that perioperative staff provide is consistent and able to meet the changing needs of the patient, there is a requirement to ensure that individuals and teams are appropriately prepared. Both the individual and the organisation share this responsibility. Professionally there is an expectation placed upon practitioners that they will enhance their knowledge throughout their career; however, this process can be helped or hindered by the organisation as a whole or the perioperative environment specifically that the individual works in.

Historically there has been a perception that staff could learn everything that they required in their initial training or by 'sitting next to Nelly'. This is no longer true. The advent of technology and the rate of change that is a common fact of life in the 21st century dictate that perioperative staff are involved in lifelong learning. Lifelong learning is something of a current hot topic. However it is not a fad that will fade, but one of the fundamental principles that underlies continuing professional development. This position is further strengthened, as continuing professional development is one of the cornerstones of the clinical governance agenda (DOH 1999).

This chapter will explore what is meant by the term personal and professional development and the various methods to achieve it. Clarification of various related terms will also be undertaken, as there are currently a plethora of confusing terms in use. Furthermore they are often utilised interchangeably by authors. The methods that are pertinent to team leaders in creating an appropriate and conducive environment will be highlighted. The latter part will explore aspects pertinent to the individual. This natural progression reflects the shared responsibility for personal and professional development that both the organisation and the individual have.

EXPERIENCE, LEARNING AND DEVELOPMENT

These three terms are in common use but are they the same? Or are they all very different? Experience is a term that is utilised frequently, though its meaning is context specific. Watson (1991) identified that there are four ways in which the term experience is used:

1 A situation, event or emotion
2 Exposure to a situation, an emotion or to information
3 Length of time spent in practice
4 Knowledge that has been gained over a period of time.

There can be occasions where the use of the term experience can be indicative of learning. That is to say that experience equals learning, but this may not be the case. For example you could have worked with a colleague who has a number of years' service, but they have less insight and abilities than someone who has served less time. These are the individuals who have five years' service, but they have no more than one year's experience served five times.

Experience does have a part to play in learning. The significance of experience in learning is made explicit in the process of reflective practice. Reflection in and on practice is explored further on p. 218.

Neary (2000) defines learning as:

... a process that allows us to move on an upward spiral of growth, change and continuous improvement. (p. 19)

It is interesting to note that it is not a vertically linear process but a gradual incline that may on occasions take a step backwards in order to go forwards. Learning is a deliberate and conscious activity that has three aspects or domains (see Box 9.1).

Traditionally assessment for courses has had a tendency to focus on the first two domains at the expense of the third. Importantly it is in the complex fusion of all three aspects of learning where personal development occurs (McGill and Beaty 1995).

Development and learning are thus interlinked. Importantly, learning can also occur without the ensuing personal growth, but the reverse is not true. Professional development is the fostering of an attitude to life and work that encourages a responsible, innovative and proactive approach to practice. It is therefore important that you take ownership of your development needs. There is a need for self-awareness to identify where you are starting from. The agenda for development, although reflecting the needs of the service, must be fundamentally based around your needs, as you know what is best for you.

Box 9.1 The three domains of learning

- Cognitive = knowing
- Conative = doing
- Affective = feeling.

It can therefore be seen that experience, learning and development are fundamentally connected and progressive in nature. However there is a requirement for a conscious and active progression along the continuum.

Lifelong learning and continuing professional development

Lifelong learning has been a term that many people have heard, but they may not be confident that they can provide a consistent definition for it (Wallace 1999). It is the recognition that we must all continue to learn throughout our life; it does not stop at the end of a period of formal education. As knowledge and evidence change, skills and practices become obsolete. Therefore as accountable practitioners there is a need to ensure that we have the skills and knowledge to deliver a responsive service.

The concept of lifelong learning is based on the notion that learning is deliberate and intentional. The learner has a specific goal to achieve and therefore there is a specific reason for undertaking the learning, which has long-term relevance. Within the sphere of perioperative practice the concept of lifelong learning manifests itself as continuing professional development.

Continuing professional development has been advocated in a number of arenas both professional and political. The advent of the Post Registration Education and Practice (PREP) Standard (UKCC 1990) and its inclusion in the First Class Service Paper (DOH 1999) heralded its importance. Both of these ensured that continuing professional development is firmly at the centre of the drive for clinical governance and hence improvements in the quality of patient care.

Clinical governance dictates that appropriately educated and trained people deliver patient care. Furthermore, there is a necessity to document when and where this learning has taken place. This process requires structure and a necessity to ensure all grades of staff are appropriately prepared to undertake their role. Hence there is a need for each individual to demonstrate competence in the tasks that they undertake. It is this continual update and extension of both knowledge and skills that demonstrates professional practice. The Bristol Royal Infirmary Inquiry Report (2001) points out that:

Continuing Professional Development must be part of the process of lifelong learning for all healthcare professions – its purpose is to help professionals care for patients. (p. 340)

The PREP standard (UKCC 1990) dictates that nurses undertake 35 hours of learning activity in the three years between re-registration. This is easily achievable and one could argue that it is minimal given the complexity of patient care today. The difficulty for nurses is in actively maintaining their professional portfolio. At the moment there is no statutory requirement placed on ODPs, but this will no doubt change with the advent of statutory registration.

Competence

The UKCC (1999) in the Fitness for Practice document defined competence as:

... the skills and ability to practice safely and effectively without the need for direct supervision. This concept of competence is fundamental to the autonomy and accountability of the individual practitioner. (p. 35)

This is what may be thought of as a threshold competence. Lockhart (1992) suggests that there are three levels of competence.

- Threshold competence enables the individual to perform at a basic level.
- Specialised competence defines a greater depth and complexity in the manifestation of skills.
- Generic competence means that there is adaptability to a wide range of situations.

This development of competence is related to the expansion of abilities to undertake new roles and jobs. Figure 9.1 relates the levels of competence to specific roles in the operating department.

It can be seen that full competence in each post provides the gateway to competence at the next level. Competence can thus be defined as:

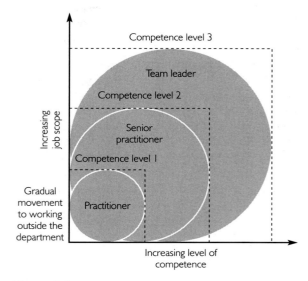

Figure 9.1 The levels of competence in relation to role (adapted from Edis, 1995)

... a broad range of knowledge, attitudes and observable patterns of behaviour which together account for the ability to deliver a specified professional service.

Neary (2000) p. 50

The measurement of competence in the clinical environment has not been without its problems. The drive towards a competency-based framework for role assessment that the agenda for change programme has developed may introduce some clarity (DOH 2002). Whether this is specific enough to be transferable across the whole healthcare arena will become clearer as time progresses.

The personal, professional and practice development debate

While exploring the literature it is apparent that there is confusion around the various forms of development. This confusion is exceptionally acute when considering the tensions between the terms professional and practice in the context of development. These two terms are often transposed within the literature and in the practice setting, where a variety of job titles are apparent. Although the concepts are fundamentally different they are all extrinsically linked.

Personal development is about gaining insight into your self (self-awareness) and growing as a person, improving the way that you are able to interact with others. This is about creating a 'rounded person', someone who has built a repertoire of skills to deal with life generally. Professional development is inherently concerned with the acquisition of sound knowledge, skills and values. Consequently it is also concerned with the individual (Mallett *et al.* 1997).

Practice development is about utilising the elements of professional development to facilitate the delivery of quality care (Joyce 1999). McCormack *et al.* (1999) have provided a definition of practice development as a:

> ...continuous process of improvement towards increased effectiveness in patient-centred care. (p. 256)

From this definition it can be seen that there is a natural progression, a sequence of events. In spite of this it is clear that at each juncture there is a need for positive action on the part of the individual and the organisation if the ultimate goal of a truly patient-centred approach to care is to be realised. Undertaking an academic course should develop the individual on a professional level and also potentially on a personal level, but there may not be an improvement in patient care due to the climate that exists in the clinical environment. For practice development to occur it requires certain contributing factors. Garbett and McCormack (2000) identified the following:

> Practice development ... is brought about by helping healthcare teams to develop their knowledge and skills and transform the culture and context of care. It is enabled and supported by facilitators committed to systematic, rigorous continuous processes of emancipatory change that reflect the perspectives of service users. (p. 88)

Therefore, innovation requires the correct environment, an environment that fosters support and where challenge of the status quo is readily accepted (Martin 2000). Likewise in order to ensure that appropriate personal and professional development occurs then the correct learning culture needs to be fostered (Gerrish 2001).

CREATING A LEARNING CULTURE

Culture is a difficult concept to quantify or measure as it contains many subconscious elements. Ekvall (1991) when talking about organisational culture identifies layers, the deepest being culture, which manifests itself on a more superficial level as climate. As Ekvall (1991) says:

> Climate has to do with behaviour, attitudes and feelings which are fairly easily observed. Culture, on the other hand, refers to the more deep-rooted assumptions, beliefs and values which are often on a preconscious level, things that are taken for granted. If we include climate in the culture concept, we can look on climate as a manifestation, on a more superficial level, of the deepest basic culture element. (p. 74)

How does this definition of culture relate to learning? Achieving a learning culture requires a commitment and willingness from everyone. In a learning culture there is an expectation that people will continue to learn and share their knowledge. Every opportunity is taken to teach and learn. It is not an add-on undertaken when time permits. A further element is the assumption that everyone has something to contribute to the learning agenda. The expectation of contribution is made irrespective of the individual's grade or professional background. A just culture that supports openness and critical debate is a pre-requisite to forming a sustainable learning culture.

The creation of a learning culture recognises a humanistic approach to learning which values the individual and recognises the unique requirements that adults have when learning (Quinn 2002). Knowles (1970) advocates that there are four main elements to effective adult learning:

- Adults already have a wealth of experience on which to build
- They exhibit a willingness to learn
- They have a need to be self directive in their learning

- They have an ability to undertake problem centred learning.

The practical application of this theory is that within the clinical area 'teachers' need to utilise facilitation skills to empower the learner. The process is not about a blanket approach to everyone, but the identification of knowledge gaps. The 'teacher' in this arena has as much to learn from the learner as the learner does from the teacher.

In order to ensure that staff have optimum prospects of expanding their practice the environment in which they work must be conducive to learning. This statement would appear obvious, and indeed it is. However the task at hand is not. The creation of a learning environment was much discussed and researched in the 1980s (Orton 1981; Fretwell 1982; Ogier 1982, 1986; Pembrey 1980). The elements of a good learning environment are identified in Box 9.2, and in themselves they are not difficult. The complexity is created by the current health-care environment that we work in and embedding them in the units philosophy.

Operating theatres have constantly struggled to recruit and retain staff. This is not a new problem. Comparison of the Lewin (DHSS 1970) and Bevan (NHSME 1989) reports identifies marked similarities. Both attempted to overcome the difficulties of delivering a quality service with insufficient staff; more importantly they were produced almost two decades apart. When one scrutinises the number of perioperative jobs currently advertised in various journals it is apparent that this position remains the same today. Considering the purpose of the operating theatre and its staff, the delivery of operations is the

order of the day. This then becomes of paramount importance and the main focus. It can be easy to see how professional and personal development can become sidelined in the push to maintain throughput. This really is a short-term approach as it creates problems for the future. Operating departments that offer educational and development opportunities are able to recruit and more importantly retain their staff (Baxter 1997).

The role of the clinical leaders in fostering the correct learning environment is paramount. This position has been highlighted across the decades and continues today. Leadership is seen as the solution to managing change which is a constant in today's health-care arena (Wedderburn-Tate 1999). It is the clinical leader that sets the tone or climate of a unit and consequently they are pivotal to the process of staff reaching their full potential (Gerrish 2001). As previously identified, a positive climate is paramount in facilitating learning. Hart and Rotem (1995) identified the six elements that promote professional development as:

- Autonomy and recognition
- Job satisfaction
- Role clarity
- Quality of supervision
- Peer support
- Opportunities for learning.

From Hart and Rotem's (1995) work it can be seen that a culture that does not recognise the individual's contribution and is oppressive will not encourage personal growth. The empowerment of practitioners to take ownership and hence responsibility for their practice is fundamental in the promotion of professional development.

An individual who gains no sense of fulfilment or achievement from their job will not be in a position to motivate others. Likewise if a practitioner lacks confidence in their own ability, and they are unsure of what is expected of them, they will be unable to help others define their role. It is therefore imperative that everyone is treated as an individual and that their unique needs are met.

Box 9.2 Elements of a good learning environment

- A motivated and enthusiastic theatre manager
- A motivated and enthusiastic theatre team
- A manageable workload
- A sufficient number of staff who have the ability to teach and assess
- Committed learners
- Time to teach and assess.

215

When developing an effective and efficient theatre team, it is vital that the organisational culture encourages everyone. This culture thus enables individual team members to support each other.

Appropriate support is vital when individuals are pushing their own personal boundaries. The greatest growth in a person is when they step out of their comfort zone. This can be a scary time and the help of another person to offset the loneliness and provide encouragement is essential. The various methods of support and the timing of their utilisation are explored later. A positive culture is therefore paramount in order to achieve personal and professional development. Significantly it is reliant on the contribution of both individuals and the organisation as a whole.

The importance of remembering the range of learning opportunities that exist cannot be emphasised enough. Traditionally academic courses have been the form of learning that is instantly recognisable. The positive reinforcement of this belief has been compounded by their link to promotional opportunities. However this is only a fragment of the picture. The operating department is overwhelmed with a wealth of learning opportunities. The range spans both the formal and informal, the traditional and the modern. Learning can take a number of guises from private study, to workplace learning, to academic courses, to e-learning. In reality experiential learning is how we gain a significant proportion of our knowledge. Therefore it is imperative that the unit culture and individuals recognise all forms of learning and the contribution that each makes. The skill in managing personal and professional development and ultimately patient-centred care is in achieving the correct balance between all the opportunities.

DEVELOPING A DEPARTMENTAL EDUCATIONAL STRATEGY

In order to create a flexible and responsive workforce one needs to have a vision of the goal. This can at times feel like 'crystal ball gazing' and it is not always easy. However if you do not know where you want to be, how do you know when you have got there? The practical reality is that evolution is better than revolution and that evolution is continuous. We live in a constantly changing world and no single solution will solve all the problems that exist in a complex environment like an operating department. There has in the past been a tendency to send people down a similar and regimented route. This approach does not acknowledge the needs of the individual or provide a sufficiently diverse knowledge base. The result is a workforce that is unable to respond innovatively to the demands that are placed upon it.

The rationale for producing an educational strategy is to clarify the purpose and meaning for everyone and to provide direction. It gives people a vision of where they are going, thereby providing some stability in the present and assisting in managing the change process. The fact that the process is evolving contributes to an enabling culture that facilitates and appreciates everyone's contribution. A good strategy will build on the strengths of the department and reduce the effects of any weaknesses.

The formation of a strategy feeds into the course commissioning process with the local Workforce Development Confederation (WDC). It also enables the service side to constructively contribute into the academic course revalidation process. If the service side is clear about where it is going, then the vision can be articulated. This enables a shared approach to the academic underpinning that formal courses provide.

PRACTICE EXEMPLAR 9.1:

Manley (2000) articulated the impact of a consultant nurse on a critical care unit. The unit had previously failed an educational audit, so it could no longer support students. The consultant nurse became a focal point, she motivated others and provided support with both education and research.

Who is your focal point? Who inspires you? When was the last time you inspired someone?

Managing staff development

In order to ensure that adequate development programmes can be formulated there needs to be role clarity and an understanding of what is expected at each grade or level. Newly qualified practitioners require a programme that will develop their clinical competence and ensure the transition from student to accountable practitioner is as smooth as possible. The focus in this group is very clinical with the emphasis being placed on developing the skills, knowledge and attitudes to deliver quality patient care in the perioperative environment.

In order to ensure that there is documentation and a standard that can be identified and replicated there is a requirement to produce a competency document. The pace at which operating departments now work dictate that the in depth underpinning knowledge is delivered away from the clinical environment. This approach would enable the learner to gain knowledge in a less pressured and stressful situation. A further bonus is the reduction in the risk of preceptor overload. This is a real problem with the large number of learners that are on various placements in the operating department. However it is important to affirm that this does not relinquish the responsibility to teach that is inherent in our professional position (NMC 2002a; AODP 2001). This approach would ensure that there is a demonstrable level of teaching that has taken place and it would be open to scrutiny and evaluation in the event that an audit or review was called for.

PRACTICE EXEMPLAR 9.2:

When is a junior no longer a junior?

It is important to remember that people mature and that as professionals we have to enable and facilitate others to grow and develop. Recently I read a reference that said someone was a junior staff nurse. They actually had two years' post-registration experience and a perioperative course.

Were they really a junior?

As staff increase in experience and begin to gain promotion, their educational and development requirements also change. Previously the focus was specifically on the clinical aspects of knowledge, the 'how and why knowledge'. The emphasis now moves to gain leadership skills. This form of knowledge enables the practitioner to shape the delivery of service that patients receive. These skills are based around developing confidence and assertiveness. Consequently there is a need to advance the understanding of current issues within the perioperative environment. The development of critical thinking skills is fundamental to the development of the ability to appraise evidence. These attributes enhance the ability to deliver evidence-based care. The attainment of a post-basic course in a relevant specialism can be a springboard for the development of these skills and hence competence in this aspect of professional growth.

The previously advocated approaches are uniform, but from this point onwards there are numerous options. The route that individuals take will be determined largely by the career path that they have chosen. For those who will be entering the clinical management route there is a need to develop people management skills. This is an area that has often been neglected, but there is now some evidence that this is being redressed with the advent of 'G grade development' courses (Gould *et al.* 2001). For individuals who wish to enter the education route there is a need to gain enhanced clinical skills and also skills in facilitation to enable others to develop.

The gradual progression through this process replicates the levels of competence identified by Lockhart (1992). It is important to reaffirm the central role of lifelong learning at every level; this is vital to the promotion of staff development. From an organisational perspective there is a need to ensure that learning resources are available. Generally the greatest challenge is finding space for resource rooms. Once this challenge is overcome, access to books, journals and importantly computers (for Internet access) also needs to be gained. Providing easy access to knowledge will contribute significantly to the fostering of a culture that promotes perioperative staff development.

Academic opportunities

The university has become the predominant centre for academic opportunities. However there are also distance learning options and the utilisation of e-learning initiatives. Although currently restricted, access will increase with the inauguration of the National Health Service University (NHSU). The specific options that are offered vary dependent on the institute so for specifics it would be necessary to contact your respective provider, although there are commonalties among all providers. The provision of full and part-time courses that are modular enables you to access elements that are relevant to you, in a time scale that is manageable.

There has also been an explosion of clinical degrees at both first and Masters levels. The preponderance of these types of degree has had the benefit of reducing the theory practice gap. They have also been instrumental in contributing to the definition of specialist and advanced practice.

The demise of the National Boards has added a perceived level of confusion around post-registration courses. Previously perioperative courses were referred to by their board number, e.g. ENB 183. This led people to assume that there was a common understanding of what the number meant, a common standard. The reality though is that this gave a false sense of security. There was a great deal of flexibility in the guidance given. Hence courses with the same numbers could appear very different. It is unclear at the moment how courses will transfer around the country, especially when their content is often relevant and specific to local need. The reality, though, is that in time loss of the numbers will be no more noteworthy than is a change of name.

Another significant advancement has been the move towards shared learning. This move is especially significant in the field of perioperative practice due to the appointment of nurses and operating department practitioners to similar roles. Shared learning reduces gaps in knowledge and understanding. It also creates a shared view of acceptable practice. Anecdotally there has been a disparity between nurses and operating department practitioners (ODPs) when accessing post-basic courses. There was traditionally also a difference in the routes accessed. Nurses travelled a clinical route whereas ODPs attended management courses. The different entry level that the two groups had compounded this situation. This position is now in transition with the advent of diploma education for ODPs and the promotion of degrees in the perioperative field. It will be interesting to see if there is now a cultural shift towards professional development that is clinically focused for both groups.

Formal learning as represented by courses is only part of the opportunities to learn. Experiential learning which manifests itself in reflective practice affords a significant opportunity.

Reflective practice

The concept of reflection is not new; Dewey defined it in 1933 as:

> ... *active, persistent and careful consideration of any belief or supposed form of knowledge in light of the grounds that support it and the further conclusions to which it tends.* (p. 9)

Boud *et al.* (1985) continued to refine the definition by identifying that reflection is:

> *A generic term for those intellectual and affective activities in which individuals engage to explore their experiences in order to lead to new understanding and appreciation.* (p. 3)

Reflection is a deliberate activity which requires time and energy in order to learn from experience. Reflection is, therefore, central to experiential learning theory (Kolb 1984; Boud *et al.* 1985) and adult learning theories (Knowles 1970; Mezirow 1981). What is more, our current experience is measured and related to our previous experiences.

Schon (1991) advocated that reflection is the means to identifying professional knowledge. He identified that there are two forms of reflection. These are reflection in and on action. 'Reflection-in-action' is closely allied to expert practice as identified by Benner (1984). This is the ability to reframe situations so that a solution can be formed from similar previous experiences. This is almost a subconscious activity which is closely allied to intuition and which the practitioner may not be able to articulate (Conway 1994).

'Reflection-on-action' is a retrospective activity that Jarvis (1992) defines as:

The process of turning thoughtful practice into a potential learning situation and significantly enough, it is the utilisation of good theory in practice. (p. 178)

From this definition it can be seen that reflective practice can contribute significantly to the development of competence. Also it facilitates the emergence of empowered and accountable practitioners because practice and decisions can be justified as they are grounded in theory.

The nursing and educational literature identifies several models that can facilitate reflection-on-action (Atkins and Murphy 1994; Driscoll 1994; Ghaye *et al.* 1996; Gibbs 1988; Johns 1996). Reviews on reflective practice are also available in the nursing literature (Atkins and Murphy 1993; Clarke *et al.* 1996).

A detailed exploration is not within the remit of this book. However there are a number of generalist aspects that warrant closer scrutiny. Most approaches are cyclic in nature and they include the following aspects:

- A description of an experience including what was felt at the time, both positive and negative feelings.
- Analysis of the event to determine what learning has occurred.
- An action plan for the future and integration of theory into practice.

The benefit of reflection is that it makes explicit what is implicit. It has been argued that non-reflective practice is ritualistic and habitual (Williams 2001). In order to ensure continued competence in the complex world of perioperative practice, practitioners must engage in reflection. It is through reflection that the wealth of learning opportunities can be truly accessed. Ultimately reflection leads to emancipation and empowerment of practitioners, because they are able to articulate their learning from experience.

Reflective practice requires skill in self-awareness, self-assessment and critical thinking. These are higher level attributes that not all practitioners possess; however, they can be learnt (Dobrzykowski 1994). Time and energy must therefore be invested in practitioners to afford them the opportunity to develop these skills. Clinical supervision is the arena where reflective skills can be fostered and honed.

THE PRACTICALITIES OF SUPPORT

In order that we can develop and grow we all require support. The type of support that is necessary will depend on the position we hold within our career (see Figure 9.2).

However it is important to recognise that some form of support is always required. If people are only in a position of giving, then they risk over-stretching themselves and the potential of burnout. There is always a need for reciprocation. This process has been likened to a bank account where it is necessary to make withdrawals and deposits in order to maintain emotional stability and function at an optimum level (Covey 1989).

The process of support can be both formal and informal. The informal approach can be seen when a colleague or friend provides words of encouragement in the rest room following a rather difficult session. This however is only half the picture; there is also the need to have formal support mechanisms. There is a confusing plethora of terms that have been formulated. They appear interchangeable and they may not reflect the process that is being undertaken.

Clinical assessors

This supervisory role is related to the facilitation and assessment of learning of people who are undergoing some form of formal course. Previously this role may have been termed mentor; however this has received heavy criticism for being a misappropriation. Clinical assessors are involved in the assessment of competence against identified outcome-based criteria. The relationship can be time-limited, for example to

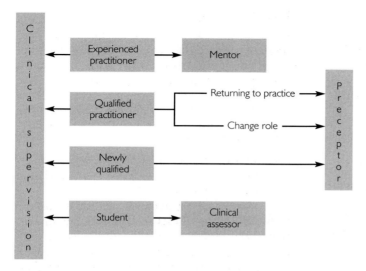

Figure 9.2 Types of support (adapted from Reid 2000)

the duration of a placement in the case of pre-registration learners. It can also be a variation on an already established professional relationship as in the case of qualified staff undertaking post-registration courses. However, irrespective of the learner, the main focus is the facilitation of learning and the assessment of competence.

Preceptorship

The recognition that the transition from learner to qualified practitioner, or a return to practice following an extensive break, are times that require specific support, were heralded by the NMC (2002b). The process of preceptorship is fundamentally different to that of clinical assessor. Preceptorship is a supportive process between a preceptee (inexperienced practitioner) and a preceptor (experienced practitioner); it is not an extension to the period of pre-registration education (NMC 2002b). The preceptee is a qualified practitioner and as such is accountable. However this period is an opportunity to gain specific competence in the field of perioperative practice.

The support of staff though role transition and new clinical experiences ensures that the standard of patient care is maintained. Preceptorship enables practitioners to consolidate knowledge

and apply it in practice. It also utilises the experience of another practitioner to guide the preceptee though areas of concern. The process should and must be used when any role transition is undertaken, for example when a practitioner is rotating to gain skills in more than one aspect of perioperative practice.

Mentorship

Mentorship is based around the idea of a senior and wise person guiding and facilitating the growth of a more junior person. The process is viewed as long term and it is focused on support-

PRACTICE EXEMPLAR 9.3:

Preceptorship is like trying to teach someone to ride their bike without the stabilisers on. If you hold on to them too tightly they will still not be riding the bike. The trick is letting them wobble a bit, making sure that they do not fall off. Encouraging preceptees to take control of their practice, while offering guidance when needed, will facilitate the transition from student to qualified practitioner.

ing and developing the individual. This is not about achieving a short-term goal like completing a course, but about helping the mentee to achieve their full potential. Mentoring is about providing guidance, support and practical help through life crises, or into a new stage of personal and professional development.

The attributes of a mentor are:

- A willingness and desire to assist in the development of others.
- Extensive experience in the skills being mentored.
- The ability to appraise the strengths and weaknesses of the mentee and to help them identify and access developmental and remedial activities.
- The ability and necessary interpersonal skills to build an effective relationship with the mentee.

When considering the attributes, the relevance of mentorship to long-term development is apparent. However it is not clear from the literature whether the process is commonplace in the NHS. Anecdotally it would appear that senior managers are the most likely to access this form of support. There remains a clear need for all clinical leaders to do so.

PRACTICE EXEMPLAR 9.4:

Mentorship enables personal growth because it exposes hidden areas. During a session a mentee said that she was an unmitigating disaster, a comment that was a half truth. The mentor response was: why do you see yourself in such a negative light? They then reiterated occasions from previous meetings when other derogatory comments were made. This challenged the mentee to reflect on their self-image. The mentee has since built her confidence and is now more positive about herself.

Clinical supervision

Clinical supervision has its roots in the fields of midwifery, counselling and social work, where it has been utilised to monitor and improve practice. Nicklin (1994) defines clinical supervision as:

> ... a process of professional support and learning which enables practitioners to develop knowledge and competence. (p. 58)

This definition encompasses the three aspects of Proctor's interactive model of supervision (Proctor 1986) (see Box 9.3).

When considering personal and professional development this model is of particular importance. The model covers the three aspects of learning, cognitive, conative and affective, and it is within a complex fusion of these three that development occurs. It has already been identified that reflection is vital to learning from experience. A clinical supervision session is the necessary time for practitioners to stop and consider their practice.

Undertaking clinical supervision requires the application of specific skills. The necessary skills are greater than just interpersonal skills. There is a need to achieve the correct balance between a number of opposing elements. The art of clinical supervision is in challenging assumptions while supporting the practitioner. This process is undertaken in an environment that is conducive to reflection, also ensuring that the supervision

Box 9.3 Interactive model of supervision

- **Formative or educational** – this aspect is concerned with the continual development of skills, abilities and understanding of the practitioner.
- **Restorative or supportive** – this aspect is concerned with how practitioners cope and deal with the stresses of clinical practice.
- **Normative or managerial** – this aspect is concerned with sustaining and evaluating the effectiveness of practice ensuring compliance with rules.

session moves gracefully through the various aspects. Due to the complexity of these skills it has been advocated that clinical supervision courses should be practical in nature (Coleman 1995). This allows the supervisor to perfect their skills in a safe and supportive environment.

It is important for supervisors to receive supervision to support and develop their competence (Korner 1994). It has been stated that supervision is the right of all nurses irrespective of their position (UKCC 1996). It should however be the right of all perioperative staff especially as its ultimate purpose is to improve patient care. There are a number of methods for achieving the successful implementation of clinical supervision. It is not possible to discuss them here but suggestions for further reading can be found at the end of the chapter.

APPRAISAL AND PERSONAL DEVELOPMENT PLANS

The process of appraisal is about identifying and assessing how a practitioner is performing against clearly identified criteria. These criteria are found within the individual's job description and the espoused values of the unit and organisation. Further elements of this process are identification of development needs and support of the individual to achieve the set objectives. The purpose of appraisals is highlighted in Box 9.4.

Box 9.4 Purpose of appraisal

- Clarity about what is expected in a role
- Feedback on performance
- Identification of problems with practice
- Better understanding between team leader and the individual
- Identification of training and development needs
- Identification of objectives
- Career planning
- To assess future potential and promotion ability.

In order for the process to be effective there is a need for open and effective communication between the appraiser and the appraisee. The process has to be shared and consequently there is a necessity to ensure that contributions are fair and equal. If a change in practice is to be sustained and internalised then the individual must own it.

Appraisals have not always been well-received in practice (Northcott 1997). It would appear that for nurses in particular to value them, there must be a strong emphasis on professional development. Therefore if the correct balance is achieved then the process of appraisal can afford a significant contribution to the professional development of a practitioner by providing a formal arena for the process to occur. The single largest contribution is the personal development plan (PDP) that is produced. The formation of a personal development plan is a cyclic process (see Figure 9.3). It utilises an action planning process that identifies areas for improvement, the resources that are available and the journey that is undertaken.

It is important to note that personal development plans do not have to only be produced during the appraisal process. Their function is to identify areas for development and how these can be achieved. This can occur any time someone wants to undertake a review of where they are and where they would like to be.

Career planning

What is career planning? And more to the point why do it? There is no longer a job for life. Indeed it could be argued that people would not want one. The diversity of opportunity that exists for health-care staff in today's health-care arena is immense. In Chapter 1, discussion has taken place around the roles that have expanded outside the 'theatre doors'. The options for perioperative staff are more than merely rising through the ranks and waiting for 'dead man's shoes'. Traditionally there was development up the hierarchy, which culminated in a management position or moving into education. The explosion of clinical roles and the opportunities that also exist in clinically based education that

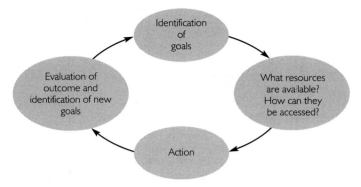

Figure 9.3 Personal development planning cycle

have occurred within the last ten years have revolutionised this position.

This plethora of opportunity is potentially the single most important reason to career plan. The pace of life is such that it would be foolhardy not to have a plan for where you would like to be. The prospect of planning for the next five years can seem daunting. It is important to remember that the plan is not set in stone; it must be flexible. Another salient point is that a career can move horizontally as well as vertically (Coombes

2003). The various options have some elements that cross over, almost like junctions; these are where choices can be made.

The process of career planning is a cycle of action planning (see Figure 9.4). Teasdale (1991) identified four stages to rational career planning.

The process involves self-awareness and identifying what is important to you as an individual. Knowing what is available is the second element. There may be times when the specific direction is not apparent nor what is required in a specific

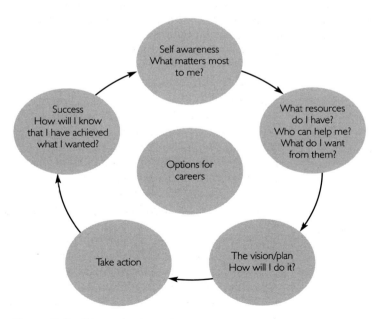

Figure 9.4 Career planning cycle

role clearly understood. A simple action is to explore the job advertisements and, for any that appeal, send for the packs. This will enable you to appraise what is required and identify any deficits that you have in your repertoire. This knowledge will then directly inform the personal development planning process. The third key stage is the merging of these two areas of knowledge and the making of an appropriate decision. The final stage is dealing with the inherent stress that any transition causes.

The process of change always has a positive and negative effect on individuals and those who are close to them. Consequently it is imperative that contingency plans are formulated to help cope with the effects. A useful tool can be reflection around how you have dealt with change previously, and critical appraisal of what techniques were particularly constructive which may be useful again. Once a definite route has been chosen, the final aspect is to ensure that there is always a plan B. The identification of a secondary plan is especially important the more senior you are, where the threat of redundancy is very real. Or it may be that the job is not what you expected.

CONCLUSION

The process of managing personal and professional development is shared between the individual and the organisation. The goal is ultimately the delivery of patient-centred care that is of the appropriate quality. The currency of skills and knowledge is in the here and now, therefore the emphasis must be on current and future learning. Emphasis on past learning is not the basis of professional practice.

There is a need to recognise all forms of learning and that reflection is a means to unlocking the hidden learning that occurs from experience. Development is a complex mix of the three domains of learning and as such requires effort and action in order to be achieved. The need for support during any form of learning is vital. The specificity of certain aspects of support to particular times during a career is also important. All of these factors contribute to the formation of a learning culture, where the needs of an organisation can be met through the development of individuals.

Finally there are significant gains to be made by an individual through planning, whether it is a personal development plan or career plan. These processes enable the individual to grow and develop, but they also demonstrate valuing by the organisation.

REFERENCES

Association of Operating Department Practitioners (2001) *Code of Conduct*. England: AODP.

Atkins S and Murphy K (1993) Reflection: A review of the literature. *Journal of Advanced Nursing* 18(8): 1188–1192.

Atkins S and Murphy K (1994) Reflective practice. *Nursing Standard* 8(39): 50–54.

Baxter B (1997) Operating department staffing – a business manager's perspective. *British Journal of Theatre Nursing* 7(7): 11, 14, 16–17.

Benner P (1984) *From Novice to Expert:Excellence and Power in Clinical Nursing Practice*. California: Addison-Wesley.

Boud D, Keogh R and Walker D (1985) *Reflection: Turning Experience into Learning*. London: Kogan Page.

Bristol Royal Infirmary Inquiry (2001) *Learning from Bristol: The report of the public inquiry into children's heart surgery at the Bristol Royal Infirmary 1984–1995*. London: The Stationery Office.

Clarke B, James C and Kelly J (1996) Reflective practice: reviewing the issues and refocusing the debate. *International Journal of Nursing Studies* 33(2): 171–180.

Coleman M (1995) Using workshops to implement supervision. *Nursing Standard* 9(50): 27–29.

Conway J (1994) Reflection, the art and science of nursing and the theory practice gap. *British Journal of Nursing* 3(3): 114–118.

Coombes R (2003) *Get The Best From Your Career*. London: Emap Healthcare.

Covey SR (1989) *The 7 Habits of Highly Effective People*. London: Simon and Schuster.

Department of Health and Social Security (1970) *The organisation and staffing of operating departments. The Lewin Report*. London: HMSO.

Department of Health (1999) *A first class service: quality in the new NHS.* London: HMSO.

Department of Health (2002) *Agenda for change.* London: HMSO.

Dewey J (1933) *How we Think.* Boston DC: Health and Co.

Dobrzykowski T M (1994) Teaching strategies to promote critrical thinking skills in nursing staff. *Journal of Continuing Education in Nursing* 25(6): 272–276.

Driscoll J (1994) Reflective practice for practice – a framework of structured reflection for clinical areas. *Senior Nurse* 14(1): 47–50.

Edis M (1995) *Performance Management and Appraisal in Health Service.* London: Kogan Page.

Ekvall G (1991) The organisational culture of idea management: a creative climate for management of ideas. In: Henry J and Walker D (eds) *Managing Innovation.* London: Sage, pp. 73–79.

Fretwell J (1982) *Sister and the Learning Environment.* London: RCN.

Garbett R and McCormack B (2000) *A Concept Analysis of Practice Development: An Executive Summary.* London: RCN.

Gerrish K (2001) A pluralistic evaluation of nursing in practice development units. *Journal of Advanced Nursing* 10(1): 109–118.

Ghaye T, Cuthbert S, Danai K and Dennis D (1996) *An Introduction to Learning Through Critical Reflective Practice.* UK: Pentaxion.

Gibbs G (1988) *Learning by Doing: A Guide to Teaching and Learning Methods.* Oxford: Further Education Unit, Oxford Polytechnic.

Gould D, Kelly D, Goldstone L and Maidwell A (2001) The changing training needs of clinical nurse managers: exploring issues for continuing professional development. *Journal of Advanced Nursing* 34(1): 7–17.

Hart G and Rotem A (1995) The clinical learning environment – nurses' perceptions of professional development in clinical settings. *Nurse Education Today* 15(1): 3–10.

Jarvis P (1992) Reflective practice and nursing. *Nurse Education Today* 12(3): 174–181.

Johns C (1996) Using a model of nursing and guided reflection. *Nursing Standard* 11(2): 34–38.

Joyce L (1999) Development of practice. In: Hamer S and Collinson G (eds) *Achieving Evidence-Based Practice: A Handbook for Practitioners.* Edinburgh: Bailliere Tindall, pp. 109–128.

Knowles M (1970) *The Modern Practice of Adult Education: Pedagogy to Androgogy.* Cambridge: Cambridge Book Company.

Kolb D (1984) *Experiential Learning: Experience as a Source of Learning and Development.* New Jersey: Prentice Hall.

Korner N (1994) *Clinical Supervision in Practice.* London: Kings Fund Centre.

Lockhart J (1992) *Effective Performance Management.* London: Kogan Page.

Mallett J, Cathimoir D, Hughes P and Whitby E (1997) Forging new roles ... professional and practice development. *Nursing Times* 93(18): 38–39.

Manley K (2000) Organisational culture and consultant nurse outcomes: Part 2. Nurse outcomes. *Nursing Standard* 14(37): 34–38.

Martin V (2000) Helping your staff to be creative. *Nursing Management* 7(7): 32–35.

McCormack B, Manley K, Kitson A, Tichen A and Harvey G (1999) Towards practice development – a vision in reality or a reality without vision? *Journal of Nursing Management* 7(5): 255–264.

McGill I and Beaty L (1995) *Action Learning: A Guide for Professional, Management and Educational Development.* London: Kogan Page.

Mezirow J (1981) A critical theory of adult learning and adult education. *Adult Education* 31(1): 3–24.

Neary M (2000) *Teaching, Assessing and Evaluation for Clinical Competence: A Practical Guide.* Cheltenham: Stanley Thornes.

NHSME (1989)*The management and utilisation of operating departments.* London: NHSME.

Nicklin P (1994) Clinical supervision. *Professional Update* 2(8): 58–59.

NMC (2002a) *Code of conduct.* London: Nursing and Midwifery Council.

NMC (2002b) *Supporting nurses and midwives through life long learning.* London: Nursing and Midwifery Council.

Northcott N (1997) Reflections on appraisal. *NT Research* 2(2): 136–145.

Ogier M (1982) *An Ideal Sister.* London: RCN.

Ogier M (1986) An 'ideal' sister – seven years on. *Nursing Times Occasional Papers* 82(2): 54–7.

Orton H (1981) Ward learning climate and student nurse response. *Nursing Times Occasional Papers* 77 (suppl 17): 65–68.

Pembrey S (1980) *The Ward Sister – Key to Care.* London: RCN.

Proctor B (1986) Supervision: a co-operative exercise in accountability. In: Marken M and Payne M (eds) *Enabling and Ensuring Supervision in Practice*. Leicester: National Youth Bureau Council for Education and Training in Youth and Community, pp. 21–34.

Quinn F (2002) *Principles and Practice of Nurse Education*, 4th edn. Cheltenham: Stanley Thornes.

Reid J (2000) Education in practice. In: Hind M and P Wicker (eds) *Principles of Perioperative Practice*. Edinburgh: Churchill Livingstone, pp. 51–65.

Schon DA (1991) *The Reflective Practitioner: How Professionals Think in Action*. Avebury: Arena.

Teasdale K (1991) A structured way to fulfil ambition: how to make rational career plans. *Professional Nurse* 6(11): 644–646, 648.

UKCC (1990) *The report of the Post-Registration Education and Practice Project (PREPP)* London: United Kingdom Central Council for Nursing Midwifery and Health Visiting.

UKCC (1996) *Position statement on clinical supervision for nursing and health visiting*. London: United Kingdom Central Council for Nursing Midwifery and Health Visiting.

UKCC (1999) *Fitness for practice*. London: United Kingdom Central Council for Nursing Midwifery and Health Visiting.

Wallace M (1999) *Lifelong Learning: Prep in Action*. Edinburgh: Churchill Livingstone.

Watson S J (1991) An analysis of the concept of experience. *Journal of Advanced Nursing* 16(9): 1117–1121.

Wedderburn-Tate C (1999) *Leadership in Nursing*. Edinburgh: Churchill Livingstone.

Williams B (2001) Developing critical reflection for professional practice through problem based learning. *Journal of Advanced Nursing* 34(1): 27–34.

FURTHER READING

Burns S and Bulman C (2000) *Reflective Practice in Nursing: The Growth of the Professional Practitioner*, 2nd edn. Oxford: Blackwell Scientific.

Driscoll J (2000) *Practising Clinical Supervision: A Reflective Approach*. Edinburgh: Bailliere Tindall.

Hamer S and Collinson G (1999) *Achieving Evidence Based Practice*. Edinburgh: Bailliere Tindall.

Nicklin PJ and Kenworthy N (2000) *Teaching and Assessing in Nursing Practice: An Experiential Approach*, 3rd edn. Edinburgh: Bailliere Tindall.

Quinn FM (1998) *Continuing Professional Development*. Cheltenham: Stanley Thornes.

Useful websites

www.athensams.net/myathens/ – Password required for NHS staff to access a number of databases.

www.doh.gov.uk – links to a number of sites including POINT for publications and COIN for all circulars from the Department of Health.

www.natn.org.uk – membership of the organisation need to access e-learning site.

www.nelh.nhs.uk – National electronic library for health has links to a number of sites.

www.nmc-uk.org – access to publications from the NMC can be found on this website.

www.nhsu.nhs.uk – the website for the university with links to e-learning site.

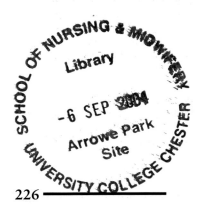

INDEX